Hiatal Hernia Surgery

Muhammed Ashraf Memon
Editor

Hiatal Hernia Surgery

An Evidence Based Approach

Springer

Editor
Muhammed Ashraf Memon
Faculty of Health Sciences and Medicine, Department of Surgery
University of Queensland Mayne Medical School
Brisbane, Queensland
Australia

ISBN 978-3-319-64002-0   ISBN 978-3-319-64003-7 (eBook)
https://doi.org/10.1007/978-3-319-64003-7

Library of Congress Control Number: 2017957714

Printed on acid-free paper

This Springer imprint is published by Springer Nature
The registered company is Springer International Publishing AG
The registered company address is: Gewerbestrasse 11, 6330 Cham, Switzerland

Contents

List of Contributors

Ciro Andolfi Department of Surgery, The University of Chicago Pritzker School of Medicine, Chicago, IL, USA

Daphne Ang Department of Gastroenterology, Changi General Hospital, Singapore, Singapore

Emanuele Asti Division of General Surgery, Department of Biomedical Sciences for Health, IRCCS Policlinico San Donato, University of Milano School of Medicine, Milano, Italy

Ralph W. Aye Swedish Thoracic and Esophageal Surgery, Seattle, WA, USA

Luigi Bonavina Division of General Surgery, Department of Biomedical Sciences for Health, IRCCS Policlinico San Donato, University of Milano School of Medicine, Milano, Italy

Dustin Carlson Division of Gastroenterology and Hepatology, Department of Medicine, Feinberg School of Medicine, Northwestern University, Chicago, IL, USA

Bernard Dallemagne IRCAD and Institute of Image Guided Surgery (IHU Strasbourg), 1 place de l'Hôpital, Strasbourg, France

Francesca M. Dimou Department of Surgery, University of South Florida, Tampa, FL, USA

Marco P. Fisichella Department of Surgery, Brigham and Women's Hospital and Boston VA Healthcare System, Harvard Medical School, Boston, MA, USA

Mark Fox Department of Gastroenterology, Abdominal Center, St. Claraspital, Basel, Switzerland

Neurogastroenterology and Motility Research Group, Department of Gastroenterology and Hepatology, University Hospital Zürich, Zürich, Switzerland

Candace Gonzalez Department of Surgery, University of South Florida, Tampa, FL, USA

Jon C. Gould Division of General Surgery, Department of Surgery, Medical College of Wisconsin, Milwaukee, WI, USA

Hans Gregersen Department of Surgery, Prince of Wales Hospital, Shatin, NT, Hong Kong

Ludovica Guerriero IRCAD and Institute of Image Guided Surgery (IHU Strasbourg), 1 place de l'Hôpital, Strasbourg, France

Maamoun Harmouch Department of Surgery, McGovern Medical School, University of Texas Health Science Center at Houston, Houston, TX, USA

Ilmo Kellokumpu Department of Surgery, Central Hospital of Central Finland, Jyväskylä, Finland

Geoffrey P. Kohn Melbourne Upper Gastrointestinal Surgical Group, Melbourne, QLD, Australia

Eastern Health Clinical School, Monash University, Melbourne, QLD, Australia

Christiane Kulinna-Cosentini Department of Biomedical Imaging and Image-guided Therapy, Medical University of Vienna, Vienna, Austria

Alfonso Lapergola IRCAD and Institute of Image Guided Surgery (IHU Strasbourg), 1 place de l'Hôpital, Strasbourg, France

Barry McMahon Trinity Academic Gastroenterology Group, Trinity College, Dublin, Ireland

Breda Memon South East Queensland Surgery (SEQS) and Sunnybank Obesity Centre, McCullough Centre, Sunnybank, QLD, Australia

Muhammed Ashraf Memon South East Queensland Surgery (SEQS) and Sunnybank Obesity Centre, McCullough Centre, Sunnybank, QLD, Australia

Mayne Medical School, School of Medicine, University of Queensland, Brisbane, QLD, Australia

Faculty of Health Sciences and Medicine, Bond University, Gold Coast, QLD, Australia

Faculty of Health and Social Science, Bolton University, Bolton, Lancashire, UK

School of Agricultural, Computing and Environmental Sciences, International Centre for Applied Climate Sciences and Centre for Health Sciences Research, University of Southern Queensland, Toowoomba, QLD, Australia

S. Mittal Creighton University Medical Center, Omaha, NE, USA

Peter Nau Department of Surgery, Carver College of Medicine, University of Iowa, Iowa City, IA, USA

Brant K. Oelschlager Division of General Surgery, Department of Surgery, UW Medical Center, University of Washington, Seattle, WA, USA

Courtney Olmsted Department of Surgery, Carver College of Medicine, University of Iowa, Iowa City, IA, USA

John Pandolfino Division of Gastroenterology and Hepatology, Department of Medicine, Feinberg School of Medicine, Northwestern University, Chicago, IL, USA

Jeffrey Ponsky Cleveland Clinic, Department of Surgery, University Hospitals Case Medical Center, Case Western Reserve University, Cleveland, OH, USA

Giuspeppe Quero IRCAD and Institute of Image Guided Surgery (IHU Strasbourg), 1 place de l'Hôpital, Strasbourg, France

John H. Rodriguez Cleveland Clinic, Department of Surgery, University Hospitals Case Medical Center, Case Western Reserve University, Cleveland, OH, USA

Shinil K. Shah Department of Surgery, McGovern Medical School, University of Texas Health Science Center at Houston, Houston, TX, USA

Michael E. DeBakey Institute of Comparative Cardiovascular Science and Biomedical Devices, Texas A&M University, College Station, TX, USA

Manjunath Siddaiah-Subramanya Department of General Surgery, Logan Hospital, Brisbane, QLD, Australia

Eero Sihvo Department of Surgery, Central Hospital of Central Finland, Jyväskylä, Finland

Kathleen Simon Division of General Surgery, Department of Surgery, Medical College of Wisconsin, Milwaukee, WI, USA

Andrea Sironi Division of General Surgery, Department of Biomedical Sciences for Health, IRCCS Policlinico San Donato, University of Milano School of Medicine, Milano, Italy

George Triadafilopoulos Stanford Multidimensional Program for Innovation and Research in the Esophagus (S-MPIRE), Division of Gastroenterology and Hepatology, Stanford University School of Medicine, Stanford, CA, USA

Kenan Ulualp Division of General Surgery, Department of Surgery, Medical College of Wisconsin, Milwaukee, WI, USA

Vic Velanovich Department of Surgery, University of South Florida, Tampa, FL, USA

Peter A. Walker Department of Surgery, McGovern Medical School, University of Texas Health Science Center at Houston, Houston, TX, USA

Jeffrey R. Watkins Swedish Thoracic and Esophageal Surgery, Seattle, WA, USA

Erik B. Wilson Department of Surgery, McGovern Medical School, University of Texas Health Science Center at Houston, Houston, TX, USA

Vivien Wong Department of Surgery, Prince of Wales Hospital, Shatin, NT, Hong Kong

Monica T. Young Division of General Surgery, Department of Surgery, UW Medical Center, University of Washington, Seattle, WA, USA

The original version of this book was revised. The First name of the Editor was misspelled and this has now been corrected to Muhammed Ashraf Memon.
An erratum to this chapter can be found at https://doi.org/10.1007/978-3-319-64003-7_20

Chapter 1
Utility of Endoscopy in the Diagnosis of Hiatus Hernia and Correlation with GERD

Francesca M. Dimou, Candace Gonzalez, and Vic Velanovich

1.1 Introduction

A hiatal hernia is a condition involving herniation of abdominal contents into the mediastinum via the diaphragmatic hiatus. Anatomically, there is proximal displacement of the gastroesophageal junction causing the intrinsic sphincter to lie proximal to the esophageal hiatus; this is likely secondary to weakening or disruption of the phrenoesophageal ligament (fascia of Laimer) [1] and widening of the diaphragmatic crura. The true prevalence of hiatal hernias is difficult to discern because many individuals are asymptomatic and, therefore, never diagnosed and the diagnostic criteria are somewhat subjective. Estimated prevalence in studies range widely from 10% to 80% in the United States [2], but is generally correlated with obesity and increasing age. Although, hiatal hernias may remain asymptomatic in most patients and diagnosed incidentally, if at all; they are frequently associated with gastroesophageal reflux disease as an incompetent lower esophageal sphincter may be a consequence of a hiatal hernia. Other patients, in whom paraesophageal hernias develop, may progress to significant symptoms including obstruction, ischemia, bleeding, and volvulus. In the asymptomatic patient, pursuing a diagnosis of hiatal hernia is not indicated, but those experiencing symptoms warrant evaluation and possible surgical intervention. Understanding the risk factors and types of hiatal hernias are vital in managing patients once they are diagnosed.

F.M. Dimou, M.D., M.S. • C. Gonzalez, M.D. • V. Velanovich, M.D. (✉)
Department of Surgery, University of South Florida, 5 Tampa General Circle, Suite 740, Tampa, FL 33606, USA
e-mail: vvelaov@health.usf.edu

M.A. Memon (ed.), *Hiatal Hernia Surgery*,
https://doi.org/10.1007/978-3-319-64003-7_1

1.2 Risk Factors

Although, the underlying cause of hiatal hernias are not well understood; elevated body mass index, higher abdominal pressure, and other aspects of sedentary lifestyle have been reported as contributing factors [3]. In fact, studies have shown that patients with a body-mass index (BMI) exceeding 25 are far more likely to be diagnosed with a hiatal hernia [4]. Thoracic deformities (kyphosis, osteoporosis, scoliosis) that occur in older patients and that cause an increase in anterior-posterior diameter of the thorax also correlate with the occurrence of hiatal hernias [5]. Furthermore, with increasing age there becomes an increased laxity of the phreno-esophageal ligament resulting in an increased risk of developing a hiatal hernia [4]. Congenital defects in children are the most common cause and sometimes may be associated with other embryologic anomalies such as intestinal malrotation [4].

1.3 Classification

Hiatal hernias can be described as either sliding hernias or paraesophageal hernias. They are classified into four types, I–IV (Table 1.1; Fig. 1.1a–d). Type I hiatal hernia is the sliding hernia in which the gastroesophageal junction is displaced proximally superior to the diaphragm; it accounts for about 95% of hiatal hernias [6]. This occurs when there is widening of the esophageal hiatus and laxity of the phreno-esophageal ligament. Type II hiatal hernias are the classic "paraesophageal hernias," with widening of the diaphragmatic hiatus resulting defect in the anterior and lateral aspect of the phrenoesophageal membrane, but with the gastroesophageal junction still fixed in the abdomen. The fundus or body of the stomach herniates through this defect while the cardia of the stomach and the gastroesophageal junction do not [7]. This is a relatively rare hernia, accounting for less that 1% of all hiatal hernias. Type III hiatal hernia is the most common of the paraesophageal hiatal hernias and they compromise approximately 5% of all hiatal hernias [8]. Type III has features of both type I and type II hernias. The phrenoesophageal membrane is lax and stretched, the esophagogastric junction is displaced into the chest as in a sliding hiatal hernia, and there is a defect in the anterolateral portion of the membrane that allows the stomach to rotate into the mediastinum as in a paraesophageal hernia [6]. Type IV hiatal

Table 1.1 Classification of hiatal hernia with regards to gastroesophageal junction location (GEJ) and symptomatology associated with each type

Type	Location of GEJ	Incidence	Symptoms
I	Above diaphragmatic hiatus	>90%	Asymptomatic or GERD
II	Normal anatomic position	<1%	Asymptomatic but may become strangulated or incarcerated
III	Above diaphragmatic	5%	Reflux and possible incarceration
IV	Above diaphragmatic hiatus	<1%	Risk of volvulus, obstruction and/or bleeding

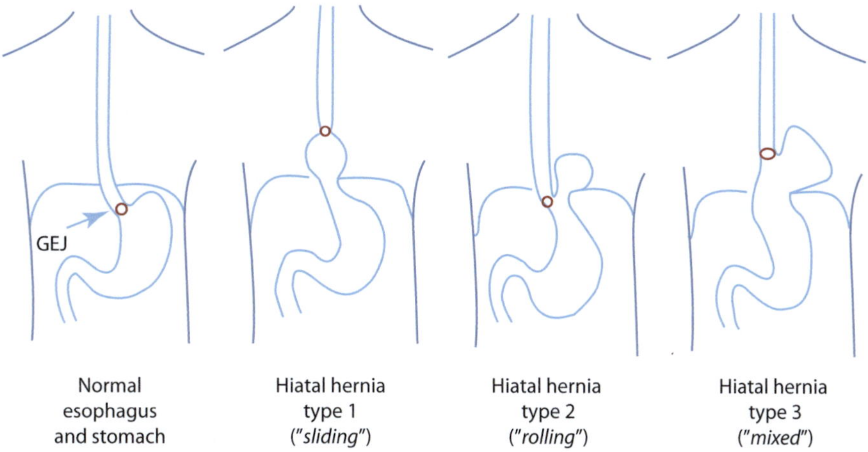

Fig. 1.1 The definitions of the four types of hiatal hernias

hernias are the least common, accounting for about 0.1% hiatal hernias [8]. They are characterized by a large defect in the diaphragmatic hiatus and an excessive laxity of the phrenoesophageal membrane. In addition to the stomach, other intra-abdominal organs are herniated into the chest [8]. Small and large intestine with associated omentum are the most common organs herniated in a type IV paraesophageal hernia; the spleen, pancreas and liver have also been found. Herniation of the stomach, specifically, can result in gastric volvulus. Rotation of the stomach along the long axis of the stomach is known as organoaxial rotation and occurs in approximately 60% of cases. Rotation in the short axis of the stomach is known as mesenteroaxial rotation where the greater curvature of the stomach is flipped anterior to the cardia and fundus and is sometimes referred to as an "upside-down" stomach [9].

Any symptomatic hiatal hernia should be considered for surgical repair, including Type I hernias that are associated with GERD. The symptomatic hernia should be repaired especially if there are obstructive symptoms or volvulus [10]. Anemia can occur in up to 20% of patients with paraesophageal hernias, especially in the presence of Cameron's lesions, and should also be an indication for repair [11]. There is debate whether an asymptomatic hiatal hernia or those causing only minimal symptoms should be repaired; considerations for surgical repair in these patients should include overall clinical presentation, patient's co-morbidities, and age.

1.4 Endoscopy in the Evaluation of Hiatal Hernia and GERD

The use of endoscopy in evaluation of the upper gastrointestinal tract has become commonplace. Its use in the diagnosis of hiatal hernia is not necessarily mandatory, as contrast radiographic images can be used to evaluate patients with suspected hiatal hernias. However, given the increased utilization of endoscopy, hiatal hernias are frequently found when endoscopy is done for other symptoms and/or conditions. Hiatal hernias are associated with GERD and this can lead to other esophageal pathology for which endoscopy can determine the presence and extent. Endoscopy can determine the size of the hiatal hernia, extent of esophagitis, presence of neoplasia and suggest the existence of delayed gastric emptying. Specifically, understanding these clinical components and using endoscopy as a tool for diagnosis and management will better help the physicians devise a management plan of their patients.

1.5 Endoscopic Assessment of Hiatal Hernia

Despite increased use of endoscopy as an adjunct in evaluating patients with a hiatal hernia, the diagnostic criteria remain unclear. The most commonly accepted definition in the literature is identification of proximal dislocation of the gastroesophageal junction (GEJ) >2 cm above the diaphragmatic indentation. This definition seems to provide a systematic method of diagnosing and reporting size of a hiatal hernia, but the confusion lies in the reference mark for the GEJ.

There are three anatomic possibilities used to assess the position of the GEJ: the squamocolumnar junction (SCJ), the upper margin of the gastric folds, and the distal margin of the palisade zone. Clarification of the endoscopic reference for the GEJ needs to be undertaken for several reasons. The SCJ, also known as the transition zone or "Z-line" is not consistent across all patients [11]. The contour and length varies, especially in those with Barrett esophagus because the junction extends cranially and is, thus, unreliable in these patients. This is important given many patients with hiatal hernias may have Barrett esophagus and may affect the estimation of the axially dimension of the hernia. Identification of the upper gastric folds is another marker that has been used as a reference of the GEJ, but may be difficult to clearly define if the stomach is not fully insufflated and anatomy is not clearly delineated endoscopically. Studies have demonstrated operator variability with regards to this measurement for hiatal hernias even in healthy individuals [12].

Another proposed system for assessing the GEJ is the Hill classification [13]. This approach evaluates the GEJ and hiatal integrity based on a "flap-valve" mechanism which is also used to predict reflux [13]. In this classification scheme, grade I flap-valve is consider the "normal" configuration. It demonstrates close adherence of the SCJ to the shaft of the endoscope with a "ridge" of tissue corresponding to the angle of His. There is no hiatal hernia (Fig. 1.2a). In grade II, the adherence of the GEJ to the endoscope is less well-defined and there is effacement of the angle of His ridge (Fig. 1.2b). Hill grade III flap valve demonstrates incomplete closure of the GEJ around the endoscope, with esophageal mucosa frequently visible and complete effacement of the angle of His ridge (Fig. 1.2c). These are frequently associated with sliding hiatal hernias. Lastly, Hill grade IV is always associated with a hiatal hernia with the diaphragmatic hiatus seen making and extrinsic compression

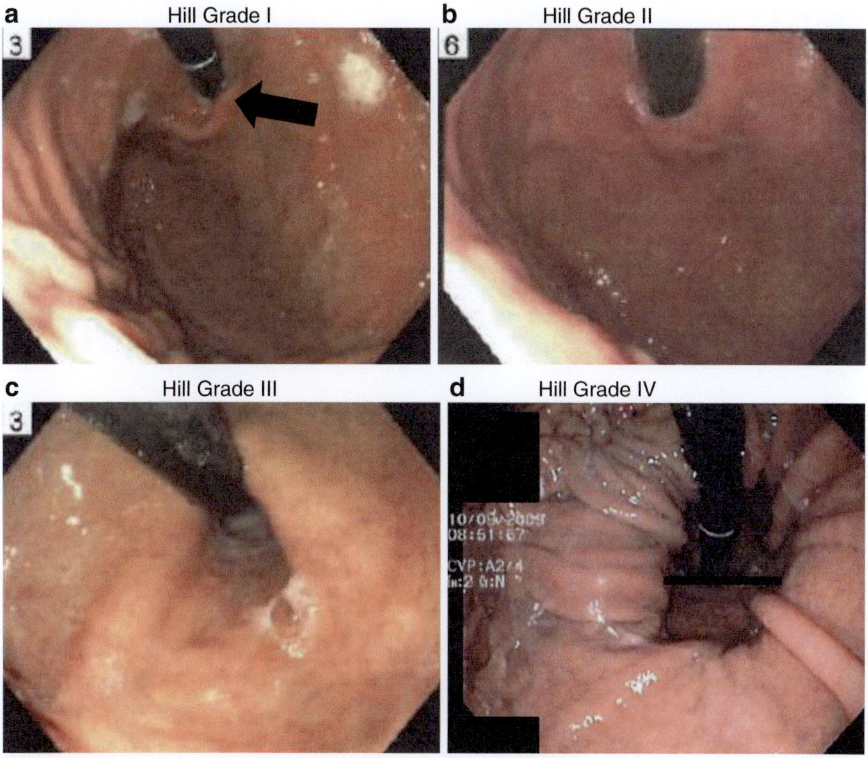

Fig. 1.2 The Hill classification of the gastroesophageal junction flap valve. *Black arrow* in (**a**) shows a normal angle of His ridge of a competent valve. *Black line* in (**d**) shows the transverse diameter of the hiatal hernia

on the gastric mucosa. There no GEJ adherence to the shaft of the endoscope and the squamous epithelium of the distal esophagus can be readily seen (Fig. 1.2d). A population-based study evaluating the concordance with hiatal hernia size and Hill classification included 334 subjects and demonstrated the Hill classification was slightly better at measuring a hiatal hernia but was not necessarily a stronger predictor [12]. The reproducibility of these results in an objective, accurate manner have yet to be elucidated.

Once it is determined that a hiatal hernia is present, there are two dimensions that determine its size. One is the axially dimension as measured from the GEJ to the "pinch" of the diaphragmatic hiatus around the stomach (Fig. 1.3). The other is the transverse dimension, as measured from the impression of the left crura against the herniated stomach to the impression of the right crura against the herniated stomach. These are measurements that are frequently not made during routine endoscopy. In patients with paraesophageal hernias, a twisting of the stomach within the hernia may be seen suggesting volvulus (Fig. 1.4).

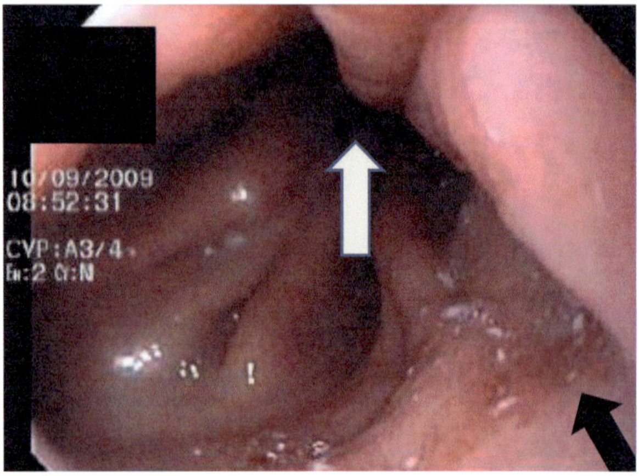

Fig. 1.3 The determination of the axial length of a sliding (type I) hiatal hernia from the Z-line (gastroesophageal junction, *black arrow*) to the "pinch" of the diaphragmatic hiatus around the stomach (*white arrow*). In conjunction with the transverse diameter (Fig. 1.2d), the size of the hiatal hernia can be determined

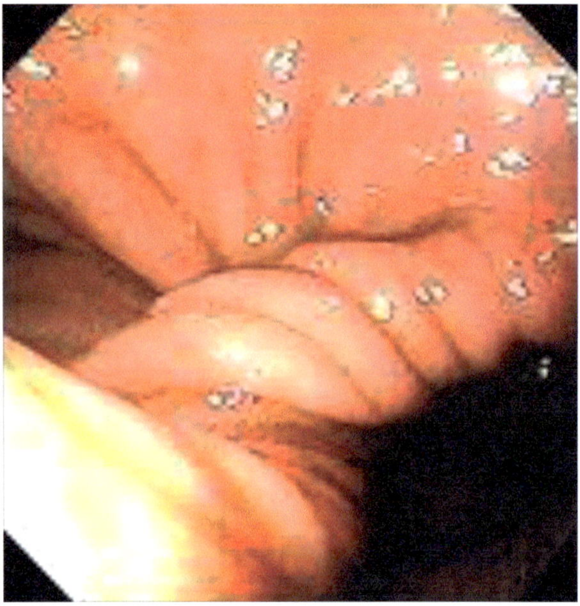

Fig. 1.4 Twisting of the stomach within a paraesophageal hernia suggesting gastric volvulus

1.6 Endoscopic Evaluation of the Esophageal Mucosa

1.6.1 Esophagitis

When evaluating patients for hiatal hernia it is also important to note the esophageal mucosa and any abnormalities. Specifically, the presence of erosive or non-erosive esophagitis needs to be determined. The severity of erosive esophagitis is graded based on the Los Angeles Classification (LA Classes) [14]. Grade A is the presence of one or more mucosal breaks that are ≤5 mm in length; Grade B is the presence of one or more mucosal breaks that are >5 mm; Grade C includes one or more mucosal breaks that

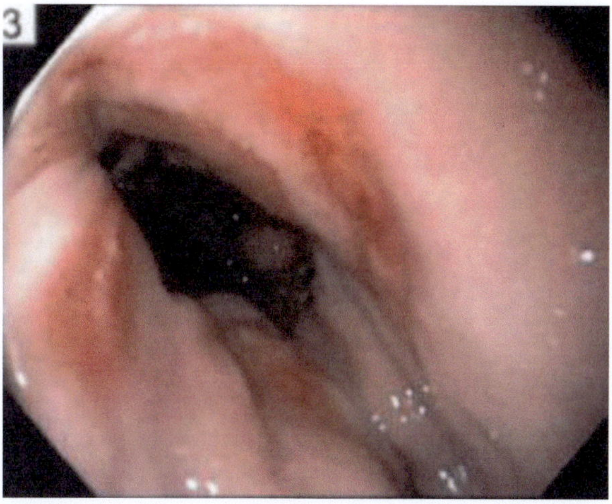

Fig. 1.5 An example of Los Angeles grade D esophagitis. Description of grades A, B and C in text

interconnect between the apices of two or more mucosal folds, but encompass <75% of the esophageal circumference. Grade D is the most extensive and includes continuous breaks within the mucosa that exceeds 75% of the esophageal circumference (Fig. 1.5). Biopsies of the area of esophagitis, in the absence of suspicion for neoplasia, appear not to have any additional value to endoscopic examination [15].

Conversely, non-erosive esophagitis is more difficult to diagnose via endoscopy and primarily diagnosed via biopsy. The presences of eosinophils, lymphocytes, balloon cells, and polymorphonuclear leukocytes have been seen on microscopy but have poor sensitivity and specificity if only one of these histologic abnormalities is identified. Specificity is increased if there are three or more of these abnormalities on microscopy but, consequently, sensitivity is decreased [16]. Nonetheless, the routine use of endoscopic biopsies in the setting of otherwise normal appearing esophageal mucosa is not recommended.

1.6.2 Barrett Esophagus

Barrett esophagus is defined as a change in the normal mucosa of the esophagus from squamous epithelium to metaplasia columnar epithelium. Barrett esophagus is a result of damage to the esophageal mucosa from persistent reflux disease. Under endoscopic visualization, it appears as salmon colored mucosa projecting proximally into the distal esophagus from the normal SCJ (Fig. 1.6a). With narrow-band imaging there is enhanced visualization of the GE junction in addition to mucosal abnormalities such as Barrett metaplasia (Fig. 1.6b). Suspicious areas seen on endoscopy and/or narrow-band imaging must be biopsied to confirm or rule out mucosal abnormalities; specifically, biopsies need to determine the presence of intestinal metaplasia and goblet cells. In the presence of esophagitis, patients need to be treated with proton pump inhibitors to enhance histologic evaluation of the Barrett metaplasia.

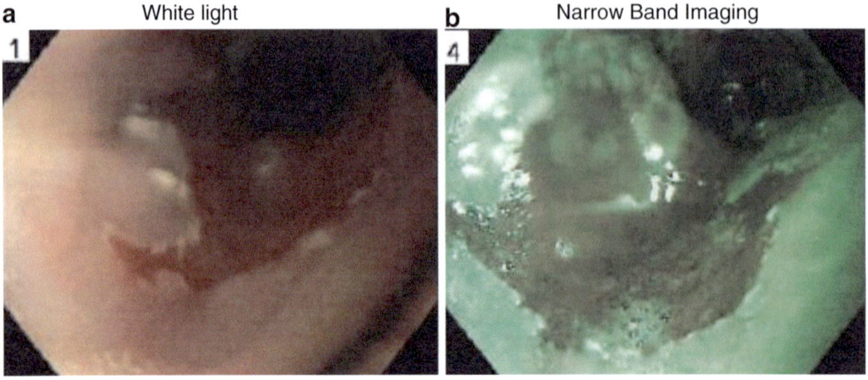

Fig. 1.6 Barrett esophagus as seen by white light (**a**) and narrow band imaging (**b**). Narrow band imaging enhances the difference between the area of normal squamous epithelium and metaplastic epithelium

Obtaining endoscopic biopsies of the esophagus that are concerning for Barrett esophagus typically follow the Seattle protocol; this is defined as four quadrant biopsies taken every 1 cm over the length of the Barrett esophagus [17]. The extent or severity of Barrett's is then further classified based on the Prague classification. This incorporates then length of circumference (Denoted as "C") of Barrett and the total length of the esophagus that includes Barrett's (Denoted as "M") [18]. For example, if a 2 cm circumferential portion of esophagus was involved and included 5 cm non-circumferential Barrett, this would be documented as C2M5.

The length and circumference is an important classification system for Barrett, but the presence of the type of metaplasia and/or dysplasia is also clinically important. Non-nodular Barrett or flat dysplasia is typically biopsied; depending on size and grade of dysplasia this is commonly managed with endoscopic eradication. This applies in the case of nodular metaplasia as well. Ulceration of the columnar epithelium and/or Barrett segment can be found in up to 60% of patients [19]. These are typically found incidentally, but may be complicated by bleeding or even perforation. There have been rare reports of fistula formation due to ulceration of Barrett esophagus [19]. Development of these findings is concerning for underlying malignancies and if seen endoscopically should be managed as such.

1.6.3 Esophageal Neoplasia

Endoscopy certainly plays a curative role in treating select patients with esophageal carcinoma. Primarily, endoscopic therapy is used for mucosal cancers. Endoscopic approaches can be divided into ablative and resection techniques. In the latter, endoscopic mucosal resection (EMR) offers the advantage of obtaining

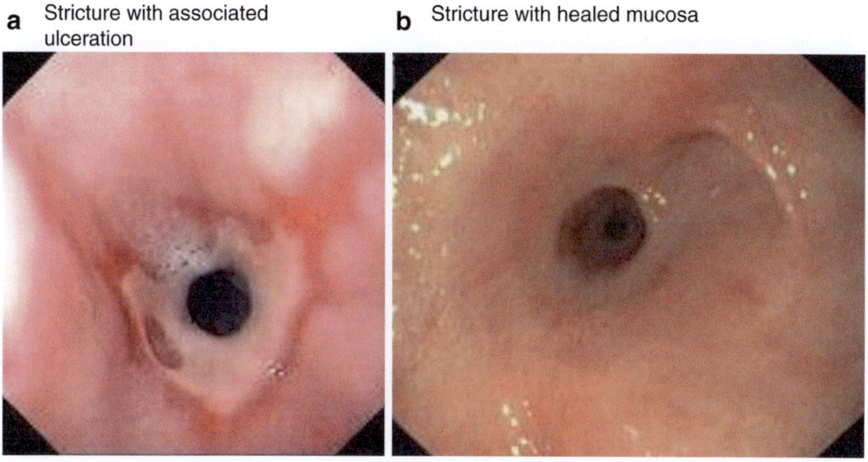

Fig. 1.7 Esophageal peptic stricture with (**a**) and without (**b**) ulceration

more tissue for appropriate cancer staging and even adequate treatment (Fig. 1.7a, b). EMR is primarily used in nodular Barrett's esophagus, T1a esophageal adenocarcinoma lesions, and in some instances, flat Barrett's esophagus with high-grade dysplasia [20]. Curative rates for EMR have reported ranges between 60% and 100%; one of the largest studies included 349 patients with high grade neoplasia or mucosal adenocarcinoma; with a follow-up of 5 years reported long-term eradication was 95% [21]. Although there has been no comparison to surgical resection, EMR offers a promising alternative to minimally invasive resection of these lesions. Complications of this intervention includes bleeding, perforation, and stricture formation.

Ablation techniques include photodynamic therapy, cryotherapy, argon plasma coagulation, heater probe treatment, and radiofrequency ablation. These techniques may be used alone or in combination with EMR. Successful treatment of Barrett esophagus or intramucosal carcinomas have been reported using ablative techniques, however, these are primarily limited to small case series and likely biased secondary to patient selection [20].

For malignancies that are greater than T1a or encompass larger areas of the esophagus, another possible endoscopic therapy is endoscopic submucosal dissection (ESD). Specifically, ESD is used for areas of dysplasia >2 cm or T1b lesions that are confined to the submucosa [20]. A recent study reported on ESD in 46 patients wither either HDG or intramucosal adenocarcinoma and a curative resection of 70%; similar curative rates have been reported [22]. However, it is important to note that this technique can be difficult given the piecemeal dissection/resection of these lesions. ESD solely for curative purposes can be done in highly selected patients, but larger sample sizes are necessary to determine its full utility.

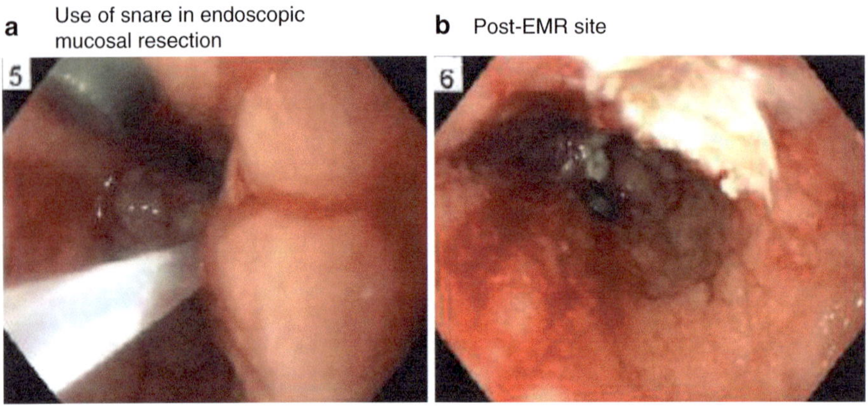

Fig. 1.8 An example of endoscopic mucosal resection of a T1a esophageal adenocarcinoma within a nodule of Barrett esophagus with high-grade dysplasia

1.6.4 Esophageal Peptic Stricture

Esophageal peptic strictures primarily occur secondary to repetitive exposure of the esophagus mucosa to stomach acid. Reportedly 7–23% of patients with reflux esophagitis develop peptic stricture [23]. Endoscopically, these strictures are defined as narrowing at the esophagus near the squamocolumnar junction and typically measure 1–4 cm in length (Fig. 1.8). This may result in esophageal narrowing up to 13 mm. Typically these strictures result in dysphagia and when visualized on endoscopy should be biopsied to ensure there is no underlying malignancy.

1.7 Intraoperative Evaluation of Newly Constructed Fundoplications

1.7.1 Perforation

Use of intraoperative endoscopy is a valuable tool for surgeons who routinely do minimally invasive foregut surgery. Trans-illuminating the gastroesophageal junction with the endoscope can help the surgeon identify the esophagus and stomach during difficult cases, such as re-do fundoplications. After the fundoplication is constructed, the endoscope is typically passed into the esophagus and stomach following creation of a fundoplication. There is visualization of the esophagus as the scope enters into the stomach. Time is also taken to visualize the GEJ to ensure no mucosal abnormalities. Once the scope is passed into the stomach, the scope is retroflexed and the GEJ is visualized as well as the newly created fundoplication. Tears or perforations may be seen with small mucosal slits or tears (Fig. 1.9). This can be either seen via the endoscope or light from the endoscope is visualized within the abdomen, which would signify a perforation. Once diagnosed, the perforation can be repaired primarily intraoperatively.

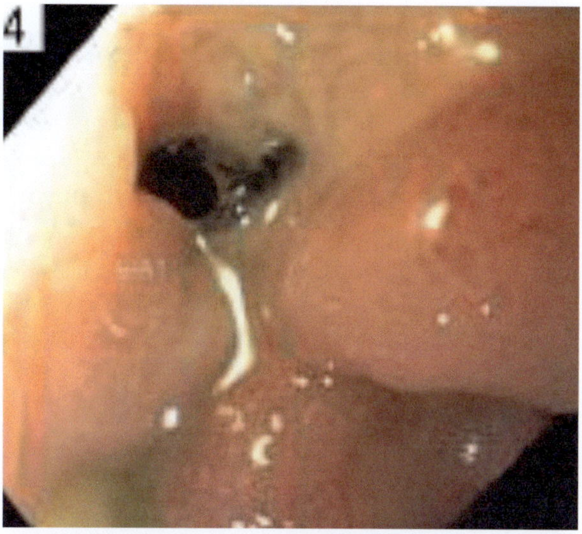

Fig. 1.9 An esophageal perforation as identified by endoscopy

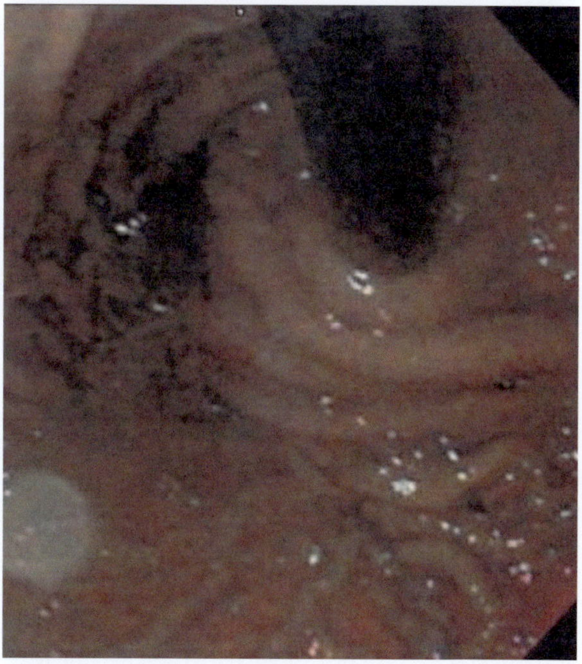

Fig. 1.10 An example of a normally constructed fundoplication immediately visualized intraoperatively. Note the "stacked coils" appearance of the wrap

1.7.2 Fundoplication Construction

The ideal construction of a fundoplication is commonly classified based on the definition derived from Jobe et al. [24] This includes: tight adherence to the scope, circumferences of the cardia <35 mm, no cardia dilatation, valve length 3–4 cm, nipple or coil type, and an intra-abdominal location of the stomach. The wrap should have a "stacked coils" appearance (Fig. 1.10). If these criteria are not met, there is concern for failed fundoplication construction and intraoperative evaluation of the newly constructed wrap should be undertaken to ensure there were no technical errors made.

1.8 Endoscopic Evaluation of Postoperative Adverse Events

Although antireflux surgery has high success rates, recurrent symptoms do occur approximately 5% of the time and may be disabling [25]. Conversely, anatomic abnormalities have been described in as many as 25% of cases with the use of endoscopy [25]. Therefore, endoscopy is important in determining the etiology for a patient's recurrent symptoms and whether their symptomology is a result of surgical failure.

1.8.1 Perforation

Perforation postoperatively is not a common event, but can happen and have severe consequences to the patient resulting in peritonitis, sepsis, and even death. Timely diagnosis is of the utmost importance and endoscopy aids in a timely diagnosis. Visualization of a tear or perforation can be seen within the mucosa on endoscopy (Fig. 1.9). Depending on the stability of the patient and severity of the tear, perforations may be repaired via endoscopic interventions including endoscopic clips, negative therapy devices, and esophageal stents. Success of these interventions has been reported to be above 80% from small case series, but with appropriate patient selection it may provide a minimally invasive treatment alternative for treating this postoperative complication.

1.8.2 Tight Fundoplication

A tight fundoplication typically refers to obstruction of the distal esophagus when the wrap was made either too tight or too long. This results in dysphagia, bloating, or regurgitation that persists several weeks after the procedure. This would be seen with a narrowing at the level of the distal esophagus and can be treated with esophageal dilation. If this fails, surgical revision may be necessary. In a normal fundoplication, the gastric mucosa is seen wrapped circumferentially around the shaft of the endoscope whereas a tight wrap results in the gastric mucosa being stretched and wrapped tightly around the shaft without laxity or visibility of the gastric folds (Fig. 1.11a).

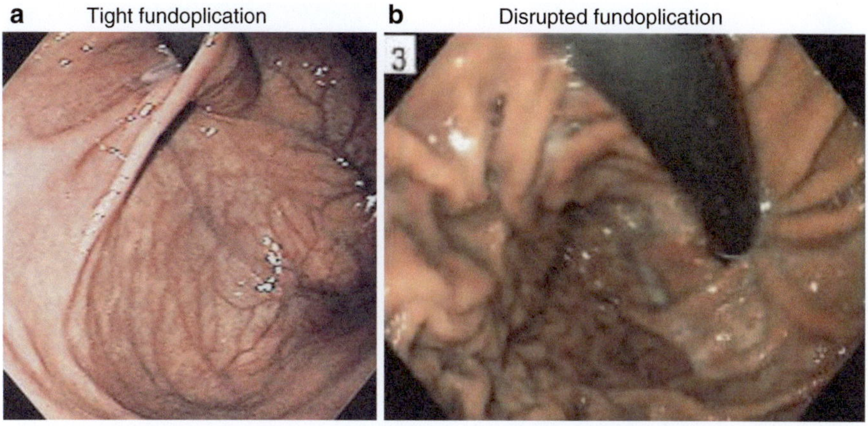

Fig. 1.11 Examples of postfundoplication problems. (**a**) a tight wrap causing dysphagia. Note the tethering of the gastric mucosa. (**b**) a disrupted wrap. Note that the mucosal folds have lost the stacked coils appearance

1.8.3 Disrupted/Loose Fundoplication

Disruption of the fundoplication involves partial or complete breakdown of the wrap; disruption commonly results in recurrence of a hiatal hernia. This complication may be secondary to inadequate suture technique and/or insufficient mobilization of the stomach fundus. Endoscopically, the gastric mucosal folds are not well-adhered to the shaft of the endoscope and essentially no evidence of a wrap is present on endoscopy, again indicating a loose or disrupted fundoplication (Fig. 1.11b).

1.8.4 Slipped Fundoplication

In the case of stomach slippage, the wrap remains below the level of the diaphragm but the proximal stomach slips and enters the chest. This may be otherwise referred to as an hourglass deformity because the stomach resides both above and below the newly created fundoplication. The herniated stomach may then become compressed by the diaphragmatic crura or a recurrent paraesophageal hernia may develop. Slippage may be secondary to breakdown of sutures or incorrect placement of the wrap around the esophagus. Conversely, slippage of the proximal stomach through an unbroken wrap creates a pouch below the diaphragm without development of a recurrent hiatal hernia. This is seen when the location of the wrap is inferior the level of the Z-line, indicating migration of the gastroesophageal junction superior to the wrap into the thoracic cavity (Fig. 1.12a).

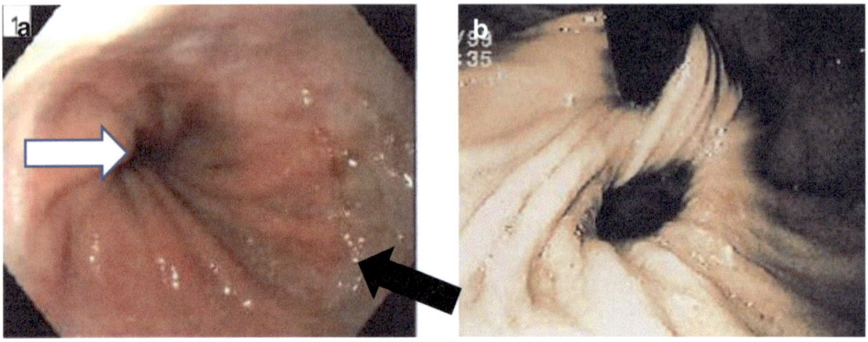

Fig. 1.12 Examples of recurrent hiatal hernias. (**a**) shows an esophageal view of a slipped Nissen fundoplication. The *black arrow* shows the gastroesophageal junction and the *white arrow* the position of the wrap. (**b**) shows a recurrent paraesophageal hernia with the wrap being pulled into the hernia

1.8.5 Recurrent Hiatal Hernia

Recurrence of a hiatal hernia is another possible surgical failure following antireflux surgery. In this case, through retroflexion a herniated pouch of stomach is typically seen next to the fundoplication fold indicating the presence of a recurrent hiatal hernia (Fig. 1.12b).

1.8.6 Twisted or Malconstructed Fundoplication

A twisted or malconstructed fundoplication may occur secondary to improper mobilization of the gastric fundus (lack of mobilizing the fundus, not ligating the short gastric vessels). Lack of mobility of the stomach fundus causing tension on the GEJ that ultimately causes rotation of the esophagus and fundoplication. Endoscopically there is a spiral-type of deformity that is seen when the scope is retroflexed to visualize the wrap.

1.9 Conclusions

Hiatal hernias occur when there is a herniation of abdominal contents in to the mediastinum via the diaphragm. Their prevalence is correlated with increasing age and obesity. Many times they are asymptomatic while other times they can have significant symptoms some of which include GERD, dysphagia, obstructive symptoms, to volvulus. Hiatal hernias are classified as either sliding or paraesophageal and are further classified into four subtypes. Symptomatic hernias need to be repaired and there is still an ongoing debate on whether an asymptomatic hernia requires repair. Although the relationship between hiatal hernias and GERD has long been debated, there is indeed a relationship between the two. One of the main clinical concerns that hiatal hernias pose is the progression to high grade dysplasia and carcinoma as a result of progression from Barrett's esophagus. Endoscopy can be an invaluable tool in the evaluation of hiatal hernias as well as postoperative evaluation in patients who may be experiencing complications following antireflux surgery.

Current Knowledge and Future Directions

- Endoscopy is an important tool that aids in the diagnosis of hiatal hernia and reflux disease
- Endoscopic criteria for measuring hiatal hernias remain vague and further studies should be done to determine a clear consensus for diagnosing and measuring hiatal hernias
- Endoscopic mucosal resection offers a minimal invasive intervention for Barrett esophagus but efficacy and curative rates are limited to small single institution studies
- Complications following fundoplication can be diagnosed and treated using endoscopy in select patients
- Larger studies comparing endoclips, vacuum devices, and other approaches are needed to determine the best management approaches for patients with complications following fundoplication construction
- Endoscopy offers a variety of options for managing patients with foregut pathology and understanding its utility provides the surgeon with a powerful diagnostic and treatment tool

References

1. van Herwaarden MA, Samsom M, Smout AJPM. The role of hiatus hernia in gastro-oesophageal reflux disease. Eur J Gastroenterol Hepatol. 2004;16(9):831–5.
2. Roman S, Kahrilas PJ. The diagnosis and management of hiatus hernia. BMJ. 2014;349:g6154. https://doi.org/10.1136/bmj.g6154.
3. Wu AH, Tseng C-C, Bernstein L. Hiatal hernia, reflux symptoms, body size, and risk of esophageal and gastric adenocarcinoma. Cancer. 2003;98(5):940–8. https://doi.org/10.1002/cncr.11568.
4. Menon S, Trudgill N. Risk factors in the aetiology of hiatus hernia: a meta-analysis. Eur J Gastroenterol Hepatol. 2011;23(2):133–8. https://doi.org/0.1097/MEG.0b013e3283426f57.
5. Masaoka A, Kondo S, Yano M, Araki Y, Nobutomo M. Thoracic deformity and hiatal hernia (intrathoracic stomach) in the elderly. J Thorac Imaging. 2012;27(6):372–5. https://doi.org/10.1097/RTI.0b013e3182698e99.
6. Abbara S, Kalan MMH, Lewicki AM. Intrathoracic stomach revisited. AJR Am J Roentgenol. 2003;181(2):403–14. https://doi.org/10.2214/ajr.181.2.1810403.

7. Kahrilas PJ, Kim HC, Pandolfino JE. Approaches to the diagnosis and grading of hiatal hernia. Best Pract Res Clin Gastroenterol. 2008;22(4):601–16. https://doi.org/10.1016/j.bpg.2007.12.007.
8. Krause W, Roberts J, Garcia-Montilla RJ. Bowel in chest: type IV hiatal hernia. Clin Med Res. 2016;14(2):93–6. https://doi.org/10.3121/cmr.2016.1332.
9. Rashid F, Thangarajah T, Mulvey D, Larvin M, Iftikhar SY. A review article on gastric volvulus: a challenge to diagnosis and management. Int J Surg. 2010;8(1):18–24. https://doi.org/10.1016/j.ijsu.2009.11.002.
10. Kohn GP, Price RR, DeMeester SR, et al. Guidelines for the management of hiatal hernia. Surg Endosc. 2013;27(12):4409–28. https://doi.org/10.1007/s00464-013-3173-3.
11. Wallner B, Sylvan A, Janunger K-G. Endoscopic assessment of the "Z-line" (squamocolumnar junction) appearance: reproducibility of the ZAP classification among endoscopists. Gastrointest Endosc. 2002;55(1):65–9. https://doi.org/10.1067/mge.2002.119876.
12. Hansdotter I, Björ O, Andreasson A, et al. Hill classification is superior to the axial length of a hiatal hernia for assessment of the mechanical anti-reflux barrier at the gastroesophageal junction. Endosc Int Open. 2016;4(3):E311–7. https://doi.org/10.1055/s-0042-101021.
13. Hill LD, Kozarek RA, Kraemer SJ, et al. The gastroesophageal flap valve: in vitro and in vivo observations. Gastrointest Endosc. 1996;44(5):541–7.
14. Genta RM, Spechler SJ, Kielhorn AF. The Los Angeles and Savary-Miller systems for grading esophagitis: utilization and correlation with histology. Dis Esophagus. 2011;24(1):10–7. https://doi.org/10.1111/j.1442-2050.2010.01092.x.
15. Nandurkar S, Talley NJ, Martin CJ, Ng T, Adams S. Esophageal histology does not provide additional useful information over clinical assessment in identifying reflux patients presenting for esophagogastroduodenoscopy. Dig Dis Sci. 2000;45(2):217–24.
16. Narayani RI, Burton MP, Young GS. Utility of esophageal biopsy in the diagnosis of nonerosive reflux disease. Dis Esophagus. 2003;16(3):187–92.
17. Levine DS, Haggitt RC, Blount PL, Rabinovitch PS, Rusch VW, Reid BJ. An endoscopic biopsy protocol can differentiate high-grade dysplasia from early adenocarcinoma in Barrett's esophagus. Gastroenterology. 1993;105(1):40–50. https://doi.org/10.1016/0016-5085(93)90008-Z.
18. Vahabzadeh B, Seetharam AB, Cook MB, et al. Validation of the Prague C & M criteria for the endoscopic grading of Barrett's esophagus by gastroenterology trainees: a multicenter study. Gastrointest Endosc. 2012;75(2):236–41. https://doi.org/10.1016/j.gie.2011.09.017.
19. Milind R, Attwood SE. Natural history of Barrett's esophagus. World J Gastroenterol. 2012;18(27):3483–91. https://doi.org/10.3748/wjg.v18.i27.3483.
20. ASGE Standards of Practice Committee, Evans JA, Early DS, et al. The role of endoscopy in the assessment and treatment of esophageal cancer. Gastrointest Endosc. 2013;77(3):328–34. https://doi.org/10.1016/j.gie.2012.10.001.
21. Pech O, Behrens A, May A, et al. Long-term results and risk factor analysis for recurrence after curative endoscopic therapy in 349 patients with high-grade intraepithelial neoplasia and mucosal adenocarcinoma in Barrett's oesophagus. Gut. 2008;57(9):1200–6. https://doi.org/10.1136/gut.2007.142539.
22. Yang D, Coman RM, Kahaleh M, et al. Endoscopic submucosal dissection for Barrett's early neoplasia: a multicenter study in the United States. Gastrointest Endosc. 2016; https://doi.org/10.1016/j.gie.2016.09.023.
23. Schlachta CM, Poulin EC, Mamazza J, Seshadri PA. Peptic strictures of the esophagus. BMJ. 2001;349:g6154.
24. Jobe BA, Kahrilas PJ, Vernon AH, et al. Endoscopic appraisal of the gastroesophageal valve after antireflux surgery. Am J Gastroenterol. 2004;99(2):233–43.
25. Braghetto I, Korn O, Csendes A, Valladares H, Davanzo C, Debandi A. Radiologic and endoscopic characteristics of laparoscopic antireflux wrap: correlation with outcome. Int Surg. 2012;97(3):189–97. https://doi.org/10.9738/CC120.1.

Chapter 2
The Role of MRI in GERD

Christiane Kulinna-Cosentini

2.1 Summary

The current diagnosis of GERD is based on a combination of endoscopy, pH monitoring, manometry, and imaging tools, such as a barium study [1]. The most sensitive technique for the assessment of gastroesophageal reflux is 24-h pH monitoring [2, 3], as well as manometry to evaluate esophageal motor disorders and functional disorders of the gastro-esophageal sphincter [4–6]. Catheters and probes for these examinations are uncomfortable, time-consuming, and not generally available.

Endoscopy is capable of detecting advanced esophagitis, but lacks sensitivity in determining pathological reflux, which is a particular limitation, as many patients with GERD do not display macroscopic erosions [7] at endoscopy.

Barium studies allow the visualization of esophageal and gastro-esophageal morphology and the alterations during physiological events with good specificity, but with a sensitivity of about 40% [8] and significant amounts of ionizing radiation [9].

With the introduction of ultrafast MR sequences with increasing temporal resolution to the subsecond level, dynamic MR fluoroscopy has become a reality for the assessment of morphological and functional imaging of the esophagus [10–13]. MRI swallowing is a completely non-invasive procedure, without ionizing radiation. Therefore, it can be implemented in pediatric patients [14] and pregnant women without danger, as an initial examination or as a follow-up examination after therapy, i.e., after anti-reflux surgery [15]. At present, MR fluoroscopy has been effectively used in oropharyngeal imaging [9, 12] and for the assessment of esophageal motility disorders, GERD [13, 16], as well as for post-surgery patients after narrow gastric tube reconstruction in esophagectomy [17].

C. Kulinna-Cosentini
Department of Biomedical Imaging and Image-Guided Therapy, Medical University of Vienna, Waehringer Guertel 18-20, 1090 Vienna, Austria
e-mail: christiane.kulinna-cosentini@meduniwien.ac.at

M.A. Memon (ed.), *Hiatal Hernia Surgery*,
https://doi.org/10.1007/978-3-319-64003-7_2

Recent advances in magnetic resonance imaging (MRI) have led to the development of a fast and accurate technique for monitoring the dynamics of the physiological processes of the gastroesophageal region in real-time, as well as evaluating surrounding structures. Due to the short examination protocol, it can be easily integrated into the clinical routine.

2.2 Impact of MRI in Diagnosing GERD

Gastroesophageal reflux disease (GERD) occurs when the reflux of gastric content into the esophagus provokes mucosal injury, often combined with typical symptoms like heartburn, acid regurgitation, globus sensation, or dysphagia due to an ineffective antireflux barrier between the esophagus and the stomach [18]. The pathophysiology of GERD is multifactorial and overlaps with other functional disorders of the esophagus and stomach, such as esophageal motility disorders [19]. To diagnose GERD, many invasive and non-invasive techniques, such as endoscopy, manometry, 24-h-pH monitoring, impedance measurements, and barium esophagram, are available. Each of these methods covers only a part of some aspect of this disease and a standardized diagnostic procedure has not yet been established.

Videofluoroscopy or barium swallow are the most common radiographic methods, which allow an assessment of the morphology and functionality of the esophagus and the GEJ. However, these techniques cannot display surrounding structures, and requires ionizing radiation exposure. Due to the radiation exposure, a short examination time is required and the procedure cannot be repeated arbitrarily.

The beneficial aspects of MRI include excellent soft-tissue contrast without exposure to ionizing radiation. Study results [7, 10, 11, 13, 14, 16, 20] have demonstrated the feasibility of dynamic swallowing MRI in healthy volunteers [20], the assessment of esophageal motility [13, 14], as well as the evaluation of bolus transit and reflux events [14] in patients with GERD.

Compared to videofluoroscopy, MRI swallowing offers the possibility of multiplanar imaging in every desired plane. Thus, an exact measurement of the size of a hiatal hernia, which is strongly associated with GERD [5, 6], is possible in various views (Fig. 2.1) [14]. The size of the hernia shows a strong correlation with the grade of reflux [14]. Approximately 60–80% of patients with reflux esophagitis have a hiatal hernia, whereas only 3–7% of patients without a hiatal hernia show signs of reflux esophagitis [5, 6, 21, 22]. The clinical importance of the size of a hiatal hernia was described by Jones et al. [23] as well. An increased hernia size is significantly correlated with total esophageal acid exposure, acid clearance time, and esophagitis severity [23]. A correlation between the prevalance of Barrett's esophagus and the size of a hiatal hernia has also been reported by [24], as well as the increased risk of esophageal cancer [25] in patients with hiatal hernia.

Dynamic MR imaging of reflux events requires an image plane that should be oriented through the GEJ. Thus, sagittal and coronal double-oblique angulated planes are preferred [14]. An axial orientation is favored for the detection and measurement of an axial hiatal hernia (Fig. 2.2).

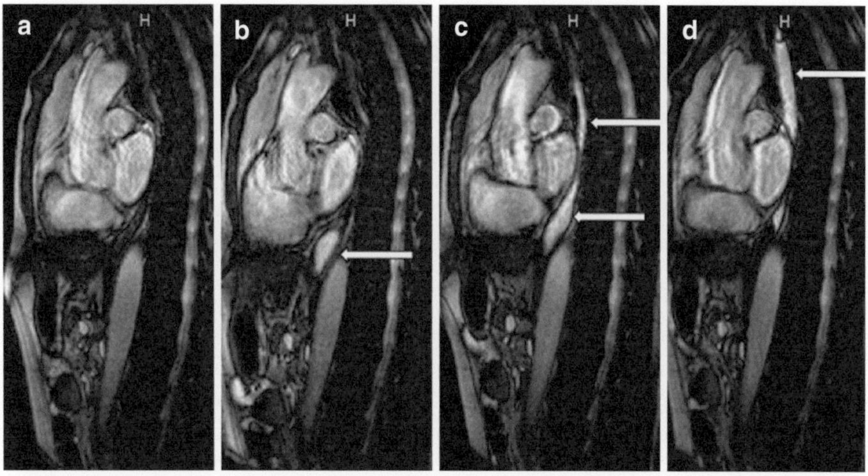

Fig. 2.1 Dynamic FFE pulse sequence in the sagittal view shows spontaneous gastroesophageal reflux (*arrows*) with typical caudo-cranial propagation of the bolus **(a–d)**

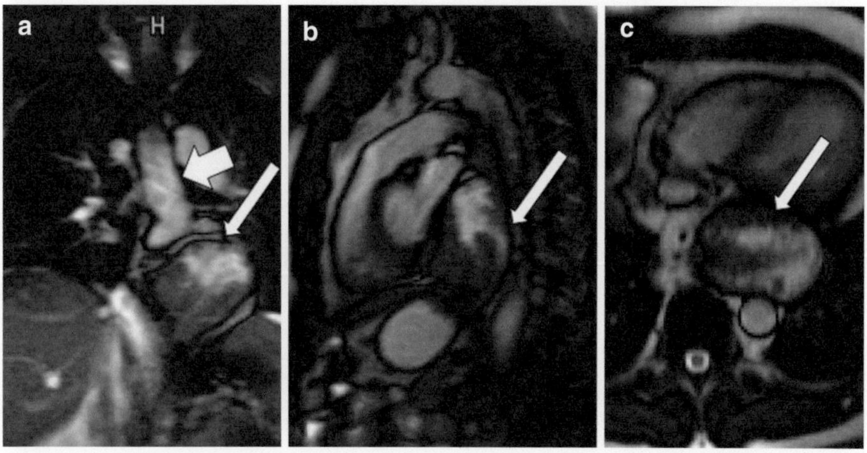

Fig. 2.2 Dynamic B-FFE pulse sequence shows a fixed axial hernia filled with buttermilk-gadolinium (*arrows*) in the coronal (**a**), sagittal (**b**), and axial views (**c**). A spontaneous gastroesophageal reflux from the hiatal hernia is demonstrated (*thick arrow*)

These orientations, in combination with the use of three contiguous slices for better coverage of the entire esophagus, which is the main challenge in this examination, promise a good correlation between reflux events in MRI and pathologic DeMeester score in pH-metric studies [14]. Another publication did not report any correlation between reflux events in MRI and grade of reflux with endoscopic findings and Carlson's questionnaire score [16]. Gastroesophageal reflux, detected on MRI, correlated to a Demeester score >14.7, which is indicative of gastroesophageal reflux, was diagnosed in 11 of 12 patients in a study by Zhnag et al. [7]. When comparing functional parameters between healthy volunteers and patients, statistically significant differences between healthy volunteers and patients could be evaluated based on diaphragm-to-sphincter distance, sphincter length, and sphincter transit time [7]. There was no significant difference of the HIS angle between healthy volunteers and patients, which is contrary to the longstanding hypothesis that a smaller HIS angle forms an anatomical antireflux barrier by a flap valve mechanism [26, 27].

The use of a simple and quick MR protocol, in combination with a good visible contrast medium, is mandatory to integrate this examination into the clinical routine.

The MRI is usually performed in the supine position on a 1.5 T or 3 T MRI, provided the patient is not at risk of aspiration. A body phased-array coil should be placed upon the chest. After a reference scan, a coronal T2-weighted, single-shot Turbo-Spin-Echo-sequence (TSE) or a T2-weighted half-Fourier-acquired, single-shot turbo spin echo (HASTE) sequence for orientation of the course of the esophagus and the gastro-esophageal junction (GEJ) should be performed. Then, a sagittal and an axial plane are obtained. After the "anatomical" static T2-weigthed sequences, a sagittal, oblique B-FFE (Balanced Fast Field Echo Sequence) or TrueFisp sequence (True Fast Imaging with steady state precession) with three contiguous slices is centered on the lower esophagus in the coronal view of the T2-weighted image according to these sequence parameters (Fig. 2.3). An additional coronal plane then is planned in the sagittal view. During these dynamic series, a buttermilk-gadolinium mixture (Dotarem®, gadoterate meglumine, Guerbet, Germany) at a dilution of 40:1 is placed in a cup with a long plastic tube in the MR gantry. The other end of the plastic tube is placed into the patient's mouth. Patients then are instructed to take a bolus in their mouth and swallow in a single gulp to prevent repetitive swallowing. If the coverage of the esophagus and the GEJ is inadequate, the pulse sequence is repeated in a slightly different angulation. Since there is increased awareness of the possible side effects of gadolinium or possible interaction between gadolinium and

Tabelle 1. MR Sequence parameter

Parameter	HASTE	B-FFE
Repetition time (ms)	1800	2.9
Echo time (ms)	100	1.5
Flip angle °	150	60
Acquisition matrix	256x256	256x256
Field of view (mm)	350x350	375x375
Slice thickness (mm)	5	15
Intersection gap (mm)	–	0.4
Aquisition time (s/image)	1	1
Aquisition cycle (s)	–	60
Slice orientation	1. Coronal	1. Sagittal oblique
	2. Sagittal	2. Coronal oblique
	3. Axial	3. Axial

Fig. 2.3 Sequence parameter our routinely used MRI protocol

gastric acid, which has not, as yet, been verified, we have changed the oral contrast medium to Lumivision® (Bender Group, b.e. imaging, Baden-Baden, Germany). Lumivision® is a natural liquid contrast for oral application in MRI and contains different special fruit juices like pineapple, agave, and black currant. Patients with a hypersensitivity to these fruits, as well as patients with fructose malabsorption, should avoid taking this contrast medium. Diabetic patients must adjust their medication according to the sugar content (6.5BE per bottle of 250 ml Lumivision®).

Real-time MRI offers a new perspective for a robust anatomic visualization combined with functional assessment of gastroesophageal reflux in patients. Another advantage is the possibility to directly view the surrounding structures, which is not possible with conventional examination techniques, for example, and represents a reliable tool with which to identify extraluminal findings. As a consequence, this non-invasive and non-ionizing approach has already shown great promise for the characterization of complex motions during swallowing, which could be of particular interest in pregnant and young patients. This method cannot replace ph-metry and manometry as measurable tools for the identification of reflux events and motility problems, but it could be a worthwhile method in pregnant patients, children, and other patients in whom a ph-metric/manometric tube cannot be placed.

2.3 The Role of MRI in Patients After Fundoplication

After a fundoplication procedure, radiologic work-up plays an important role in identifying possible problems.

The impact of a routinely conducted postoperative swallowing examination has been discussed controversially [28]. However, 2–17% of patients need a postoperative diagnostic clarification of their new or recurrent clinical symptoms, such as recurrent heartburn, regurgitation, or dysphagia. During the last several decades, a wide range of diagnostic modalities, such as endoscopy, pH monitoring, manometry, and barium swallow, were used to solve the possible problems. However, the modalities cover only a partial aspect of potential postoperative failure and are inaccurate in up to 40% of cases [29] in explaining the reason for dysphagia.

Because these patients are often young, a functional and morphologic imaging method without ionizing radiation was introduced in [15]. This study analyzed the role of MRI for the evaluation of anatomical and functional disorders after Nissen fundoplication compared to intraoperative findings in 29 patients. MRI was able to determine the position of the fundoplication wrap in 93% (Fig. 2.4), and correctly identified 67% of all malpositions of the wrap. Intrathoracic migration of the wrap, in particular, can be detected very well (Fig. 2.5). All wrap disruptions (Fig. 2.6), as well as all stenosis could be identify by MRI. In three cases, stenosis were caused by too-tight crural sutures, and, in two cases, by too-tight wraps. Stenosis that are shorter than 1 cm in length are usually caused by too-tight crural sutures. A stenosis measuring 2–3 cm in length is usually caused by a too-tight (Fig. 2.7) or too-long wrap (>3 cm).

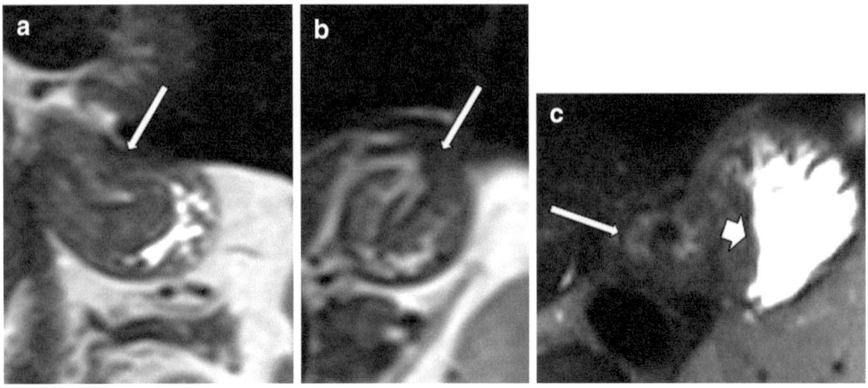

Fig. 2.4 Normal postoperative appearance after Nissen fundoplication on MRI. The coronal (**a**) and sagittal (**b**) view shows the correct position of the wrap under the diaphragm. A ring-like "pseudotumor" (*long arrow*) of the fundoplication, and a well-defined smooth defect in the fundus (*short arrow*) acquired in the axial plane (**c**)

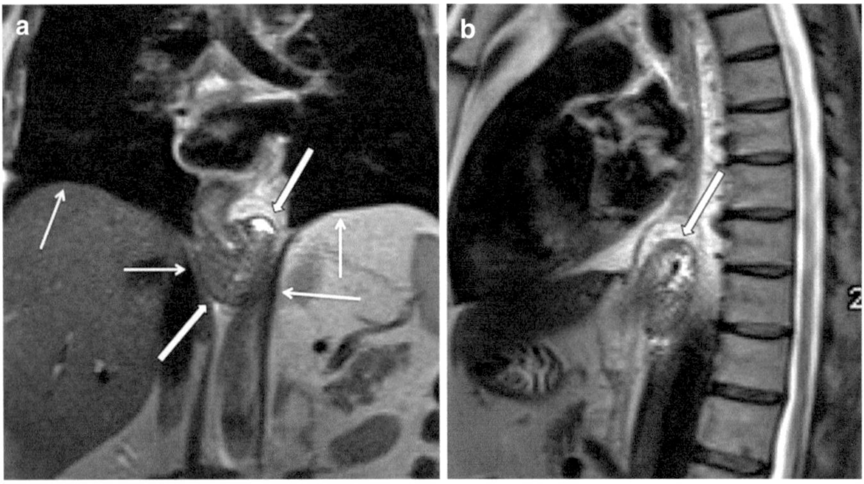

Fig. 2.5 Intrathoracic wrap migration. T2w HASTE sequences in the coronal view were performed to demonstrate the integrity of the wrap (*long arrow*) (**a**), but the wrap was detected above the esophageal hiatus and above the diaphragms (*thin arrows*) (**b**)

When abnormal esophageal motility is present before surgery, there is a greater likelihood of dysphagia developing after fundoplication [30]. The prolonged mechanical obstruction of the distal esophagus by the fundoplication wrap, with loss of peristalsis above the wrap, could be the cause of so-called secondary achalasia, even if there was normal esophageal motility before surgery.

Thus, the examination of peristalsis and esophageal motility in patients with dysphagia after Nissen fundoplication is mandatory. Usually, this condition is observed

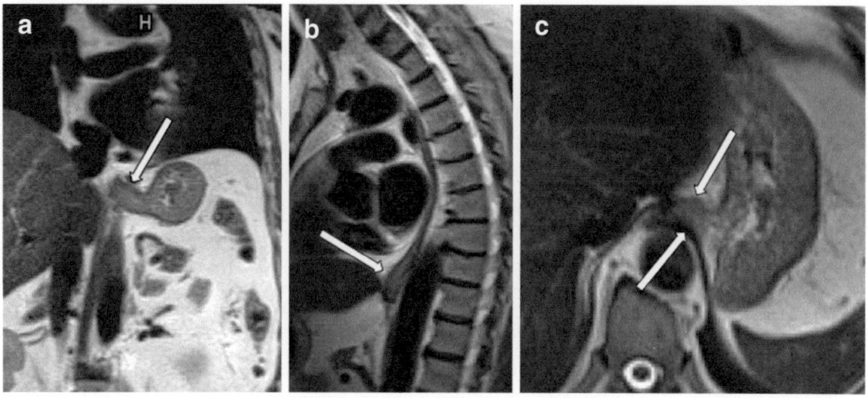

Fig. 2.6 Complete wrap disruption. Complete wrap disruption obtained in a patient with symptoms of recurrent reflux. The typical "pseudotumor" is missed on the coronal, sagittal and axial (*arrows*) view (**a–c**)

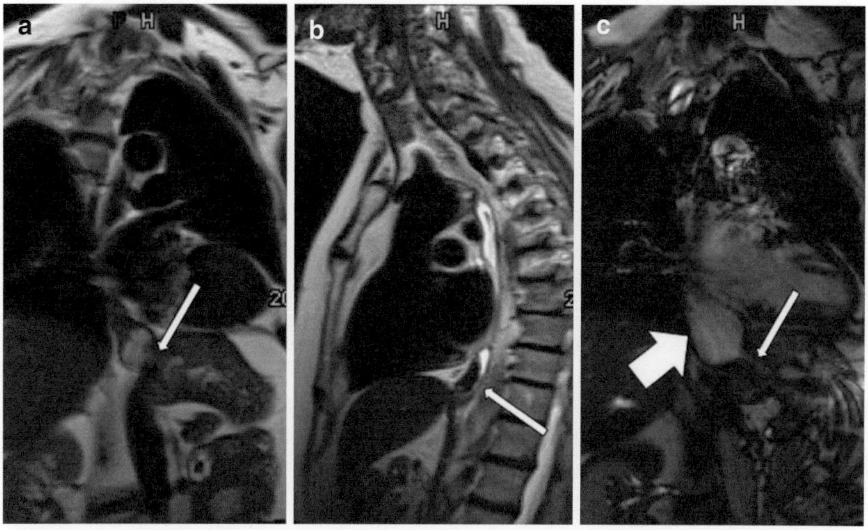

Fig. 2.7 Stenosis at the gastroesophageal junction. If the stenosis measures less than 1 cm in length (*thin arrow*) on the coronal and *sagittal view*, it strongly suggests too-tight crural sutures as the cause of dysphagia (**a**, **b**). A ballooning of the distal esophagus can be shown in the *coronal view* of the dynamic FFE pulse sequence (*thick arrow*) (**c**)

by manometry and barium swallow, the latter of which has the disadvantage of ionizing radiation. A delayed bolus transit of more than 20 s and a lack of propulsive peristalsis was found in MRI swallowing in our study in three patients. The diagnosis of secondary motility disorder was confirmed by manometry. Another study by Covotta et al. showed a sensitivity of 87.5%, with a specificity of 100% in MRI, compared to manometry, for the detection of motility alterations in 24 patients who presented with dysphagia and specific and non-specific motor disorders [31]. There is a lack of other MRI studies after esophago-gastric operations, except for one study by Panebianco et al. This paper evaluated the functionality and morphology of a neo-esophagus with narrow gastric tube reconstruction (NGT) after radical esophagectomy [17] using MRI. MRI was able to properly invesitgate the peculiar alterations that developed after this kind of intervention [17]. These authors showed the strong association between an increased NGT caliber and poor NGT functionality.

A short examination protocol in symptomatic patients after antireflux surgery should include HASTE sequences for clarifying the wrap situation and dynamic sequences for excluding a secondary motility disorder:

Starting with a single-shot sequence, such as a T2-weighted half-Fourier-acquired single-shot turbo spin echo (HASTE) sequence, a good overview of the postoperative hiatal anatomic situation can be obtained. The HASTE sequence is first performed in the coronal, then in the sagittal and axial views.

This sequence serves to depict the wrap, its exact location, and any possible slipping. A slipping or telescope phenomenon indicates that a part of the stomach slips through the wrap into the thoracic area.

The HASTE sequence in the coronal and sagittal views can also depict the complete course of the esophagus. The best views for depicting the position of the fundoplication wrap are the coronal and sagittal views. The axial view is preferred for estimating the integrity of the wrap with a typical "ring-like pseudotumor" appearance (Fig. 2.4c), as well as for evaluating a possible recurrent hernia.

The HASTE sequence is very helpful in depicting the correct position for the dynamic double-angulated B-FFE or TrueFisp sequences, which is performed next. A sagittal, oblique B-FFE sequence is performed as a pulse sequence with three contiguous slices for better coverage of the entire esophagus, and is centered on the lower esophagus.

This dynamic sequence, in particular, enables an evaluation of persitalsis and the bolus transit time of the esophagus, including the lower esophageal sphincter. In most patients, it is also possible to assess the passage through the fundoplication wrap, even though this occurrence often can be evaluated better with a coronal view, which is performed after the sagittal view. The coronal view should be centered on the course of the lower esophagus and the wrap. A dynamic axial view has no advantages and is rarely executed in routine clinical practice.

With the introduction of dynamic MRI in symptomatic patients after fundoplication, it is now possible to visualize not only luminal structures, such as with a barium esophagogram, but also to illustrate structural details of the esophagus and stomach, as well as the surrounding structures. Thus, rupture or malposition of the fundoplication wrap, as well as other anatomical problems in the hiatal position, can also be detected, as well as motility disorders The short examination protocol of about 30 min provides the possibility to include this examination into normal clinical routine.

2.4 Summary

Swallowing MRI is coming of age. Until now several publications of swallowing MRI in healty patients, as well as in patients with GERD and in symptomatic after antireflux surgery could give novel insights into this disease without ionizing radiation. Not only luminal structures but also anatomical as well as functional structures in one diagnostic method can now be identified.

The development of more uniformed analysis methods in future will aid translation into clinical routine. Therefore further work validating this method is needed.

What Is the Current Knowledge and What Future Direction Is Required

1. With the introduction of ultrafast MR sequences with increasing temporal resolution, dynamic MR swallowing has become reality for the assessment of morphological and functional imaging of the esophagus.
2. MRI swallowing is a completely non-invasive procedure, without ionizing radiation.
   Due to the short examination protocol, it can be easily integrated into the clinical routine.
3. The beneficial aspects of MRI include excellent soft-tissue contrast and the possibility to directly view the surrounding structures, which is not possible with conventional examination techniques, for example, and represents a reliable tool with which to identify extraluminal findings.
4. MR swallowing cannot replace ph-metry and manometry as measurable tools for the identification of reflux events and motilty problems, but it could be a worthwhile method in patients in whom a ph-metric/manometric tube cannot be placed.
5. After antireflux surgery a rupture or malposition of the fundoplication wrap, as well as other anatomical problems in the hiatal position, can also be detected, as well as secondary motility disorders
6. The implementation of uniformed analysis methods and scoring systems are need to translate MR swallowing into clinical routine.

References

1. Gordon C, Kang JY, Neild PJ, et al. The role of hiatus hernia in gastro-oesophageal disease. Aliment Pharmacol Ther. 2001;20:719–32.
2. Leite LP, Johnston BT, Barrett J, et al. Ineffective esophageal motility (IEM): The primary finding in patients with nonspecific esophageal motility disorder. Dig Dis Sci. 1997;42:1859–65.
3. Streets CG, DeMeester TR. Ambulatory 24-hour esophageal pH monitoring: why, when and what to do. J Clin Gastroenterol. 2003;37:14–22.
4. Kahrilas PJ. Beyond the motor elements of swallow. Gastroenterology. 1994;107:879–81.

5. Van Herwaarden MA, Samsom M, Smout AJ. The role of hiatus hernia in gastro-oesophageal reflux disease. Eur J Gastroenterol Hepatol. 2004;16:831–5.
6. Wright RA, Hurwitz AL. Relationship of hiatal hernia to endoscopically proved reflux esophagitis. Dig Dis Sci. 1979;24:311–3.
7. Zhang S, Joseph AA, Gross L, Ghadimi M, Frahm J, Beham AW. Diagnosis of gastroesophageal reflux disease using real-time magnetic resonce imaging. Sci Rep. 2015;15(5):12112.
8. Thompson JK, Kohler RE, Richter JE. Detection of gastroesophageal reflux: value of barium studies compared with 24-hr pH monitoring. AJR Am J Roentgenol. 1994;162(3):621–6.
9. Crawley MT, Savage P, Oakley F. Patient and operator dose during fluoroscopic examination of swallow mechanism. Br J Radiol. 2004;77:654–6.
10. Barkhausen J, Goyen M, von Winterfeld F, Lauenstein T, Arweiler-Harbeck D, Debatin JF. Visualization of swallowing using real-time TrueFISP MR fluoroscopy. Eur Rad. 2002;12:129–33.
11. Curcic J, Fox M, Kaufman E, Forras-Kaufman Z, et al. Gastroesophageal junction: structure and function as assessed by using MR imaging. Radiology. 2010;257:115–24.
12. Hartl DM, Kolb F, Bretagne E, Marandas P, Sigal R. Cine magnetic resonance imaging with single-shot fast spin echo for evaluation of dysphagia and aspiration. Dysphagia. 2006;21:156–62.
13. Panebianco V, Tomei E, Anzidei M, et al. Functional MRI in the evaluation of oesophageal motility: feasibility, MRI patterns of normality, and preliminary experience in subjects with motility disorders. Radiol Med. 2006;111:881–9.
14. Kulinna-Cosentini C, Schima W, Lenglinger J, et al. Is there a role for dynamic swallowing MRI in the assessment of gastroesophageal reflux disease and oesophageal motility disorders? Eur Radiol. 2012;22:364–70.
15. Kulinna-Cosentini C, Schima W, Ba-Ssalamah A, Cosentini EP. MRI patterns of Nissen fundoplication: normal appearance and mechanisms of failure. Eur Radiol. 2014;24(9):2137–45.
16. Manabe T, Kawamitsu H, Higashino T, et al. Observation of gastro-esophageal reflux by MRI: a feasibility study. Abdom Imaging. 2009;34:419–23.
17. Panebianco V, Francioni F, Anzidei M, Anile M, Rolla M, Pasariello R. Magnetic resonance-fluoroscopy as longterm follow-up examination in patients with narrow gastric tube reconstruction after radical esophagectomy. Eur J Cardiothorac Surg. 2006;30:663–8.
18. Tack J. Gastric motor disorders. Best Pract Res Clin Gastroenterol. 2007;21:633–44.
19. Quigley EM. Bacteria: a new player in gastrointestinal motility disorders–infections, bacterial overgrowth, and probiotics. Gastroenterol Clin North Am. 2007;36:735–48.
20. Kulinna-Cosentini C, Schima W, Cosentini EP. Dynamic MR imaging of the gastroesophageal junction in healthy volunteers during bolus passage. J Magn Reson Imaging. 2007;25:749–54.
21. Berstad A, Weberg R, Froyshov Larsen I, et al. Relationship of hiatus hernia to reflux esophagitis. Scand J Gastroenterol. 1986;21:55–8.
22. Petersen H, Johannessen T, Sandvik AK, et al. Relationship between endoscopic hiatus hernia and gastroesophageal reflux symptoms. Scand J Gastroenterol. 1991;26:921–6.
23. Jones MP, Sloan SS, Jovanovic B, et al. Impaired egress rather than increased access: an important independent predictor of erosive oesophagitis. Neurogastroenterol Motil. 2002;14:625–31.
24. Cameron AJ. Barrett's esophagus: prevalance and size of hiatal hernia. Am J Gastroenterol. 1999;94:2054–9.
25. Chow WH, Finkle WD, McLaughin JK, et al. The relation of gastroesophageal reflux disease and its treatment to adenocarcinomas of the esophagus and gastric cardia. JAMA. 1995;274:474–7.
26. Hill LD, et al. The gastroesophageal flap valve: in vitro and in vivo observations. Gastrointest Endosc. 1996;44:541–7.
27. Kahrilas PJ, et al. Esophageal peristaltic dysfunction in peptic esophagitis. Gastroenterology. 1986;91:897–904.
28. Hogan BA, Winter DC, Broe D, Broe P, Lee MJ. Prospective trial comparing contrast swallow, computed tomography and endoscopy to identify anastomotic leak following oesophagogastric surgery. Surg Endosc. 2008;22(3):767–71.

29. Hashemi M, Peters JH, DeMeester TR, et al. Laparoscopic repair of large type III hiatal hernia: objective followup reveals high recurrence rate. J Am Coll Surg. 2000;190:553–60.
30. Wehrli NE, Levine MS, Rubesin SE, Katzka DA, Laufer I. Secondary achalasia and other esophageal motility disorders after laparoscopic Nissen fundoplication for gastroesophageal reflux disease. AJR Am J Roentgenol. 2007;189:1464–146.
31. Covotta F, Piretta L, Badiali D, Laghi A, Biondi T, Corazziari ES, Panebianco V. Functional magentic resonce in the evaluation of oesophageal motility disorders. Gastroenterol Res Pract. 2011;2011:5. Article ID 367639. https://doi.org/10.1155/2011/36763.

Chapter 3
Utility of Ambulatory Esophageal pH and High-Resolution Manometry in the Diagnosis of Gastro-Esophageal Reflux Disease and Hiatal Hernia

Daphne Ang and Mark Fox

3.1 Introduction

The esophagogastric junction (EGJ) is the major defense against reflux of gastric contents into the esophagus; however, normal EGJ function is crucial also for normal esophageal swallowing and venting of air (belching). These represent opposing demands and the complex structure and function of the EGJ reflects this need to allow bolus passage whilst preventing excessive reflux of gastric contents [1]. It follows that EGJ pathology, for example the presence of hiatus hernia, will either impair the passage of food and fluid from the esophagus into the stomach or increase the risk of gastroesophageal reflux.

Gastroesophageal reflux disease (GERD) is very common in the community and symptoms impact on quality of life [1]. The prevalence of GERD and its complications, including esophageal adenocarcinoma, is rising; a trend that has been linked to the increasing age of the population and increasing prevalence of obesity over time [2]. Age is associated with a an increased prevalence of hiatus hernia and impaired esophageal motility [3]. Obesity has been linked to mechanical and neurohormonal effects on EGJ function, both of which can increase acid exposure of the distal esophagus [4–6].

Medical treatment with proton pump inhibitors (PPI) is the mainstay of therapy in GERD; however, acid suppression does not correct the underlying pathology of this condition and the frequency of reflux events is unchanged [7]. Persistent

D. Ang
Department of Gastroenterology, Changi General Hospital, Singapore, Singapore

M. Fox (✉)
Department of Gastroenterology, Abdominal Center, St. Claraspital, Kleinriehenstrasse 30, Basel, Switzerland

Neurogastroenterology and Motility Research Group, Department of Gastroenterology and Hepatology, University Hospital Zürich, Zürich, Switzerland
e-mail: dr.mark.fox@gmail.com

M.A. Memon (ed.), *Hiatal Hernia Surgery*,
https://doi.org/10.1007/978-3-319-64003-7_3

“weakly- and non-acid” reflux is a frequent cause of reflux symptoms in patients taking PPI therapy; [8] however, in one large series from a tertiary referral unit, only half the patients referred for further investigation have GERD confirmed on ambulatory pH-impedance studies [1]. Anti-reflux surgery, including hiatal repair and fundoplication, restores the EGJ reflux barrier and dramatically reduces the frequency of reflux and acid exposure; [9] however, a proportion of patients have persistent or recurrent symptoms after surgery related either to failure to create an effective reflux barrier or, conversely, the presence of EGJ outlet obstruction.

In this article, we review the structure and function of the EGJ in health and disease. The contribution of esophageal high-resolution manometry (HRM) and ambulatory pH-impedance monitoring to GERD diagnosis is considered. Throughout there is an emphasis on how the results of investigation in patients with suspected GERD impacts on management. Additionally, the role of physiological investigation in patients with esophageal symptoms after anti-reflux surgery is considered.

3.2 EGJ Anatomy

The esophago-gastric junction (EGJ) comprises an intrinsic component made up by smooth muscles of the lower esophageal sphincter (LES) with the clasp and sling fibers of the gastric cardia, and an extrinsic component formed by the crural diaphragm [10–15]. These two components are brought together into a functional unit by the phreno-esophageal ligament that anchors the LES to the crural diaphragm (Fig. 3.1).

In health, the lower esophageal sphincter (LES) is approximately 4 cm long extending from just above the squamo-columnar junction (Z-line) into the proximal stomach with distinct upper and lower sections. The upper section comprises relatively thick, tonically contracted esophageal smooth muscle fibers and the lower section comprises the sling and clasp muscle fibers of the gastric cardia [11, 15]. The function of the intrinsic sphincter is modulated by vagal tone such that LES pressure is higher in expiration than inspiration. The striated muscle of the crural

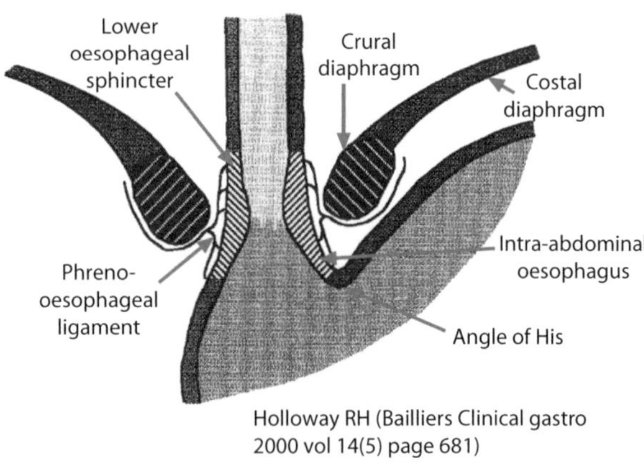

Fig. 3.1 Schematic representation of the gastroesophageal junction (GEJ)

diaphragm, which forms the esophageal hiatus, encircles the proximal 2 cm of the LES; an anatomical arrangement that increases EGJ pressure during inspiration, coughing and abdominal straining [10, 14]. Thus, the intrinsic and extrinsic components of the EGJ have complimentary effects that provide effective reflux protection throughout the respiratory cycle and during physical exertion.

3.3 EGJ Function

On pharyngeal swallowing a vagal reflex is triggered that results in "deglutitive" relaxation of the esophagus and LES to allow bolus transit from the mouth to the stomach. Repetitive swallowing results in complete relaxation of the intrinsic LES and the extrinsic crural diaphragm to facilitate rapid intake of food and fluid. During this process, relaxation of the proximal stomach ("gastric accommodation") ensures that the stomach can be filled without an important increase in intra-gastric pressure.

Ingestion of a meal is accompanied by gastric secretion that tends to collect immediately below the LES forming an "pocket" or layer of unbuffered acid overlying an ingested meal. In health, the transition from the acid to alkaline milieu occurs at the EGJ in the post prandial period [16]. However, when the EGJ barrier is weak or disrupted (e.g. in presence of hiatus hernia) the acid pocket can migrate into the distal esophagus, leading to pathological acid reflux in the distal esophagus [17]. Delayed gastric emptying [18] and acid hypersecretory states are additional downstream factors that can contribute to the esophageal reflux burden. At the same time, gastric filling is accompanied by a decrease in LES pressure and an increased frequency of spontaneous, transient LES relaxations (TLESRs) that allow air swallowed during the meal to be released (belching). Together, these events represent a major challenge to the EGJ reflux barrier and it has been shown that when the EGJ barrier is weak or disrupted, especially in the presence of hiatus hernia, the acid pocket can migrate into the distal esophagus, leading to pathological acid reflux and mucosal disease [19]. A small number of reflux events during TLESRs after meals is normal in healthy individuals; however, the number of reflux events is much higher in GERD patients. Studies using magnetic resonance imaging combined with high-resolution manometry (HRM) have shown how active contraction of the clasp and sling fibers maintains an acute angle of insertion between the esophagus and the proximal stomach (termed "angle of His" in surgical studies) [20, 21]. The presence of an acute angle of insertion allows the proximal stomach to compress the EGJ and prevents reflux of gastric contents into the esophagus [22]. This "flap-valve" effect is much less efficient if the angle of insertion is wide (obtuse) due to ineffective contraction of the clasp and sling fibers or structural disruption of EGJ anatomy, both of which are observed in GERD patients [20].

Another challenge to EGJ function occurs in the fasted state, especially at night, when powerful migrating motor complex (MMC III) contractions clear the stomach of undigested material. These contractions increase intra-gastric pressure and can trigger gastro-esophageal reflux; however, this does not occur in healthy individuals with an intact reflux barrier because LES pressure increases during MMC III contractions [23].

3.4 Mechanism of Reflux

Large studies have identified several markers from manometry studies that correlate with the severity of reflux defined by the presence of reflux esophagitis or pathological acid exposure on 24 h pH-studies. These include resting LES pressure, intra-abdominal LES length (i.e. distance between PIP and distal LES border[1]) and disorders of esophageal motility that impact on clearance function [3, 24–26]. More detailed observations after a test meal identify three main mechanisms that cause individual reflux events: [27–30].

1. Transient LES Relaxation (TLESR). In health and in patients with mild-moderate GERD most reflux occurs during TLESRs characterized by a period of complete, prolonged (10–60 s) LES relaxation that is not caused by swallowing [31]. Gastric distention, laryngeal or pharyngeal stimulation provide the afferent stimulus for the TLESR reflex, which is transmitted to the nucleus solitarius in the brainstem. A set of events from the dorsal vagal nucleus and the nucleus ambiguous mediates EGJ relaxation via the vagal efferent fibres [10].
2. Swallow-induced LES relaxations. In health about 5–10% of reflux episodes occur during swallow-induced LES relaxations [32]. The relatively low risk of reflux events during swallow-induced LES relaxations compared to TLESRs is due to incomplete and shorter relaxation of the crural diaphragm during swallowing and immediate clearance of reflux by oncoming peristalsis [32, 33].
3. Very low or absent LES pressure is an uncommon cause of reflux in health; [28, 29] however, it occurs frequently in the absence of a mechanically sufficient reflux barrier in patients with a hiatus hernia and severe GERD [30].

Manometry can identify TLESRs and other potential causes of reflux. Moreover, the presence of "common cavity pressure" (i.e. equilibration of pressure) between the stomach and the esophagus indicates the occurrence of a reflux event. The initial description of TLESRs by Dent *et al.* was based on the conventional water perfused manometry with an "sleeve sensor" to provide stable pressure measurements from the EGJ [30]. TLESRs were defined by the absence of a preceding swallow, rapid rate of relaxation, low nadir LES pressure and prolonged duration of LES relaxation [34]. Additional markers include inhibition of crural diaphragm and presence of a prominent after-contraction [35]. The inter-observer agreement for detection of TLESRs is superior for HRM compared to conventional manometry [36] and criteria for identification of TLESRs were recently validated for this advanced technology [37]. These include the occurrence of LES relaxation in the absence of swallowing

[1] In these studies hiatus hernia is defined by a negative intra-abdominal LES length

4 s before and 2 s after the onset of LES relaxation and prolonged duration of LES relaxation lasting more than 10 s with concurrent inhibition of the crural diaphragm. The introduction of combined high-resolution impedance manometry (HRiM) supports this observation by direct detection of EGJ relaxation, opening and retrograde flow of gastric contents (i.e. reflux) during TLESRs (and other events) [37, 38]. It is also possible to discriminate between reflux of air (belching) and gastric secretions based on the impedance profiles [37, 38].

Additionally, the use of HRiM facilitates the detection of rumination syndrome and supra-gastric belching in patients with persistent "reflux" symptoms on PPI medication [39, 40]. These behavioral conditions are characterized by the voluntary, albeit unconscious, contraction of abdominal and thoracic muscles resulting in the forceful return of gastric or oesophageal contents to the mouth. It is important to recognize these conditions because the mechanism of disease is not the same as GERD, cannot be corrected by standard medical treatment and can be exacerbated by anti-reflux surgery. Instead, patients can be taught to suppress these "abnormal responses" by simple exercises delivered by physiotherapists [39].

3.4.1 Motility and Reflux

After a reflux episode occurs, the refluxate is cleared most often by a primary peristaltic contraction that also neutralizes acid by bringing saliva from the mouth [41]. In many GERD patients, esophageal motor function is preserved; however, ineffective esophageal motility (IEM) can impair esophageal clearance and is associated with increased likelihood of esophagitis [26, 42, 43]. The spectrum of IEM consists of fragmented peristalsis, hypotensive peristalsis and absent contractility (all can be observed in the same patients). Patients with more severe disease are characterized by a failure to respond to the physiologic challenge of multiple repeated swallows or the solid swallows (absent "contractile reserve"). It is the frequency of ineffective esophageal contractions after reflux events that impacts on esophageal clearance and the severity of acid exposure [44, 45].

3.4.2 Obesity and Reflux

A high body mass index (BMI) and, especially, a high waist circumference is associated with an increased risk of GERD [6]. Epidemiological studies suggest that the prevalence of GERD symptoms and reflux esophagitis is significantly increased in patients with BMI $\geq$ 25 compared to normal weight subjects [46]. Obesity has effects on EGJ structure and function that increase the risk of reflux by all the mechanisms discussed above [6, 47–49]. The mechanical hypothesis proposes that obesity results in increased mechanical stress at the EGJ due to increased intra-gastric pressures and disruption of EGJ morphology (i.e. increased separation of the LES and crural diaphragm) which favors reflux [4]. Other hypotheses include the release of metabolic and humoral mediators from visceral adipose tissue that have effects on vagal activity and may well impact on the frequency of TLESRs and other key aspects of EGJ function [50–52]. Of interest, although obese subjects complain of heartburn and acid regurgitation more frequently than normal weight controls, [46] this effect is weaker than that expected and many obese subjects with GERD have only mild or occasional reflux symptoms. This lack of sensitivity and failure to seek treatment could, in part, explain the relatively high risk of GERD complications, including adenocarcinoma, in this group.

3.4.3 Hiatus Hernia

In patients with a small hiatus hernia, separation of the LES and crural diaphragm results in a twofold increase in reflux events [19] and the risk of GERD increases with the size of the hiatus hernia [3, 53, 54]. The presence of a hiatus hernia has multiple effects on EGJ structure and function. First, the wide esophageal hiatus impairs the ability of the crural diaphragm to contribute to reflux protection [55]. Indeed, in HRM studies, reduced augmentation of EGJ pressure during inspiration is an independent risk factor for GERD [56]. Second, contraction of the crural diaphragm can trap gastric contents in the hiatal sac that can then pass into the esophagus through the (weak) LES due to negative thoracic pressure during inspiration [55]. Third, the frequency of reflux events of all kinds is increased in patients with hiatus hernia [53, 54] due to mechanical effects on EGJ and proximal gastric function. Whilst TLESR remains an important cause of reflux events in this patient group, other mechanisms appear to be more important in the presence of a hiatus hernia [57]. Additionally, once reflux has occurred, ineffective esophageal motility and impaired esophageal clearance are common in patients with a large hiatus hernia [58, 59]. This results in prolonged exposure of the distal esophagus with acid gastric secretions that are thought to be a major cause of reflux esophagitis, Barrett esophagus and other complications; all of which are more common in GERD patients with hiatus hernia than those without.

3.5 Hiatus Hernia: Diagnosis

The diagnosis of a hiatus hernia is most often made on barium esophagogram or endoscopy. Features on radiology include the presence of a herniated B-ring at the squamocolumnar junction or rugal folds traversing the diaphragm [60]. On endoscopy, the distance between the squamocolumnar junction and the diaphragmatic pinch is measured to determine the length of the hiatus hernia. Recent studies indicate that both investigations lack sensitivity for small hiatus hernias and, moreover, distention of the stomach during endoscopy often triggers TLESR with EGJ opening potentially leading to false positive diagnosis or overestimation of hiatus hernia size [61].

In health and in many patients with mild-moderate GERD separation of the intrinsic (LES) and extrinsic (crural diaphragm) components of the EGJ reflux barrier is not constant but occurs intermittently [62]. HRM studies identify this spatial dissociation of the intrinsic LES and diaphragmatic sphincter, as a double peak pressure profile at the EGJ [63]. HRM provides a more prolonged and detailed analysis of EGJ pressure and this increased spatial and temporal resolution has excellent sensitivity and specificity for hiatus hernia [61]. Compared to barium fluoroscopy or endoscopy which each have a sensitivity of 73% for detection of a hiatus hernia, the sensitivity and specificity of HRM for hiatus hernia detection was 92% and 93% respectively [61].

The Chicago Classification of hiatus hernia by HRM is based on spatial separation of the two “high pressure zones” produced by the LES and diaphragmatic crus [56, 61, 64]. An EGJ pressure morphology with a single pressure peak during inspiration and expiration, indicating that the axial position of the LES coincides with the CD, is classified as EGJ Type 1 (Fig. 3.2a). In the latest iteration of Chicago Classification v3.0, [64] when LES-CD separation is observed that is <3 cm the hiatus hernia is classified as EGJ Type II (Fig. 3.2b). When there is a marked LES-CD separation ≥3 cm (typically with a nadir pressure between the two pressure peaks less than gastric pressure) then the hiatus hernia is classified as EGJ Type III. Large type III hernias can be further sub-classified according to the position of the pressure inversion point (PIP) (Fig. 3.2c, d).

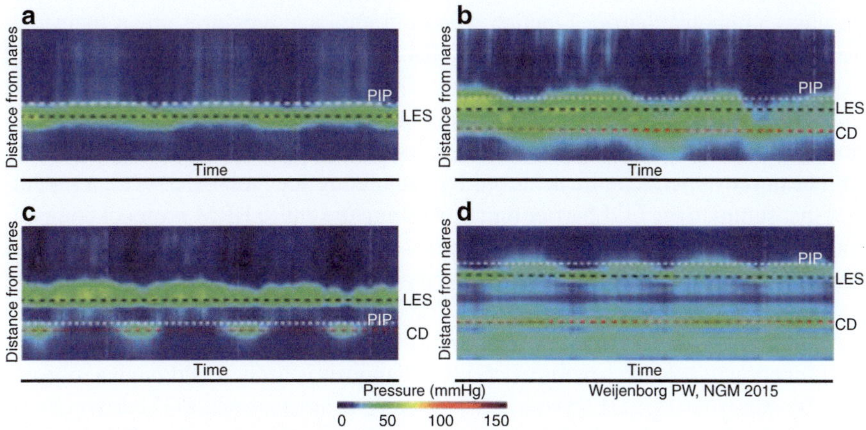

Fig. 3.2 Different types of EGJ morphology identified by esophageal pressure topography across the EGJ. Different types of EGJ morphology identified by esophageal pressure topography across the esophagogastric junction. (**a**) EGJ Type I: the LES and CD overlap both in inspiration and expiration, and the PIP is located directly above the LES. (**b**) EGJ Type II: minimal separation of LES and CD, but a nadir pressure between the peaks that is higher than gastric pressure. (**c**) EGJ Type IIIa: LES and CD separated but PIP is located at the proximal margin of the diaphragm. (**d**) EGJ Type IIIb: LES and CD separated but PIP Is located above the LES

This classification system for hiatus hernia has been validated against endoscopy and ambulatory pH-measurement. There is a positive correlation between increasing disruption of EGJ morphology with the prevalence and severity of reflux esophagitis [55, 57, 65]. In addition, esophageal acid exposure is higher in GERD patients with compared to those without hiatus hernia [66, 67]. Notwithstanding the above, other metrics derived from HRM measurements of EGJ function may provide better sensitivity and specificity for the diagnosis of GERD (see below).

3.6 EGJ Measurement

Advances in esophageal motility diagnostic tests have provided further insights into the anatomy and function of the EGJ reflux barrier [68–70]. Unlike "conventional" esophageal manometry systems with up to 12 pressure sensors, HRM systems acquire pressure measurements from closely spaced sensors and display this information as topographic (Clouse) plots that integrate time, position and pressure data. Assessment of esophageal motility by the Chicago Classification for HRM is based on objective metrics derived from these measurements [64]. The intraluminal pressure at the EGJ is referenced to the intra-gastric pressure in clinical studies. The presence of adequate resting pressure provides an indication of resistance to retrograde flow of gastric content across the reflux barrier. As discussed above, the intact EGJ barrier consists of superimposed LES and CD. The intrinsic LES can independently have a low resting tone, with values <8 mmHg during the end expiratory phase consistently abnormal [56, 64]. Inspiratory augmentation of the CD provides adjunctive barrier function when intrathoracic pressures are at their lowest; [71] an element of the EGJ barrier that is not well assessed by basal and end expiratory LES pressure measurements. The EGJ contractile integral (EGJ-CI) may overcome these drawbacks by combining EGJ anatomy, basal tone, and variation with respiration into a single metric assessing vigor of the EGJ [72, 73]. A further improvement can be achieved by calculating the "total-EGJ-CI", a parameter that summarizes EGJ barrier function during the entire HRM protocol compensating for variation in morphology and pressure over time [74]. Normative EGJ-CI and total EGJ-CI values have been described, and available data indicate that the risk of GERD is increased in the setting of abnormal results [74, 75]. Notwithstanding this finding, GERD has a complex aetiology and the ability of *any* measurement of EGJ function to provide a definitive GERD diagnosis is limited (although a robustly normal value may rule GERD out) [74]. Therefore, an abnormal EGJ barrier can be hypotensive (with reduced resting tone that can be overcome by events that increase intra-abdominal pressure), disrupted with separation of the two components of the EGJ barrier (i.e. hiatus hernia) or both. In the presence of a hiatus hernia, the resting tone of the intrinsic LES is typically hypotensive, with esophageal reflux burden higher than with either abnormality alone. Therefore, abnormalities of EGJ structure and function can coexist, and both can contribute to abnormal reflux burden.

3.7 Ambulatory Reflux Monitoring

The presence of "typical reflux symptoms" including heartburn and acid regurgitation on validated questionnaires are unreliable in the diagnosis of GERD [76]. In general, typical reflux symptoms are initially managed with an empiric PPI trial; however, this approach is also unreliable, with a specificity of only 50–60% despite sensitivity of approximately 80% in predicting erosive esophagitis or an abnormal pH study [77]. Indeed, only half of patients referred for physiological investigations have pathological acid exposure on ambulatory pH-studies [78]. These findings emphasize the need for objective evaluation of reflux prior to antireflux surgery [79]. This includes esophageal manometry to rule out achalasia and other, clinically relevant motility disorders that appear in almost every published series.

Ambulatory reflux monitoring is performed when there is a need to document esophageal reflux burden, or to define the relationship between symptom events and reflux episodes. The most common settings consist of persisting esophageal symptoms despite seemingly adequate acid suppressive therapy, i.e. a failed PPI test, or atypical symptoms (e.g. chest pain, cough, laryngeal symptoms) that may not directly implicate GERD, but could improve with GERD therapy if esophageal reflux burden is pathological. In the typical clinical scenario, ambulatory reflux monitoring has either 'rule in' or 'rule out' value in defining abnormal esophageal reflux burden. In settings where there is no independent evidence for reflux (unproven GERD), testing is performed off anti-secretory therapy for 7–10 days. Ambulatory reflux monitoring prior to anti-reflux surgery is also performed off anti-secretory therapy. When there is strong evidence for GERD (proven GERD), such as EGD evidence of severe erosive esophagitis, peptic stricture or long segment Barrett's mucosa (or prior abnormal ambulatory reflux monitoring), testing can be performed on anti-secretory therapy, where the objective is to determine if ongoing symptoms can be explained by abnormal esophageal reflux burden or linked to reflux episodes. In this setting, pH impedance monitoring needs to be employed for reflux monitoring, as pH testing alone is insufficient in describing weakly acid reflux episodes that predominate in patients on PPI therapy [7]. If suspicion for GERD is strong in the setting of negative 24 h reflux monitoring, repeating monitoring using a prolonged pH measurement can be considered, as day-to-day variation in esophageal reflux burden is present, and the finding of abnormal reflux burden can impact management direction [80–82].

The best-established method for objective diagnosis of GERD is 24-h pH-measurement with the pH-sensitive electrode mounted on an naso-esophageal catheter placed in the esophagus 5 cm above the proximal border of the LES as determined by manometry. An alternative technique using wireless pH probes is also available, and are particularly useful in patients that fail to tolerate ambulatory catheter based testing [83]. These single sensor probes are positioned 6 cm proximal to the squamo-columnar junction during endoscopy and can record and transmit distal esophageal pH data for up to 96 h. Catheter or probe placement is performed after an overnight fast, and after withholding anti-secretory therapy for at least 7 days when testing off PPI is performed (essential in pH-only studies). Patients are recommended to maintain normal activities and meals, and keep a diary of meals, recumbency periods and, crucially, symptoms. Careful instruction to record symptoms promptly ensures that not only the objective severity of disease but also the subjective association between symptoms and reflux can be assessed.

The percentage of total recording time with $pH < 4$ (i.e. acid exposure time) is the single most important parameter used in GERD diagnosis [84]. This is calculated as the percent time the pH is <4.0 in the distal esophageal (5 cm above the LES), for the duration of the ambulatory study. Total AET is considered physiologic when <4%, and pathologic when >6%; values in between are borderline and require additional clinical or physiological evidence to confirm GERD [85]. Additional information can be obtained by separately calculated AET for upright and supine periods; elevated supine AET can implicate a disrupted EGJ barrier, as TLESRs are generally suppressed during sleep. However, proximal esophageal and pharyngeal reflux monitoring have limited value in directing anti-reflux therapy [86, 87]. AET is marginally higher with the wireless probe, but the same thresholds can be employed for both modes of reflux monitoring. AET is considered more reliable and better reproducible than the composite Johnson-DeMeester score that is no longer recommended in clinical practice [85].

More recently multiple intra-luminal impedance (MII) monitoring has been combined with pH-measurement and is currently regarded as the gold standard for reflux detection [85, 88]. By measuring differences in resistance to alternating current between pairs of adjacent electrodes, MII can detect bolus movement through the esophagus and the retrograde flow of refluxate from the stomach into the esophagus. Moreover, the combination of pH and MII differentiates between acid and non-acid reflux events and the conductivity of esophageal contents can distinguish between liquid and gas reflux (belching) [89] (Fig. 3.3a, b). Thus, combined pH-impedance monitoring permits the detection of (1) anterograde and retrograde bolus movement (Fig. 3.4) (2) characterizes the nature of the refluxate (air reflux, liquid reflux or mixed air-liquid reflux) and (3) determines the pH of the refluxate (acidic [$pH < 4$], weakly acidic [$4 \leq pH < 7$] and weakly alkaline $pH \geq 7$ [89, 90] (Fig. 3.5). The number of acid and non-acid reflux events over 24-h is highly variable and is a less reliable marker of GERD than AET; [91] however, the presence of <40 reflux events is considered physiologic, and large numbers >80 are likely to be pathologic; as for AET, values in between are borderline and require additional clinical or physiological evidence to confirm GERD [85]. For example, a low median nocturnal baseline impedance (e.g. MNBI <2000 ohms) and the presence of a low post-reflux swallowed induced peristaltic wave (PSPW) index[2] derived from pH-impedance studies have been shown to predict response to medical and surgical GERD therapy [92].

---

[2] PSPW is an impedance-detected antegrade bolus propagation that passes through the esophagus within 30 seconds of a reflux event. The PSPW index is the proportion of reflux events followed by PSPW compared to all reflux events, and can be lower in erosive and nonerosive GERD compared to controls. Further, this index may distinguish hypersensitive esophagus from functional heartburn.

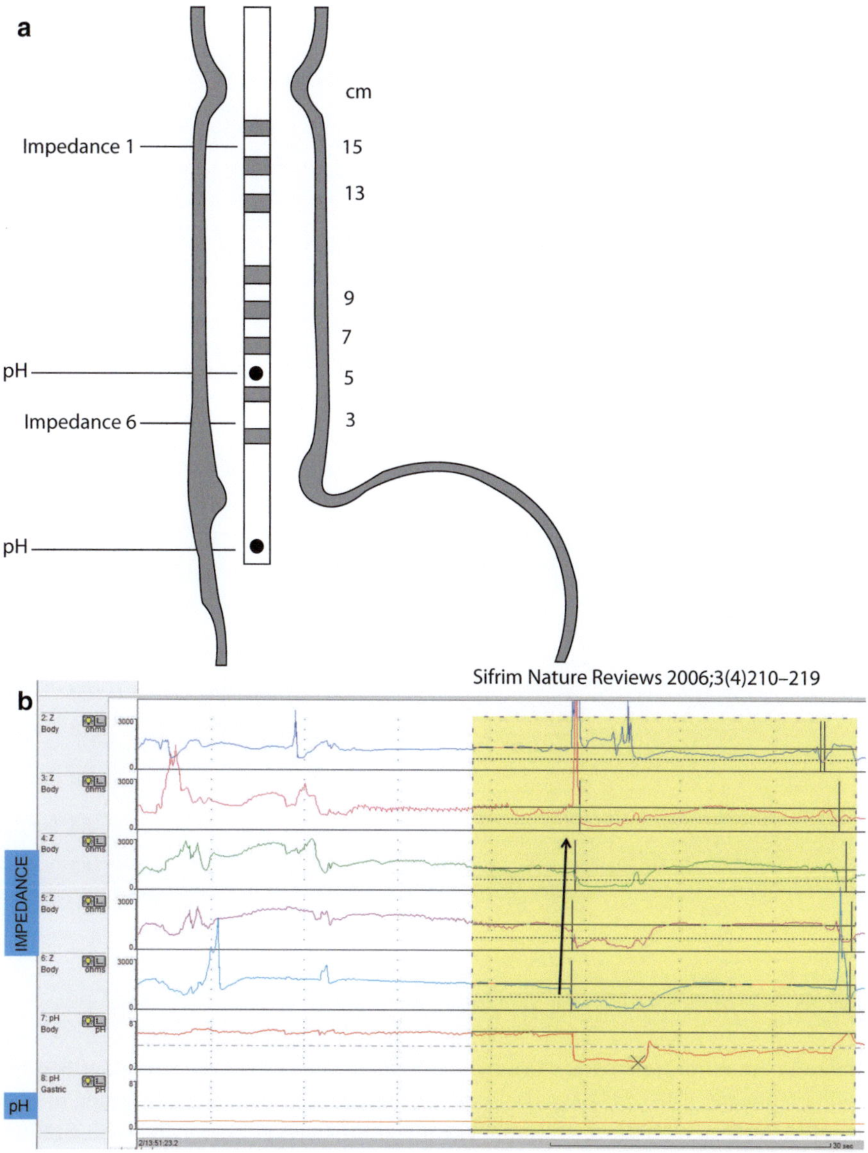

Fig. 3.3 (**a**) A combined impedance-pH catheter consisting of six impedance channels and two pH sensors. (**b**) Example of an acid reflux event detected on impedance-pH monitoring. Upper 6 channels display impedance readings in the esophageal body. The lower channel displays pH at 5 cm above the lower esophageal sphincter. Illustrative example of retrograde movement of liquid bolus during an acid-reflux event

Ambulatory reflux studies are also used to confirm (or exclude) reflux events as the cause of patient symptoms. Symptom-reflux association requires reporting of symptoms during the ambulatory study, typically using an event monitor button on

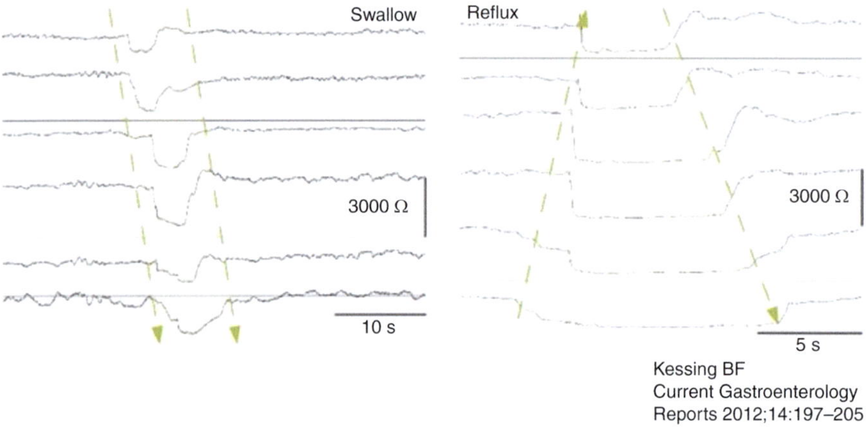

Fig. 3.4 Comparison of impedance tracings during a swallow event and a reflux event

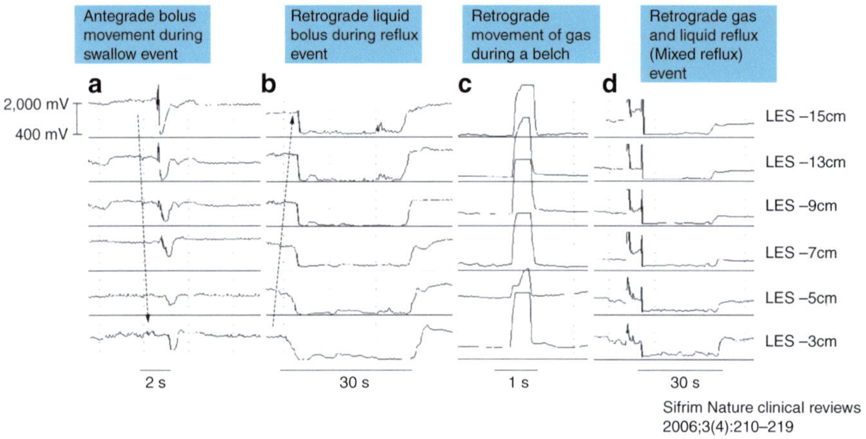

Fig. 3.5 Impedance patterns during swallow and reflux (liquid, gas, mixed liquid-gas) events

the reflux monitoring device worn by the patient. Reflux episodes are identified by reflux software, using pH drops below 4.0 or impedance-detected retrograde movement of gastric contents. A symptom event is designated as associated with a reflux episode if the symptom occurs within 2 min following the reflux episode. Studies have shown that ongoing non-acid reflux accounts for up to 50% symptoms in patients with an incomplete response to PPIs [8, 93]. A simple ratio of associated symptoms to all symptoms defines the symptom index (SI; abnormal if >50%). Symptom reflux probability (SAP) takes into account 2 min periods with and without reflux episodes and symptom events, and applies a statistical test (Fisher's exact test) to assess the probability that symptoms and reflux episodes could have co-occurred by chance (SAP positive if >95% (1-$p < 0.05$)). The yield and diagnostic value of symptom reflux association is highest when many symptoms are recorded, with the patient recording the symptom promptly upon occurrence. A positive, symptom reflux association can augment the strength of a GERD diagnosis based on borderline AET or number of reflux events. Reflux hypersensitivity is present when AET is normal but a significant symptom reflux association is present (ideally both SAP and SI are positive) [92, 94].

The metrics described above have been shown to predict reflux outcome when testing is performed off PPI therapy in unproven GERD [91, 92]. In the clinical setting, the results provide guidance as to whether reflux management should continue (if pathological reflux is identified) or if alternate mechanisms should be sought for persisting symptoms. However, as discussed above, thresholds defining pathological from physiological reflux burden are not precise, and a 'grey area' exists ("borderline reflux burden") where the clinical presentation and alternate evidence from physiological investigations (HRM, pH-impedance studies) could complement ambulatory reflux monitoring findings to support or reject GERD [85, 95] diagnosis. Reflux hypersensitivity is defined by a positive symptom-reflux association in the setting of physiologic reflux, is part of the GERD spectrum and can respond to optimal acid and reflux suppression therapy. In contrast, functional heartburn or functional chest pain is defined by normal ambulatory reflux monitoring with negative symptom reflux association and are functional conditions that are not caused by reflux events.

3.8 Impact of Esophageal Function Testing on Management and Outcome

GERD is a complex condition that is defined by mucosal disease or symptoms associated with the retrograde flow of gastric contents into the esophagus [96]. Several GERD phenotypes can be defined based on clinical assessment, endoscopy and esophageal function testing. This is helpful because identifying the appropriate GERD phenotypes can direct management and maximize therapeutic outcome. In this regard, symptoms and PPI response do not adequately phenotype GERD into reliable therapeutic categories.

Using EGD findings, GERD can be phenotyped into erosive and non-erosive disease, with clearly better symptomatic outcomes in erosive GERD compared to non-erosive GERD. Within erosive GERD, Los Angeles (LA) grades C and D provide definitive evidence for GERD, whereas LA grade B esophagitis is borderline and LA grade A esophagitis can often be encountered in healthy volunteers, and does not provide conclusive evidence for GERD. Many patients with erosive GERD will also have hiatus hernia that is obvious on endoscopy (and radiology) and this additional evidence may be sufficient for a recommendation for anti-reflux surgery.

There is limited research available describing prediction of outcomes of therapy based on manometry studies including EGJ morphology and esophageal motor function; however, the purpose of this investigation is not to diagnose GERD but to exclude a major motility disorder, rumination syndrome and similar conditions. Using ambulatory reflux monitoring, pathologic AET is a predictor of outcome from both medical and surgical antireflux therapy [91, 92]. Within abnormal AET cohorts, those with positive symptom reflux association have the highest likelihood of improvement from antireflux therapy [94]. Therefore, the strongest GERD phenotype consists of pathologic AET associated with positive symptom reflux association [97, 98]. When AET is normal or borderline but a positive symptom reflux association is recorded, antireflux management approaches (including surgery) may be successful, especially if there is evidence for EGJ disruption and hiatus hernia [99, 100]. In contrast, physiologic AET with no symptom reflux association is associated with suboptimal outcomes from anti-reflux therapy, and can overlap with functional esophageal syndromes [99, 101]. In these settings, coexisting functional syndromes (functional dyspepsia, IBS) may also predict suboptimal outcome from antireflux therapy [98, 100]. Instead, similar to other functional esophageal syndromes, these conditions may respond better to medications that modulate visceral sensitivity and perception (e.g. low-dose tricyclic antidepressants) than to antireflux therapy alone [1].

3.9 Anti-Reflux Surgery

Anti-reflux surgery prevents reflux by two main mechanisms (1) restoring the "normal" position of the stomach by reduction of a hiatal hernia and repair of the hiatal orifice, (2) reducing distensibility of the EGJ and the number of TLESRs associated with reflux by formation of a fundoplication wrap that limits EGJ opening [102–105]. In well selected patients (see above) this surgery dramatically reduces the number of reflux events and associated symptoms; however, a small proportion of patients have ongoing "reflux symptoms" or swallowing problems that can persist in the long-term [9]. Symptoms are not specific for underlying pathology and repeat physiological investigation is recommended. Ideally the HRM study should include a test meal to increase test sensitivity to EGJ outlet obstruction which is common in this patient group [106, 107].

Ongoing reflux symptoms may be related to persistent or recurrent GERD due to failure of the fundoplication wrap occasionally with reformation of a hiatus hernia; however, in clinical case series this diagnosis was confirmed only in about half of patients tested [106]. Other patients had a symptomatic motility disorder, functional heartburn or rumination syndrome. Conversely persistent dysphagia was most often attributed to an excessively "tight" fundoplication wrap (or hiatal canal repair), with a slipped wrap or trans-diaphragmatic herniation of the wrap observed less often. All these complications affect esophageal emptying and lead to dysphagic symptoms [108]. HRM with a test meal is more sensitive to symptomatic EGJ outlet obstruction than endoscopy or radiology (Figs. 3.6 and 3.7). If a clinically relevant obstruction to bolus passage was present, then a balloon dilatation to the fundoplication wrap produced symptom improvement and removed the need for re-operation in nearly two thirds of patients [107].

A further technology that could assist diagnosis in this setting is the Endoluminal Functional Lumen Imaging Probe (EndoFLIP, Cropson, Galway, Ireland) which uses high resolution impedance planimetry during volume controlled distension to measure the luminal cross-sectional area (CSA) and distensibility of the EGJ [109]. EndoFlip is not helpful for GERD diagnosis; [110, 111] however, it may assist sur-

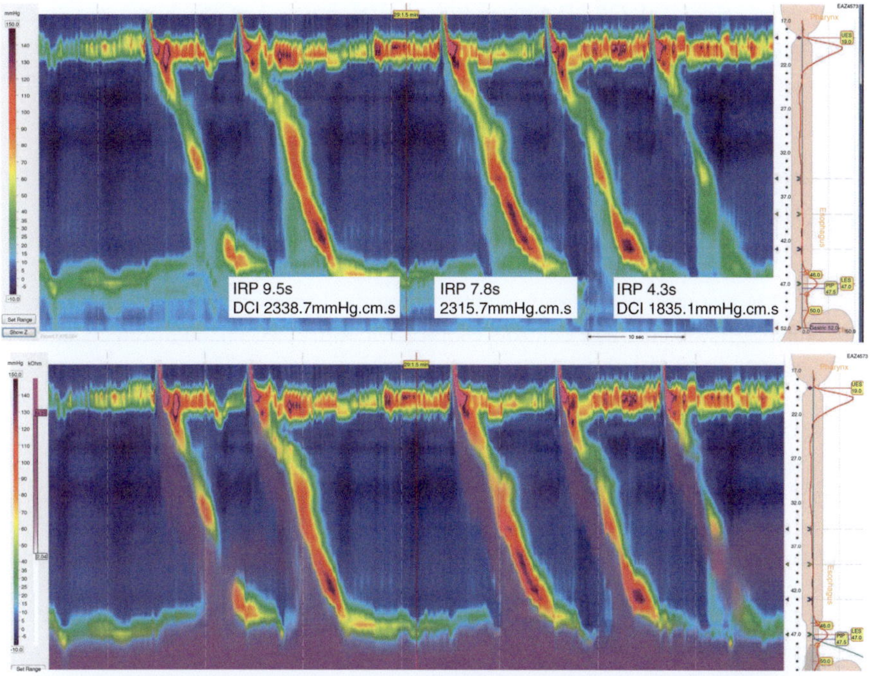

Fig. 3.6 Example of normal swallows seen on Esophageal HRM and Impedance-HRM

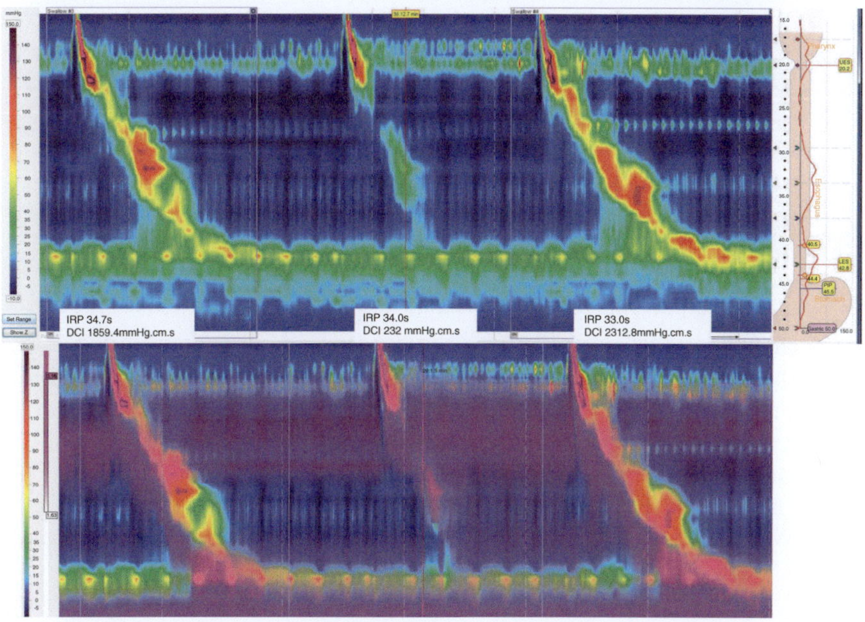

Fig. 3.7 HRM findings of esophagogastric junction (EGJ) outflow obstruction on esophageal HRM and Impedance-HRM

gical management of GERD by guiding the "tightness" of the hiatal repair and fundoplication wrap [112]. Further it may be useful in the post-operative setting to identify patients with an excessively tight fundoplication wrap; however, outcome studies are required before its use in routine practice [104].

3.10 Summary

The EGJ is a complex structure encompassing the lower esophageal sphincter and the diaphragmatic crus that controls esophageal bolus passage and protects against retrograde flow of gastric contents. Gastroesophageal reflux disease is characterized by progressive disruption of EGJ structure and function, with hiatus hernia being a marker of more severe disease. Advances in physiological measurement, including esophageal HRM and ambulatory pH-impedance monitoring has provided new insight into the mechanism of reflux protection. The same technology is now used to diagnose GERD and identify the causes of reflux symptoms. The results of investigation allow physicians and surgeons to identify specific GERD phenotypes and, based on this information, to tailor treatment to the individual patient.

What is the Current Knowledge and What Future Direction is Required

1. The esophago-gastric junction (EGJ) is the major defense against reflux of gastric contents into the esophagus. Impaired EGJ barrier function is characteristic in gastro-esophageal reflux disease (GERD).
2. The EGJ comprises an intrinsic component made up by smooth muscles of the lower esophageal sphincter (LES) with the sling and clasp fibers of the gastric cardia, plus an extrinsic component formed by the crural diaphragm.
3. In health and in patients with mild-moderate GERD most reflux occurs during Transient LES Relaxation (TLESRs) characterized by a period of complete, prolonged LES relaxation that is not caused by swallowing.
4. In patients with more severe GERD, especially in the presence of a hiatus hernia, multiple mechanisms of reflux and impaired esophageal clearance are present.
5. High Resolution Manometry has superior sensitivity and specificity for detection of hiatus hernia compared to barium fluoroscopy or endoscopy.
6. Existing parameters for manometric (and other) evaluation of EGJ barrier function do not predict gastroesophageal reflux disease (GERD) reliably.
7. The presence of "typical reflux symptoms" including heartburn and acid regurgitation on validated questionnaires are unreliable in the diagnosis of GERD.
8. Ambulatory pH-impedance provides objective measurements of acid exposure and documents the association between reflux events and patient symptoms.

References

1. Fox M, Forgacs I. Gastroesophageal reflux disease. BMJ. 2006;332:88–93.
2. Mittal RK, Balaban DH. The esophagogastric junction. N Engl J Med. 1997;336(13):924–32.
3. Lee J, Anggiansah A, Anggiansah R, Young A, Wong T, Fox M. Effects of age on the gastroesophageal junction, esophageal motility, and reflux disease. Clin Gastroenterol Hepatol. 2007;5(12):1392–8.
4. Pandolfino JE, El-Serag HB, Zhang Q, Shah N, Ghosh SK, Kahrilas PJ. Obesity: a challenge to esophagogastric junction integrity. Gastroenterology. 2006;130(3):639–49.
5. Wu JC, Mui LM, Cheung CM, Chan Y, Sung JJ. Obesity is associated with increased transient lower esophageal sphincter relaxation. Gastroenterology. 2007;132(3):883–9.
6. Anggiansah R, Sweis R, Anggiansah A, Wong T, Cooper M, Fox M. The effects of obesity on oesophageal function, acid exposure and the symptoms of gastro-oesophageal reflux disease. Aliment Pharmacol Ther. 2013;37(5):555–63.
7. Vela MF, Camacho-Lobato L, Srinivasan R, Tutuian R, Katz PO, Castell DO. Simultaneous intraesophageal impedance and pH measurement of acid and nonacid gastroesophageal reflux: effect of omeprazole. Gastroenterology. 2001;120(7):1599–060.
8. Mainie I, Tutuian R, Shay S, Vela M, Zhang X, Sifrim D, Castell DO. Acid and non-acid reflux in patients with persistent symptoms despite acid suppressive therapy: a multicentre study using combined ambulatory impedance-pH monitoring. Gut. 2006;55(10):1398–402.
9. Lundell L, Miettinen P, Myrvold HE, Pedersen SA, Thor K, Lamm M, et al. Long-term management of gastro-oesophageal reflux disease with omeprazole or open antireflux surgery: results of a prospective, randomized clinical trial. The Nordic GORD Study Group. Eur J Gastroenterol Hepatol. 2000;12(8):879–87.
10. Corley DA, Kubo A, Zhao W. Abdominal obesity, ethnicity and gastroesophageal reflux symptoms. Gut. 2007;56:756–62.
11. Brasseur JG, Ulerich R, Dai Q, Patel DK, Soliman AMS, Miller L. Pharmacological dissection of the human gastroesophageal segment into three sphincteric components. J Physiol. 2007;580(3):961–75.
12. Mittal RK, Rochester DF, McCallum RW. Sphincteric action of the diaphragm during a relaxed lower esophageal sphincter in humans. Am J Physiol. 1989;256:G139–44.
13. Kahrilas PJ, Lin S, Chen J, Manka M. The effect of hiatus hernia on gastroesophageal junction pressure. Gut. 1999;44:476–82.
14. Heine KJ, Dent J, Mittal RK. Anatomical relationship between the crural diarphagm and the lower esophageal sphincter: an electrophysiologic study. J Neurogastroenterol Motil. 1993;5:89–95.
15. Pehlivanov N, Liu J, Kassab G, Puckett J, Mittal RK. Relationship between esophageal muscle thickenss and intraluminal pressure: an ultrasonographic study. Am J Physiol Gastrointest Liver Physiol. 2001;280:G1093–8.
16. Fletcher J, Wirz A, Young J, Vallance R, McColl KE. Unbuffered highly acidic gastric juice exists at the gastroesophageal junction after a meal. Gastroenterology. 2001;121(4):775–83.
17. Beaumont H, Bennink RJ, de Jong J, Boeckxstaens GE. The position of the acid pocket as a major reflux factor for acidic reflux in healthy subjets and patients with GERD. Gut. 2010;49:441–51.
18. Boecxstaens V, Bisschops R, Blondeau K, Vos R, Scarpellini E, De Wulf D, Tack J. Modulation of the postprandial acid and bile pockets at the gastroesophageal junction by drugs that affect gastric motility. Aliment Pharmacol Ther. 2011;33(12):1370–7.
19. Kahrilas PJ, McColl K, Fox M, O'Rourke L, Sifrim D, Smout AJ, Boeckxstaens G. The acid pocket: a target for treatment in reflux disease? Am J Gastroenterol. 2013;108(7):1058–64.
20. Curcic J, Roy S, Schwizer A, Kaufman E, Forras-Kaufman Z, Menne D, et al. Abnormal structure and function of the esophagogastric junction and proximal stomach in gastroesophageal reflux disease. Am J Gastroenterol. 2014;109(5):658–67.

21. Curcic J, Schwizer A, Kaufman E, Forras-Kaufman Z, Banerjee S, Pal A, et al. Effects of baclofen on the functional anatomy of the oesophago-gastric junction and proximal stomach in healthy volunteers and patients with GERD assessed by magnetic resonance imaging and high-resolution manometry: a randomised controlled double-blind study. Aliment Pharmacol Ther. 2014;40(10):1230–40.
22. Roy S, Fox M, Curcic J, Schwizer W, Pal A. The gastro-esophageal reflux barrier: biophysical analysis on 3D models of anatomy from magnetic resonance imaging. Neurogastroenterol Motil. 2012;24(7):616–25. e269
23. Grossi L, Ciccaglione AF, Travaglini N, Marzio L. Swallows, oesophageal and gastric motility in normal subjects and in patients with gastro-oesophageal reflux disease: a 24-h pH-manometric study. Neurogastroenterol Motil. 1998;10(2):115–21.
24. Zaninotto G, DeMeester TR, Schwizer W, Johansson KE, Cheng SC. The lower esophageal sphincter in health and disease. Am J Surg. 1998;155(1):104–11.
25. Jones MP, Sloan SS, Jovanovic B, Kahrilas PJ. Impaired egress rather than increased access: an important independent predictor of erosive oesophagitis. Neurogastroenterol Motil. 2002;14(6):625–31.
26. Daum C, Sweis R, Kaufman E, Fuellemann A, Anggiansah A, Fried M, Fox M. Failure to respond to physiologic challenge characterizes esophageal motility in erosive gastro-esophageal reflux disease. Neurogastroenterol Motil. 2011;23(6):517–e200.
27. Dent J, Dodds WJ, Friedman RH, Sekiguchi T, Hogan WJ, Arndorfer RC, Petrie DJ. Mechanism of gastroesophageal reflux in recumbent asymptomatic human subjects. J Clin Invest. 1980;65:256–67.
28. Dodds WJ, Hogan WJ, Helm JF, Dent J. Pathogenesis of reflux esophagitis. Gastroenterology. 1981;81:376–94.
29. Dodds WJ, Dent J, Hogan WJ, Helm JF, Hauser R, Patel GK, Egide MS. Mechanisms of gastroesophageal reflux in patients with reflux esophagitis. N Engl J Med. 1982;307:1547–52.
30. Dent J, Holloway RH, Toouli J, Dodds WJ. Mechanisms of lower esophageal sphincter incompetence in patients with symptomatic gastroesophageal reflux. Gut. 1988;29:1020–8.
31. Mittal RK, Holloway RH, Penagini R, Blackshaw LA, Dent J. Transient lower esophageal sphincter relaxation. Gastroenterology. 1995;109:601–10.
32. Holloway RH. The anti-reflux barrier and mechanisms of gastroesophageal reflux. Baillieres Clin Gastroenterol. 2000;14(5):681–99.
33. Mittal RK, Fisher MJ. Electrical and mechanical inhibition of the crural diaphragm during transient relaxation of the lower esophageal sphincter. Gastroenterology. 1990;99:1265–8.
34. Holloway RH, Penagini R, Ireland AC. Criteria for objective definition of transient lower esophageal sphincter relaxation. Am J Physiol. 1995;268:G128–33.
35. Holloway RH, Boeckxstaens GE, Penagini R, Sifrim D, Smout AJ. Objective definition and detection of transcient lower esophageal sphincter relaxation revisited: is there room for improvement? Neurogastroenterol Motil. 2012;24:54–60.
36. Roman S, Zerbib F, Belhocine K, des Varannes SB, Mion F. High resolution manometry to detect transient lower oesophageal sphincter relaxations: diagnostic accuracy compared with perfused-sleeve manometry, and the definition of new detection criteria. Aliment Pharmacol Ther. 2011;34(3):384–93.
37. Roman S, Holloway R, Keller J, Herbella F, Zerbib F, Xiao Y, et al. Validation of criteria for the definition of transient lower esophageal sphincter relaxations using high-resolution manometry. Neurogastroenterol Motil. 2016;29(2):1–9.
38. Pandolfino JE, Shi G, Zhang Q, Ghosh S, Brasseur JG, Kahrilas PJ. Measuring EGJ opening patterns using high resolution intraluminal impedance. Neurogastroenterol Motil. 2005;17:200–6.
39. Tucker E, Knowles K, Wright J, Fox M. Rumination variations: aetiology and classification of abnormal behavioural responses to digestive symptoms based on high-resolution manometry studies. Aliment Pharmacol Ther. 2013;37(2):263–74.

40. Kessing BF, Bredenoord AJ, Smout AJ. Objective manometric criteria for the rumination syndrome. Am J Gastroenterol. 2014;109(1):52–9.
41. Anggiansah A, Taylor G, Bright N, Wang J, Owen WA, Rokkas T, et al. Primary peristalsis is the major acid clearance mechanism in reflux patients. Gut. 1994;35(11):1536–42.
42. Lin S, Ke M, Xu J, Kahrilas PJ. Impaired esophageal emptying in reflux disease. Am J Gastroenterol. 1994;89:1003–6.
43. Bredenoord AJ, Hemmink GJ, Smout AJ. Relationship between gastro-oesophageal reflux pattern and severity of mucosal damage. Neurogastroenterol Motil. 2009;21:807–12.
44. Ribolsi M, Balestrieri P, Emerenziani S, Guarino MP, Cicala M. Weak peristalsis with large breaks is associated with higher acid exposure and delayed reflux clearance in the supine position in GERD patients. Am J Gastroenterol. 2014;109:46–51.
45. Savarino E, Gemignani L, Pohl D, Zentilin P, Dulbecco P, Assandri L, et al. Oesophageal motility and bolus transit abnormalities increase in parallel with the severity of gastro-oesophageal reflux disease. Aliment Pharmacol Ther. 2011;34:476–86.
46. El-Serag HB, Graham DY, Satia JA, Rabeneck L. Obesity is an independent risk factor for GERD symptoms and erosive esophagitis. Am J Gastroenterol. 2005;100:1243–50.
47. Fisher BL, Pennathur A, Mutnick JL, Little AG. Obesity correlates with gastroesophageal reflux. Dig Dis Sci. 1999;44:2290–4.
48. Nilsson M, Lundegardh G, Carling L, Ye W, Lagegren J. Body mass and reflux oesophagitis: an oestrogen-dependent association? Scand J Gastroenterol. 2002;37:626–30.
49. Diaz-Rubio M, Moreno-Elola-Olaso C, Rey E, Locke GR 3rd, Rodriguez-Artalejo F. Symptoms of gastroesophageal reflux: prevalence, severity, duration and associated factors in a Spanish population. Aliment Pharmacol Ther. 2004;19:95–105.
50. Chung SJ, Kim D, Park MJ, Kim YS, Kim JS, Jung HC, Song IS. Metabolic syndrome and visceral obesity as risk factors for reflux oesophagitis: a cross-sectional case-control study of 7078 Koreans undergoing health check-ups. Gut. 2008;57(10):1360–5.
51. Nam SY, Choi IJ, Ryu KH, Park BJ, Kim HB, Nam BH. Abdominal visceral adipose tissue volume is associated with increased risk of erosive esophagitis in men and women. Gastroenterology. 2010;139:1902–11.
52. Tilg H, Moschen AR. Visceral adipose tissue attacks beyond the liver: esophagogastric junction as a new target. Gastroenterology. 2010;139:1823–6.
53. Kahrilas PJ, Shi G, Manka M, Joehl RJ. Increased frequency of transient lower esophageal sphincter relaxation induced by gastric distention in reflux patients with hiatal hernia. Gastroenterology. 2000;118(4):688–95.
54. van Herwaarden MA, Samsom M, Smout AJ. Excess gastroesophageal reflux in patients with hiatus hernia is caused by mechanisms other than transient LES relaxations. Gastroenterology. 2000;119(6):1439–46.
55. Sloan S, Rademaker AW, Kahrilas PJ. Determinants of gastroesophageal junction incompetence: hhiatal hernia, lower esophageal sphincter, or both? Ann Intern Med. 1992;117:977–82.
56. Pandolfino JE, Kim H, Ghosh SK, Clarke JO, Zhang Q, Kahrilas PJ. High resolution manometry of the EGJ: an analysis of crural diaphragm function in GERD. Am J Gastroenterol. 2007;102:1056–63.
57. Kaul B, Petersen H, Myrvold HE, Grette K, Roysland P, Halvorsen T. Hiatus hernia in gastroesophageal reflux disease. Scand J Gastroenterol. 1986;21:31–4.
58. Mittal RK, Lange RC, McCallum RW. Identification and mechanism of delayed esophageal acid clearance in subjects with hiatal hernia. Gastroenterology. 1987;92:130–5.
59. Sloan S, Kahrilas PJ. Impairment of esophageal emptying with hiatal hernia. Gastroenterology. 1991;100:596–605.
60. Ott DJ, Gelfand DW, Chen YM, Wu WC, Munitz HA. Predictive relationship of hiatal hernia to reflux esophagitis. Gastrointest Radiol. 1985;10:317–20.
61. Weijenborg PW, Van Hoeij FB, Smout AJPM, Bredenoord AJ. Accuracy of hiatal hernia detection with esophageal high resolution manometry. Neurogastroenterol Motil. 2015;27:293–9.

62. Bredenoord AJ, Weusten BLAM, Timmer R, Smout AJM. Intermittent spatial separation of diaphragm and lower esophageal sphincter favors acidic and weakly acidic reflux. Gastroenterology. 2006;130:334–40.
63. Bredenoord AJ, Weusten BL, Carmagnola S, Smout AJ. Double peaked high pressure zone at the esophagogastric junction in controls and in patients with a hiatal hernia. A study using high resolution manometry. Dig Dis Sci. 2004;49:1128–35.
64. Kahrilas PJ, Bredenoord AJ, Fox M, Gyawali CP, Roman S, Smout AJ, Pandolfino JE, International High Resolution Manometry Working Group. The Chicago classification of esophageal motility disorders, v3.0. Neurogastroenterol Motil. 2015;27:160–74.
65. Berstad A, Weberg R, Froyshov Larsen I, Hoel B, Hauer-Jensen M. Relationship of hiatus hernia to reflux esophagitis. A prospective study of coincidence, using endoscopy. Scand J Gastroenterol. 1986;21:55–8.
66. Kasapidis P, Vassilakis JS, Tzovaras G, Chrysos E, Xynos E. Effect of hiatal hernia on esophageal manometry and pH-metry in gastroesophageal reflux disease. Dig Dis Sci. 1995;40:2724–30.
67. DeMeester TR, LaFontaine E, Joelsson BE, Skinner DB, Ryan JW, O'Sullivan GC, et al. Relationship of a hiatal hernia to the function of the body of the esophagus and the gastroesophageal junction. J Thorac Cardiovasc Surg. 1981;82:547–58.
68. Bredenoord AJ, Weusten BL, Roelofs JM, Smout AJ. The gastroesophageal pressure inversion point revisited. Scand J Gastroenterol. 2003;38:812–8.
69. Fox M, Hebbard J, Janiak P, Brasseur JG, Ghosh S, Thumshirn M, et al. High resolution manometry predicts the success of esophageal bolus transport and identifies clinically important abnormalities not detected by conventional manometry. Neurogastroenterol Motil. 2004;16:533–42.
70. Clouse RE, Staiano A, Alrakawi A. Topographic analysis of esophageal double-peaked waves. Gastroenterology. 2000;118:469–76.
71. Nicodeme F, Lin Z, Pandolfino JE, Kahrilas PJ. Esophagogastric Junction pressure morphology: comparison between a station pull-through and real-time 3D-HRM representation. Neurogastroenterol Motil. 2013;25:e591–8.
72. Nicodeme F, Pipa-Muniz M, Khanna K, Kahrilas PJ, Pandolfino JE. Quantifying esophagogastric junction contractility with a novel HRM topographic metric, the EGJ-Contractile Integral: normative values and preliminary evaluation in PPI non-responders. Neurogastroenterol Motil. 2014;26:353–60.
73. Gor P, Li Y, Munigala S, Patel A, Bolkhir A, Gyawali CP. Interrogation of esophagogastric junction barrier function using the esophagogastric junction contractile integral: an observational cohort study. Dis Esophagus. 2016;29:820–8.
74. Jasper D, Freitas-Queiroz N, Hollenstein M, Misselwitz B, Layer P, Navarro-Rodriquez T, et al. Prolonged measurement improves the assessment of the barrier function of the esophago-gastric junction by high-resolution manometry. Neurogastroenterol Motil. 2017:29(2). https://doi.org/10.1111/nmo12925.
75. Tolone S, de Cassan C, de Bortoli N, Roman S, Galeazzi F, Salvador R, et al. Esophagogastric junction morphology is associated with a positive impedance-pH monitoring in patients with GERD. Neurogastroenterol Motil. 2015;27(8):1175–82.
76. Patti MG, Diener U, Tamburini A, Molena D, Way LW. Role of esophageal function tests in diagnosis of gastroesophageael reflux disease. Dig Dis Sci. 2001;46(3):597–602.
77. Fass R, Ofman JJ, Gralnek IM, Johnson C, Carmargo E, Sampliner RE, et al. Clinical and economic assessment of the omeprazole test in patients with symptoms suggestive of gastroesophageal reflux disease. Arch Intern Med. 1999;159:2161–8.
78. Herregods TV, Troelstra M, Weijenborg PW, Bredenoord AJ, Smout AJ. Patients with refractory reflux symptoms often do not have GERD. Neurogastroenterol Motil. 2015;27(9):1267–73.
79. Bello B, Zoccali M, Gullo R, Allaix ME, Herbella FA, Gasparaitis A, et al. Gastroesophageal reflux disease and antireflux surgery-What is the proper preoperative workup? J Gastrointest Surg. 2013;17:14–20.
80. Pandolfino JE, Richter JE, Ours T, Guardino JM, Chapman J, Kahrilas PJ. Ambulatory esophageal pH monitoring using a wireless system. Am J Gastroenterol. 2003;98(4):740–9.

81. Sweis R, Fox M, Anggiansah A, Wong T. Prolonged, wireless pH-studies have a high diagnostic yield in patients with reflux symptoms and negative 24-h catheter-based pH-studies. Neurogastroenterol Motil. 2011;23(5):419–26.
82. Penagini R, Sweis R, Mauro A, Dominques G, Vales A, Sifrim D. Inconsistency in the diagnosis of functional heartburn: usefulness of prolonged wireless pH monitoring in patients with proton pump inhibitor refractory gastroesophageal reflux disease. J Neurogastroenterol Motil. 2015;21:265–72.
83. Sweis R, Fox M, Anggiansah R, Anggiansah A, Basavaraju K, Canavan R, et al. Patient acceptance and clinical impact of Bravo monitoring in patients with previous failed catheter-based studies. Aliment Pharmacol Ther. 2009;29(6):669–76.
84. Jamieson JR, Stein HJ, DeMeester TR, Bonavina L, Schwizer W, Hinder RA, et al. Ambulatory 24h esophageal pH monitoring: normal values, optimal thresholds, specificity, sensitivity and reproducibility. Am J Gastroenterol. 1992;87:1102–11.
85. Roman S, Gyawali CP, Savarino E, Yadlapati R, Zerbib F, Wu J, et al. Ambulatory reflux monitoring for the diagnosis of gastroesophageal reflux disease: update of the Porto consensus and recommendations from an international consensus group. Neurogastroenterol Motil. 2017. https://doi.org/10.1111/nmo.13067.
86. Yadlapati R, Pandolfino JE, Lidder AK, Shabeeb N, Jaiyeola DM, Adkins C, et al. Oropharyngeal pH testing does not predict response to proton pump inhibitor therapy in patients with laryngeal symptoms. Am J Gastroenterol. 2016;111:1517–24.
87. Dulery C, Lechot A, Roman S, Bastier PL, Stoll D, de Gabory L, et al. A study with pharyngeal and esophageal 24-hour pH-impedance monitoring in patients with laryngopharyngeal symptoms refractory to proton pump inhibitors. Neurogastroenterol Motil. 2017;29(1). https://doi.org/10.1111/nmo12909.
88. Shay S, Richter J. Direct comparison of impedance, manometry and pH probe in detecting reflux before and after a meal. Dig Dis Sci. 2005;50:1584–90.
89. Sifrim D, Castell D, Dent J, Kahrilas PJ. Gastroesophageal reflux monitoring: Review and consensus report on detection and definitions of acid, non-acid and gas reflux. Gut. 2004;53:1024–31.
90. Bredenoord AJ. Impedance-pH monitoring: new standard for measuring gastro-oesophageal reflux. Neurogastroenterol Motil. 2008;20:4343–9.
91. Patel A, Sayuk GS, Gyawali CP. Parameters on esophageal pH-impedance monitoring that predict outcomes of patients with gastroesophageal reflux disease. Clin Gastroenterol Hepatol. 2015;13:884–91.
92. Frazzoni M, Savarino E, de Bortoli N, Martinucci I, Furnari M, Frazzoni L, et al. Analyses of the post-reflux swallow-induced peristaltic wave index and nocturnal baseline impedance parameters increase the diagnostic yield of impedance-pH monitoring of patients with reflux disease. Clin Gastroenterol Hepatol. 2016;14(1):40–6.
93. Boeckxstaens GE, Smout A. Systematic review: role of acid, weakly acidic and weakly alkaline reflux in gastroesophageal reflux disease. Aliment Pharmacol Ther. 2010;32:334–43.
94. Kushnir VM, Sayuk GS, Gyawali CP. Abnormal GERD parameters on ambulatory pH monitoring predict therapeutic success in noncardiac chest pain. Am J Gastroenterol. 2010;105:1032–8.
95. Gyawali CP, Roman S, Bredenoord AJ, Fox M, Keller J, Pandolfino JE, et al. Classification of esophageal motor findings in gastro-esophageal reflux disease: conclusions from an international consensus group Neurogastroenterol Motil. 2017. https://doi.org/10.1111/nmo13104.
96. Vakil N, van Zanten SV, Kahrilas P, Dent J, Jones R, Global Consensus Group. The Montreal definition and classification of gastroesophageal reflux disease: a global evidence-based consensus. Am J Gastroenterol. 2006;101(8):1900–20. quiz 1943
97. Patel A, Sayuk GS, Kushnir VM, Chan WW, Gyawali CP. GERD phenotypes from pH-impedance monitoring predict symptomatic outcomes on prospective evaluation. Neurogastroenterol Motil. 2016;28:513–21.
98. Sifrim D, Zerbib F. Diagnosis and management of patients with reflux symptoms refractory to proton pump inhibitors. Gut. 2012;61:1340–54.

99. Broeders JA, Draaisma WA, Bredenoord AJ, de Vries DR, Rijnhart-de Jong HG, Smout AJ, et al. Oesophageal acid hypersensitivity is not a contraindication to Nissen fundoplication. Br J Surg. 2009;96(9):1023–30.
100. Garros A, Mion F, Marjoux S, Damon H, Roman S. Factors associated with nonresponse to proton pump inhibitors therapy in patients referred for esophageal pH-impedance monitoring. Dis Esophagus. 2016;29(7):787–93.
101. Patel A, Sayuk GS, Gyawali CP. Prevalence, characteristics, and treatment outcomes of reflux hypersensitivity detected on pH-impedance monitoring. Neurogastroenterol Motil. 2016;28(9):1382–90.
102. Bredenoord AJ, Draaisma WA, Weusten BLAM, Gooszen HG, Smout AJ. Mechanisms of acid, weakly acidic and gas reflux after anti-reflux surgery. Gut. 2008;57(2):161–6.
103. Pandolfino JE, Curry J, Shi G, Joehl RJ, Brasseur JG, Kahrilas PJ. Restoration of normal distensive characteristics of the esophagogastric junction after fundoplication. Ann Surg. 2005;242(1):43–8.
104. Kwiatek MA, Kahrilas K, Soper NJ, Bulsiewicz WJ, McMahon BP, Gregersen H, et al. Esophaogastric junction distensibility after fundoplication assessed with a novel functional luminal imaging probe. J Gastrointest Surg. 2010;14(2):268–76.
105. Boudewijn KF, Bredenoord AJ, Schijven MP, van der Peet DL, van Berge HM, Smout AJ. Long-term effects of anti-reflux surgery on the physiology of the esophagogastric junction. Surg Endosc. 2015;29:3726–32.
106. Wang YT, Tai LF, Yazaki E, Jafari J, Sweis R, Tucker K, et al. Investigation of dysphagia after antireflux surgery by high-resolution manometry: impact of multiple water swallows and a solid test meal on diagnosis, management, and clinical outcome. Clin Gastroenterol Hepatol. 2015;13(9):1575–83.
107. Ang D, Misselwitz B, Hollenstein M, Knowles K, Wright J, Tucker E, et al. High resolution manometry with a solid test meal increases diagnostic sensitivity for clinically relevant, symptomatic esophageal motility disorders: results from a large case series. Lancet Gastroenterol Hepatol. 2017;2(9):654–61.
108. Kahrilas PJ, Lin S, Spiess A, Brasseur J, Joehl R, Manka M. Impact of fundoplication on bolus transit across esophagogastric junction. Am J Physiol. 1998;275(6Part 1):G1386–93.
109. Kwiatek MA, Pandolfino JE, Hirano I, Kahrilas PJ. Esophagogastric junction distensibility assessed with an endoscopic functional luminal imaging probe (EndoFLIP). Gastrointest Endosc. 2010;72:272–8.
110. Tucker E, Sweis R, Anggiansah A, Wong T, Telakis E, Knowles K, et al. Measurement of esophago-gastric junction cross-sectional area and distensibility by an endoluminal functional lumen imaging probe for the diagnosis of gastroesophageal reflux disease. Neurogastroenterol Motil. 2013;25(11):1–7.
111. Hirano I, Pandolfino JE, Boeckxstaens GE. Functional lumen imaging probe for the management of esophageal disorders: expert review from the clinical practice updates committee of the AGA institute. Clin Gastroenterol Hepatol. 2017;15:325–44.
112. Ilczyszyn A, Botha AJ. Feasibility of esophagogastric junction distensibility measurement during Nissen fundoplication. Dis Esophagus. 2014;27(7):637–44.

Chapter 4
Preoperative Diagnostic Workup for GERD and Hiatal Hernia: An Evidence and Experience-Based Approach

Geoffrey P. Kohn

4.1 Diagnostic Workup for GERD

4.1.1 Confirmation of the Diagnosis

A useable definition of Gastroesophageal Reflux Disease (GERD) is difficult to create but is necessary to guide management and research of this very common disorder which affects up to 20% of the population of the Western World [1–5]. The diagnosis of GERD requires more than solely the reflux of gastric contents into the esophagus; indeed, some reflux is normal in all patients. Basing the definition upon the amount of reflux would be problematic because any determined threshold between physiological reflux and pathological would be arbitrary [6]. In addressing this problem, an international consensus panel has devised the so-called Montreal definition of gastroesophageal reflux disease, requiring both the objective finding of reflux of gastric contents into the esophagus together with the subjective reporting of troublesome symptoms [7]. This is the most widely accepted definition of GERD in use today. Troublesome symptoms include the "typical" symptoms of heartburn and regurgitation, together with the "atypical" symptoms of cough, dysphonia, chest pain, epigastric pain, dysphagia, pneumonia and sinusitis and others. GERD can be the cause of all these symptoms, but there can be many other etiologies too. Defining a disease based on subjective reporting of nonspecific symptoms is problematic and assuming reflux as the cause and then treating as such, whether with lifestyle modification, antisecretory medications or by antireflux surgery, may be unhelpful in relief of symptoms where a non-GERD etiology is present. Objective evidence of GERD is therefore required, together with appropriate symptoms, before the diagnosis can be confirmed. Before considering surgery, this objective documentation of gastroesophageal reflux is mandatory [8].

G.P. Kohn, MBBS(Hons), MSurg, FRACS, FACS
Melbourne Upper Gastrointestinal Surgical Group, Melbourne, Victoria, Australia

Eastern Health Clinical School, Monash University, Melbourne, Victoria, Australia
e-mail: GKohn@uppergi.net

M.A. Memon (ed.), *Hiatal Hernia Surgery*,
https://doi.org/10.1007/978-3-319-64003-7_4

4.1.2 Confirming GERD

The reflux of acidic gastric contents into the esophagus may cause endoscopically detectable changes. Objective evidence of GERD may thus be obtained by endoscopic detection of "mucosal breaks" of the distal esophagus, Barrett's metaplasia or the reflux-related complication of peptic stricture.

4.1.2.1 Mucosal Breaks

Endoscopic visualization of any area of slough or erythema in the distal esophagus which is clearly demarcated from adjacent normal-appearing mucosa [9], a so-called "mucosal break", is considered objective evidence of gastroesophageal reflux disease in the appropriate clinical setting. This mucosal break is the minimum endoscopic lesion that is a reliable indicator of reflux esophagitis [10].

Histological examination of esophageal biopsies is not currently part of the standard diagnostic pathway for GERD, and such investigation is of unproven benefit. However, there are some emerging data suggesting that there may be some utility in recognizing the microscopic presence of inter-cellular space dilatation in the diagnosis of non-erosive reflux disease [8].

In an appropriate setting, a peptic stricture is also acceptable evidence of gastroesophageal reflux disease [11] provided malignancy has been excluded by multiple biopsies.

4.1.2.2 Barrett's Esophagus

Barrett's esophagus is the replacement of the normal squamous esophageal epithelium with a metaplastic specialized columnar epithelium with villiform appearance. The added requirement for "goblet cells" to be present is not universally accepted [12]. Barrett's metaplasia is believed to arise nearly always as a result of gastroesophageal reflux and constitutes an alternative method of esophageal repair in the setting of reflux esophagitis [13, 14]. Histological proof of Barrett's esophagus is currently also considered objective evidence of gastroesophageal reflux disease.

4.1.2.3 Contrast Esophagrams

For many years, contrast radiology studies of the esophagus were the standard for demonstration of gastroesophageal reflux. The technique of contrast esophagrams usually involves the patient swallowing a liquid or semisolid contrast bolus. Physiologically, the initiation of this swallow is expected to cause relaxation of the lower esophageal sphincter (LES) mechanism to permit bolus transport into the stomach. Thus, the "failure" of the LES mechanism is actually expected during swallowing and over-interpreting this as evidence of GERD will cause many false positive results. Ambulatory pH studies therefore have both a higher sensitivity and specificity than fluoroscopy [15–20] and have superseded contrast studies in the diagnosis of GERD.

In patients with typical symptoms and endoscopy-proven esophagitis, the diagnosis of GERD is evident and additional investigation with esophageal pH monitoring is unnecessary [8]. It is in patients with non-erosive reflux disease (NERD) where there is an absence of endoscopic evidence of GERD that esophageal pH testing remains crucial.

4.1.3 Catheter-Based pH Monitoring

Conventional catheter-based pH monitoring systems principally consist of a flexible catheter with one or more pH sensors and a data recorder. The catheter is passed through the nares and is placed with the pH sensor in the distal esophagus. It is connected to a data recorder that is carried by the patient during the study. Ambulatory catheter-based pH monitoring is generally performed over a 24-hr period, as a complete circadian cycle allows for determining the effect of physical activity and body positions on esophageal acid exposure [21, 22].

In general, esophageal pH monitoring is carried out while the patient is off acid-suppressant medication. Patients are normally instructed to discontinue the use of proton pump inhibitors at least 7 days prior, histamine H2-antagonists 3–5 days prior and simple antacids 24 hr prior to the investigation. Only when the aim of the study is to measure the esophageal acid exposure that persists during treatment should acid suppressants be continued. If such medications are continued during the study period, then the reduced gastric acid environment will result in an elevated false-negative rate and lower sensitivity of the test.

During the study patients are instructed to keep a diary and to record symptoms, mealtimes and times for supine and upright positions. Meal periods can be excluded from the analysis to avoid potential artefacts produced by acidic meal ingestion and this may improve the clinical reliability of the test [23]. The study period should probably resemble the average day of the patient, both in terms of diet and activity. However, some centers encourage the patient to attempt to exacerbate reflux by consuming "challenge meals" of refluxogenic food types such as fatty or spicy meals, alcoholic beverages, or any food recognized by the patient as precipitating symptoms (Fig. 4.1).

The catheter-based technique for esophageal pH monitoring is limited by discomfort in the patient's nose and throat, and as a consequence the test is not tolerated by all patients. Early removal of the catheter will result in an inability to compare to a normal control period, though some positive attempts have been made to reduce the measurement time to a better-tolerated 3-hr period [24].

4.1.4 Wireless pH Monitoring

In order to avoid the discomfort of the catheter-based technique of esophageal pH measurement, a catheter-free, wireless pH system (Bravo, Medtronic, MN, USA) has been developed. In addition to improved patient comfort [25], the capsule-based

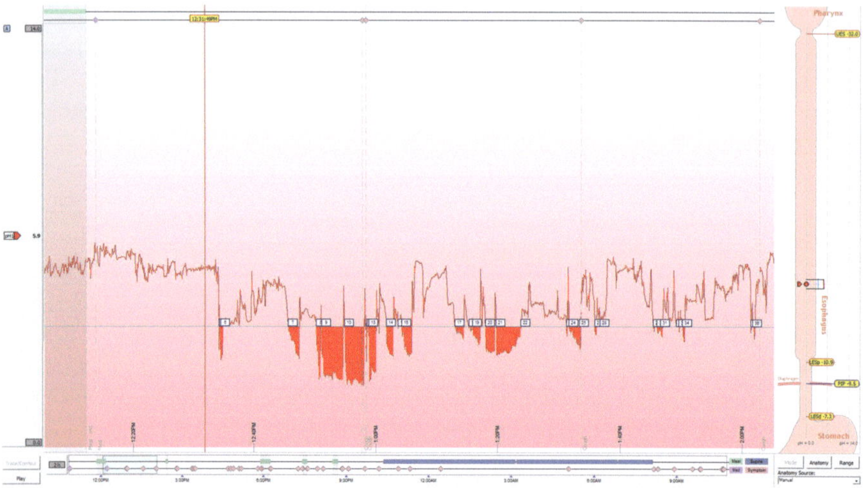

Fig. 4.1 A typical 24-hr catheter-based pH study

pH system has the potential advantages of fixed placement of the pH electrode, minimizing the risk of slipping into the stomach, and of allowing for prolonged recordings. The longer duration of pH monitoring has been suggested to increase the sensitivity of reflux monitoring in identifying patients with gastroesophageal reflux [26]. Recognized contraindications for the use of the Bravo capsule are hemorrhagic diathesis, esophageal varices, severe esophagitis, patients with a cardiac pacemaker or defibrillator, and pregnancy.

The pH system consists of a capsule and a telemetry receiver. The capsule includes a pH electrode, an internal battery and a transmitter. The capsule simultaneously measures and transmits pH data using radiotelemetry to the portable receiver. The delivery system for the pH capsule is most commonly passed transorally after completion of an upper endoscopy and attached to the mucosa of the distal esophagus. The capsule is designed to detach in 3–7 days and then pass through the gastrointestinal tract. There are reports of the probe remaining attached for longer periods usually without consequence [26] but sometimes requiring endoscopic removal [26].

Wireless esophageal pH monitoring is associated with fewer adverse symptoms and less interference with normal daily activities and is preferred by patients [27], though there are still limitations associated with the wireless technique. The wireless pH capsule is associated with thoracic discomfort in 10–65% of the patients. The severity of chest symptoms ranges from a mild foreign-body sensation to severe chest pain, although the latter is uncommon. In rare cases, the pain is so severe that endoscopic removal of the capsule is necessary [28–30].

Possible problems with the capsule-based pH system include technical problems such as premature detachment of the capsule or interruption of the radiotelemetry signal. Detachment of the pH capsule is suggested by an abrupt pH drop as the sensor dislocates into the stomach with an increasing pH reaching above 7 as gastric motility propels the pH capsule into the duodenum. In a small proportion of patients with unsuccessful recordings, pH monitoring has to be repeated as a consequence of these technical problems [21].

4.1.5 Duration of pH Monitoring

The standard duration of recording for catheter-based esophageal pH testing is 24 hr. For the wireless pH system is 48 hr, though approximately 10% of wireless probes detach prior to the completion of this period [26, 31]. The extended recording capabilities of the wireless pH system as compared with the conventional catheter-based technique appear to increase the sensitivity of the test. Studies have demonstrated that by increasing the pH recording time from 24 to 48 h, the yield of the procedure increases in capturing more abnormal pH tests or symptom-associated reflux events [28].

The 48 hr data can be interpreted using an average of the 2 days, or alternatively using only the 24-hr period with the greatest acid exposure, termed "worst day analysis". A significant increase in the sensitivity of the pH testing is seen, together with a small decrease in specificity, when using the worst day data as compared to either 24 hr data or averaged 48 hr data [21, 22].

4.1.6 pH Electrode Placement

Consistent positioning of the pH electrode is vital for obtaining reliable esophageal pH data and for comparison to normative population data values. Studies performed using catheters with multiple pH sensors for simultaneous pH recording at different levels in the esophagus have unsurprisingly shown greater acid exposure in the distal esophagus compared to more proximally [32, 33]. Consequently, esophageal acid detection will be significantly reduced when the distance from the lower esophageal sphincter (LES) to the recording level increases, and therefore accurate pH probe placement is essential for a reliable diagnosis of GERD. Typically, the pH electrode should be placed close enough to the stomach to sample the region most affected by gastroesophageal reflux without displacing into the stomach during the course of the study, noting that the gastroesophageal junction migrates approximately 2–4 cm during deglutition [34, 35]. By convention, the catheter-based pH electrode is placed 5 cm above the manometrically defined upper border of the LES [36]. Therefore, esophageal manometry must be performed prior to the pH study to ensure correct placement. Placement on the basis of the pH profile recorded on withdrawal of the electrode from the stomach has been found to be inferior to placement based on manometric LES localization [21, 37].

In wireless esophageal pH monitoring the pH sensor is most commonly placed according to endoscopic landmarks. By convention, the electrode is placed 6 cm above the squamocolumnar junction (SCJ), a position that has been derived from the findings of concurrent manometry and videofluoroscopy studies suggesting that the upper border of the LES high-pressure zone typically extends 1–1.5 cm above the SCJ [38]. Positioning the pH electrode 6 cm above the SCJ therefore approximates the standard 5 cm above the upper border of the manometrically defined LES electrode position of the catheter-based technique. Transnasal placement of the pH capsule normally requires prior manometry, as the electrode is positioned 5 cm above the upper border of the LES [39].

4.1.7 Interpretation of Esophageal pH Studies

With esophageal bicarbonate secretion and swallowed saliva, esophageal pH is normally maintained between pH 5 and pH 7. Gastric acid secretion generates a highly acidic environment within the stomach, with a pH of 1–2, and rarely more than 3. During esophageal pH monitoring, gastroesophageal reflux events are detected as abrupt declines in intra-esophageal pH. Generally, episodes where pH falls below 4 are taken as evidence of reflux events. The arbitrary choice of the cut-off of pH 4 is supported by the observation that patients with symptomatic reflux usually report heartburn at an intraesophageal pH below this threshold [40]. Physiologic acid reflux seen in healthy subjects is characterized by reflux episodes that occur in the upright position most commonly after a meal and are rapidly cleared. Physiologic acid reflux rarely occurs while supine. In patients with mild reflux disease more reflux episodes occur, especially in the upright, postprandial period. With increasing severity of GERD, acid reflux increases first in the upright position, and thereafter typically becomes bipositional with acid reflux in both the upright and supine postures [41–43]. Both the duration and number of acid reflux episodes increase, resulting in prolonged esophageal acid exposure times.

The total percentage of time the pH is <4 is the most useful single discriminator between physiologic and pathologic reflux [36]. An abnormal pH test is defined by a value greater than the 95th percentile of normal controls, though this can vary depending on the age and gender distribution of the selected control population.

Another method of presenting esophageal acid exposure data is calculation of a composite score, comprised of six measured parameters, including (1) total percent time pH < 4; (2) percent time pH < 4 whilst upright; (3) percent time pH < 4 whilst recumbent; (4) the total number of reflux episodes; (5) the total number of reflux episodes longer than 5 min; (6) the duration of the longest reflux episode. This so-called DeMeester Composite Score, named for one of its original proponents [44], is automatically calculated and reported by most commercially available pH software. The most referenced value for an abnormal DeMeester composite score is a value larger than 14.7 [44]. Regardless of whether the composite score or individual acid exposure time is used, a detailed evaluation of the pH tracing is of fundamental importance to recognize and exclude artefacts and to assess symptom association [21].

4.1.8 Symptoms Association

Reflux symptoms such as heartburn and regurgitation are very common but as these symptoms are not specific for GERD, it is important to be able to determine if there is a temporal relationship between symptoms and reflux events. Such a relationship between symptoms and reflux episodes can be expressed numerically using symptom association analysis [45]. The most frequently used indices are the Symptom Index (SI) and the Symptom Association Probability (SAP) [46].

The Symptom Index is the percentage of symptoms preceded by a drop in esophageal pH below 4 within a time window, usually selected to be 5 min, divided by the total number of symptoms. The Symptom Index can be calculated for each symptom attributable to reflux, including heartburn, regurgitation, or atypical symptoms, such as chest pain or respiratory symptoms. A positive symptom association is declared if the symptom index is ≥50% (i.e., at least half of the reported symptoms are preceded within a 5-min time window by an intraesophageal pH below 4) [47]. The Symptom Index does not consider the total number of reflux episodes and does not include the total number of symptom events. When few symptoms are reported during the study period, the Symptoms Index is less relevant.

The Symptom Association Probability is a statistical method to determine the relationship between symptoms and reflux episodes. The SAP is calculated by dividing the entire study's pH data into consecutive 2-min segments. For each of these segments, it is determined whether reflux occurred in the segment, allowing for calculation of the total number of 2-min segments with and without reflux. Subsequently, it is determined whether or not a reflux episode occurred in the 2-min period before each symptom. A 2 × 2 contingency table is constructed in which the number of 2-min segments with and without symptoms, and with and without reflux events, are tabulated. Using the Fisher exact test, a p value is calculated and the SAP index is calculated as $(1 - p) \times 100\%$ [48]. The cut-off value for a positive test is often defined as SAP ≥95%. However, even a statistically significant relationship between reflux events and symptoms does not necessarily imply causality [21]. The yield of the SI and SAP is greater when performed off- rather than on-acid suppressant therapy [22].

4.1.9 pH testing On- versus Off-Acid Suppressive Medication

An important decision has to be made by the treating physician as to whether to perform pH testing on or off acid-suppressant medications. Esophageal pH testing without medication is more accurate, and a negative result (i.e., normal distal esophageal pH with negative symptom association) is very helpful in suggesting that the symptoms are not caused by acid reflux. Testing off-therapy is therefore often recommended for patients in whom there is a low index of clinical suspicion for GERD in order to "rule out" reflux as a cause of the symptoms [22]. Off-therapy pH testing may demonstrate abnormal reflux but this does not indicate causality between the reflux and the patient's symptoms.

A positive pH test while off acid suppressant therapy does not necessarily explain why the patient is still having symptoms while taking PPIs. On-therapy testing is more commonly used to evaluate patients with refractory reflux symptoms despite medical therapy [22]. An abnormal esophageal pH test (i.e., increased amount of distal esophageal acid exposure with therapy and a positive symptom association for acid reflux) performed during therapy is helpful because it suggests that the acid suppression may be insufficient. In these situations, the use of dual pH electrodes to monitor both distal esophageal and gastric pH are sometimes recommended, especially for patients unresponsive to antireflux therapy [22]. Although intragastric pH measurement can help determine the efficacy of acid suppressive medications or suggest poor patient compliance, its clinical relevance is unclear because there is a paucity of data showing a correlation between intragastric pH and gastroesophageal reflux [49, 50]. A negative esophageal pH test while receiving therapy cannot exclude nonacid reflux being associated with the residual symptoms [21]. Combining intraluminal impedance and pH testing is postulated to be able to address this issue, but high quality data are lacking.

4.1.10 Limitations of Esophageal pH Monitoring

Ambulatory esophageal pH monitoring is not without its limitations. The sensitivity and specificity of catheter-based pH monitoring have traditionally been reported to be in the range of 87–96% and 97–100%, respectively [51, 52]. Importantly, these reports are based on studies consisting of patients with complicated reflux disease, manifested by severe esophagitis and manometrically defective lower esophageal sphincters. As there is a relationship between the severity of the disease and the discriminatory power of the test [53], the published data on sensitivity and specificity reflect the severity of reflux disease in the populations tested and may not necessarily apply to the ordinary patient with symptoms suggestive of reflux disease [46]. In more recent studies of patients with typical reflux symptoms and esophagitis, a sensitivity of 76–78% and a specificity of 93–95% were reported for the capsule-based technique of esophageal pH monitoring [26, 53]. The apparently lower discriminatory power of the capsule-based technique probably only reflects differences in the selection of the patient populations [21].

Patients most likely to benefit from an objective documentation of abnormal acid reflux are those without endoscopic evidence of GERD, who constitute up to two-thirds of all patients with typical reflux symptoms [54]. In these patients, catheter-based testing has a lower sensitivity of <71% [22] and capsule-based pH monitoring has a specificity of 93–95% and sensitivity as low as 36–42% [26, 53].

4.1.11 Proximal Esophageal pH Assessment

An association between reflux of acidic gastric contents into the larynx and laryngeal symptoms has been proposed [55]. There are multiple alternative potential causes for these respiratory and laryngeal symptoms, and establishing reflux as the cause based on symptoms alone is unreliable [56, 57]. Measurement of distal esophageal acid exposure by catheter-based or wireless pH monitoring would be expected to be less than useful in assessment of the proximal esophagus. Indeed when distal esophageal acid exposure is used as an indication for antireflux surgery to address extraesophageal manifestations of reflux such as laryngeal symptoms, outcomes are usually suboptimal, particularly in patients who have already not successfully responded to antisecretory medical therapy [58, 59].

Attempts have been made to improve operative outcomes for such atypical symptoms of reflux by preoperative assessment of proximal esophageal acidification. Normative value for upper esophageal acid exposure have been defined [57]. The total time of $pH < 4$ in the proximal esophagus in normal subjects is similar to that measured in the distal esophagus. However, the number of reflux episodes is significantly higher when measured in the proximal esophagus. The widespread clinical utility of such systems remains unclear [60, 61].

4.1.12 Multichannel Intraluminal Impedance

Multichannel intraluminal impedance (MII) is a relatively new technique for evaluating esophageal bolus transit during swallowing and for monitoring gastroesophageal reflux independent of its pH.

The presence and movement of an intraesophageal bolus is detected by MII based on measuring differences in electrical conductivity within the esophagus (Fig. 4.2) [62]. Liquid boluses are better conductors than the empty oesophagus, leading to a rapid decline in intraluminal impedance when the bolus enters the impedance measuring segment [62]. Impedance returns to baseline once the bolus has exited the segment. Multiple impedance measuring segments mounted on the same catheter allow determination of the direction of bolus movement based on the timing of changes in impedance at individual levels. Proximal to distal (antegrade) progression of impedance changes is indicative of swallowing, whereas a distal to proximal (retrograde) progression indicates reflux episodes [63].

Multiple impedance-measuring segments can be added to a regular pH probe, and when combined as such MII-pH can evaluate the presence of refluxate independent of its pH and at the same time can differentiate between acid and non-acid reflux [21].

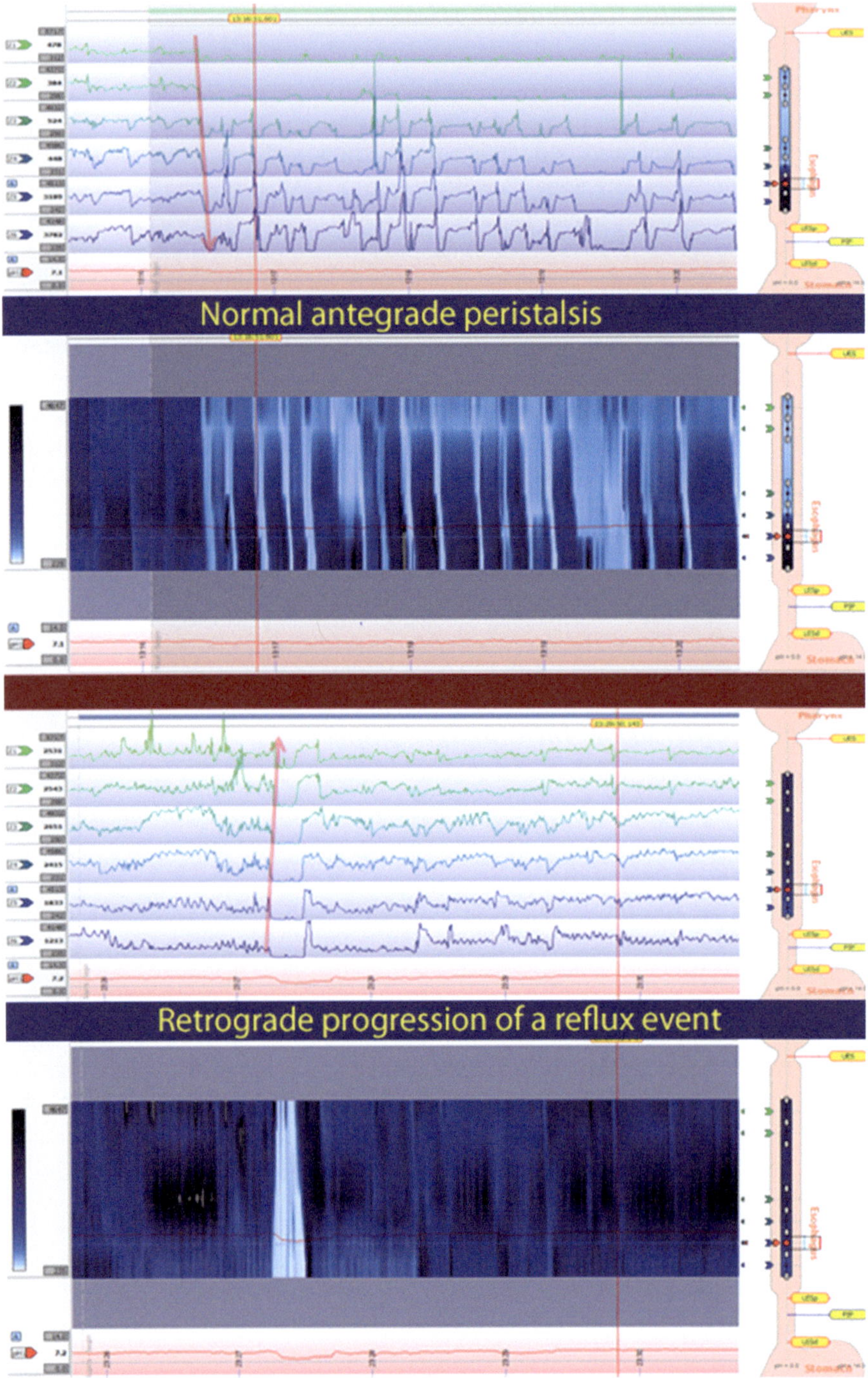

Fig. 4.2 Esophageal multichannel intraluminal impedance assessment

4.1.13 Combined Multichannel Intraluminal Impedance and pH

Impedance assessment is best added to pH measurements to give a more thorough evaluation of the function of the antireflux barrier [64].

Normal values for acid and nonacid reflux in healthy volunteers from multiple centers not receiving acid-suppressive therapy [65] have been published, as have various population-specific norms [66–68]. A hypothesis that proximal extension of the refluxate to the level of the larynx may be the cause of respiratory and laryngeal symptoms of reflux [7] is supported by MII findings [69].

MII-pH is a useful tool in expanding the group of patients expected to have a successful outcome after antireflux surgery. Prior to the introduction of MII, some patient with non-acidic reflux might have been denied surgery when in fact their symptoms might be improved by an antireflux procedure. It is now appreciated that there exists a subset of refluxers with normal pH studies but abnormal MII tests that will have good short-term outcomes after fundoplication [70].

MII-pH is now being increasingly employed in the assessment of patients with atypical symptoms of GERD [71–73]. However, the utility of this approach in patients being considered for antireflux surgery remain uncertain, with little evidence demonstrating a prognostic effect on post-surgical outcomes. There remains a paucity of studies comparing outcomes of extraesophageal symptoms of reflux disease after antireflux surgery based solely on ambulatory pH assessment as compared to studies including MII assessment. Reports are also emerging of poor correlation between pH studies and MII studies [74], where instead close correlation is expected if these studies are to be viewed as both sensitive and additive in the diagnosis of GERD.

4.1.14 Other Preoperative Tests

After confirmation of GERD, but before undertaking antireflux surgery, regular preoperative tests are recommended to assess general fitness for surgery, including basic biochemical analysis, electrocardiography on some patients and other tests determined as necessary after appropriate history and examination of the patient.

While antireflux surgery is a reasonable, safe and cost-effective option for all patients with symptomatic reflux of stomach contents into the esophagus [75], the symptoms for which patient with reflux present for medical care are not always due to GERD. For example, a symptomatic pharyngeal pouch may concomitantly be present in a patient with elevated distal esophageal acid exposure. Clearly therapy directed towards the lower esophageal sphincter mechanism will not solve all problems of concern to the patient. For this reason, many surgeons will request a contrast esophagram to evaluate the entire esophagus prior to considering antireflux surgery.

Fundoplication is the most commonly performed antireflux procedure. The role of preoperative manometric evaluation of the esophagus prior to fundoplication is debated. Amongst the possible side-effects of fundoplication are included dysphagia and gas bloat syndrome, occurring in approximately 5–8% [76–79] and up to 40% [80] respectively of post fundoplication patients. It has been postulated that preoperative manometric investigation of the esophagus will predict postoperative side effects, particularly postoperative dysphagia. It has also been thought that the "tailoring" of the extent of the fundoplication, whether 90°, 360° or an intermediate extent, would achieve superior postoperative quality-of-life and patient satisfaction. A systematic review provides evidence that this is not the case, and an operation tailored to the manometric measurements of esophageal motility is unwarranted [8]. Nonetheless, many centers do perform preoperative manometry. This is often justified as pre-emptive management of possible postoperative problems. For the postoperative patients who presents with dysphagia (again, averaging 5–8% of all postoperative patients, but much higher in the immediate postoperative period), knowledge of esophageal motility may help guide management. Moreover, certain motility disorders can mimic GERD by demonstrating the same symptomatology. For example, achalasia cardia can present with substernal burning, regurgitation and elevated distal esophageal acid exposure, but in this case the etiology is not due to incompetency of the antireflux mechanism. Antireflux surgery in such patients would result in a very poor outcome, and hence preoperative manometry will be helpful in such patients. Other preoperative tests have been examined, such as nuclear medicine gastric emptying studies [81], but there are no data to support a correlation between their results and postoperative outcomes. Gastric emptying studies may be important however in patients who require reoperation, as it may provide indirect evidence for vagal nerve injury during the original surgery [8].

4.2 Diagnostic Workup for Hiatal Hernia

The antireflux mechanism of the lower esophagus is dependent upon multiple variables; the tone of the distal esophageal musculature (lower esophageal sphincter), the actions of the diaphragmatic crura, the intra-abdominal esophageal length and the orientation of the angle of His all affect competency of the antireflux mechanism. With proximal migration of the stomach or gastroesophageal junction through the diaphragmatic hiatus, this mechanism is disrupted. Therefore, there is a close association between gastroesophageal reflux disease and hiatal hernias.

Indications for treatment of hiatal hernia include symptoms of GERD, symptoms related to gastric obstruction due to the hernia, complications due to the hernia and a desire to prevent future complications.

Hiatal hernias have been divided into various subtypes. Type I hernias, also known as sliding hiatal hernias, have the gastroesophageal junction above the diaphragm with the remainder of the stomach located remaining in the usual subdiaphragmatic position. The major clinical significance of a Type I hernia is its association with reflux disease [82]. In patients with proven gastroesophageal reflux disease, with or without a sliding hiatal hernia, antireflux surgery is an option for the management of their condition [83, 84]. The indication for repair of a sliding (Type I) hiatal hernia is gastroesophageal reflux disease. The hernia is not the indication for the procedure. Occasionally, such hernias are thought to produce symptoms of dysphagia or rarely cause gastric ulceration. While these may occur, they are rare and repair of a Type I hernia is nearly always unnecessary in the absence of gastroesophageal reflux disease. Therefore, preoperative diagnostic workup for Type I hiatal hernia is directed toward confirming GERD.

Where more than just the gastroesophageal junction lies above the diaphragm but the actual fundus or body of the stomach (and often other organs too) then this is often termed a paraesophageal hernia. Such hernia are frequently divided into subtypes dependent on the extent of herniation of abdominal contents, but the treatment is more dependent on the area of the diaphragmatic defect and the orientation of the hernia contents rather on the specific subtype. Larger defects with more herniation of contents, particularly with a degree of volvulus are more likely to be symptomatic and have a greater indication for repair [85, 86].

4.2.1 *Preoperative Diagnostic Workup for Paraesophageal Hernias*

Information regarding the anatomy of the hernia, the function of the upper gastrointestinal tract and esophageal acidification will be of use to the surgeon managing paraesophageal hernias. Relevant investigations may include the following [8, 82]:

4.2.1.1 Diagnosis of the Hernia

Plain chest radiographs: A retrocardiac air-fluid level on chest X-ray is pathognomonic for a paraesophageal hiatal hernia. Visceral gas may be seen in cases of intestinal herniation into the chest. *Contrast studies* (Fig. 4.3) are helpful to gauge the size and reducibility of the hiatal hernia and to localize precisely the gastroesophageal junction in relation to the esophageal hiatus. Contrast findings may add to suspicion of existing short esophagus [87]. This may allow for the surgeon to be prepared to address a short esophagus with a lengthening procedure if needed intraoperatively. Further, when performed as a video-esophagram, information on bolus transport is provided by the study. Given the increased aspiration risk of patients with paraesophageal hernias presenting with acute gastric outlet obstruction, ionic water soluble contrast should be generally avoided due to the risk of aspiration pneumonitis [88] Contrast studies will also evaluate the proximal esophagus to detect the presence of concomitant pathology, such as a pharyngeal pouch. *Computed tomography* (CT) scan may be useful in an urgent situation for patients with

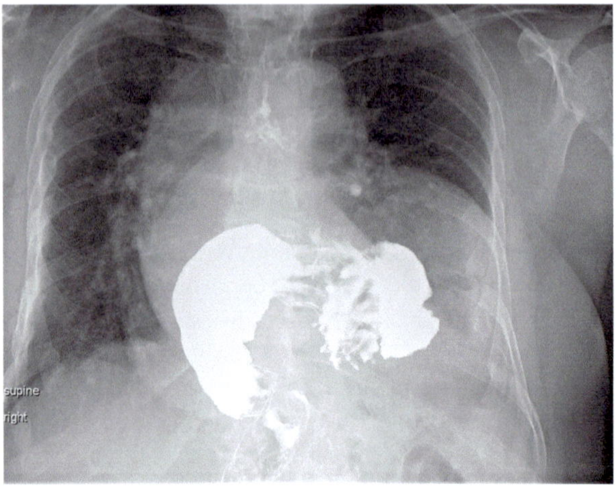

Fig. 4.3 A contrast study of a large paraesophageal hernia with organoaxial volvulus of the intrathoracic stomach

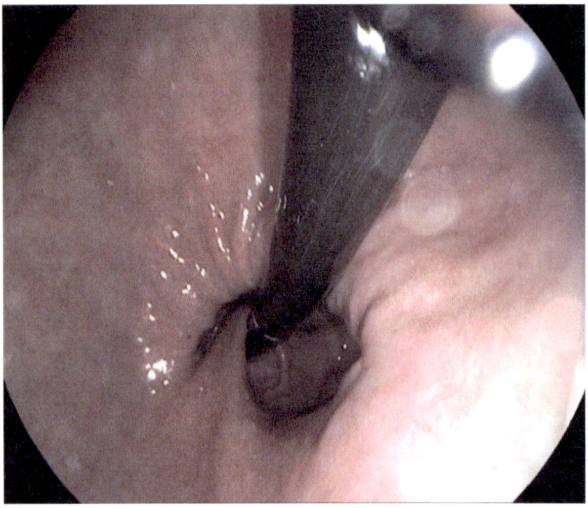

Fig. 4.4 Endoscopic retroflexed view of a hiatal hernia with the gastroesophageal junction seen to lie above the diaphragm

suspected complications from a volvulized paraesophageal hernia. The hernia site and any herniated organs within the chest cavity are clearly visualized in most cases. Rarely a hernia will be seen to be of a type different to a paraesophageal hernia, such as the congenital Bochdalek or Morgagni hernias or hernias secondary to traumatic diaphragmatic injury. If intestinal obstruction and strangulation occur, dilated intestinal segments will be visualized with air-fluid levels within the chest cavity and abdomen. Cephalad migration of the gastroesophageal junction or gastric fundus through the hiatus can be clearly visualized on oral contrast-enhanced CT images.

Esophagogastroduodenoscopy (EGD) allows for visual assessment of the mucosa of the esophagus, stomach and duodenum. The presence of erosive esophagitis, Schatzki's ring, or Barrett's esophagus can be determined. Further, the size and type of hernia can be determined (Fig. 4.4). The sensitivity of EGD in the diagnosis of large paraesophageal hernias is lower than expected. The expected anatomical landmarks, that is the diaphragmatic impressions, are often difficult to appreciate particularly in the presence of wide separation of the crura [89]. Therefore, an appreciation of the gastroesophageal junction being above the diaphragm is often missed. Evaluation of gastric viability is particularly important among patients undergoing emergency surgery for incarcerated hernias.

4.2.1.2 Evaluation of Function

Esophageal manometry can demonstrate the level of the diaphragmatic crura, the respiratory inversion point and the location of the lower esophageal sphincter. The size of the sliding component of a hiatal hernia can then be calculated, particularly with new high resolution manometry technology (Fig. 4.5). In patients with a para-esophageal hiatal hernia with volvulus placement of the manometry catheter across the lower esophageal sphincter and below the diaphragm can be difficult [90, 91]. Whether preoperative manometric evaluation of the esophagus is required is an

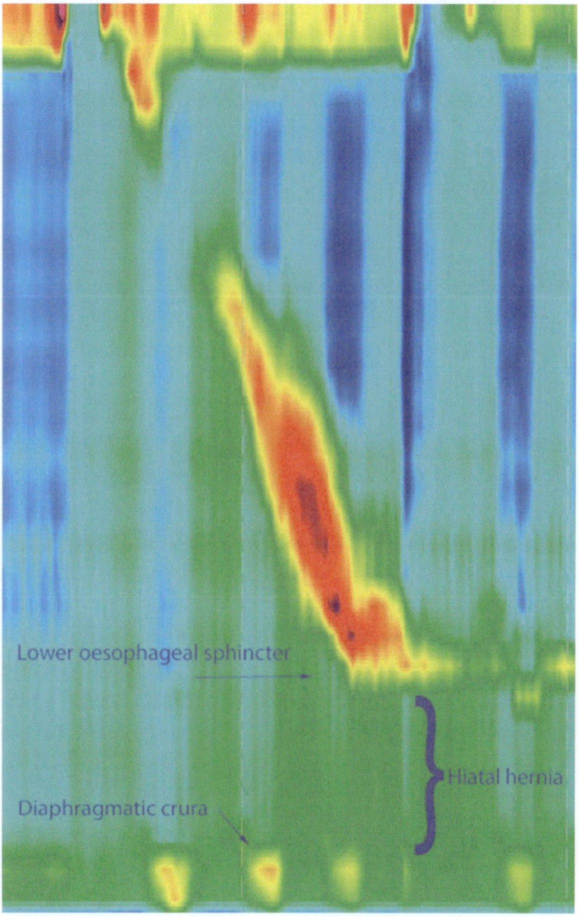

Fig. 4.5 High-resolution manometry findings of hiatal hernia

oft-debated topic [92] Similar to the situation around antireflux surgery, the role of preoperative esophageal manometry with the purpose of allowing a tailored approach to construction of the fundoplication is probably unwarranted. Moreover, the presence of a hiatal hernia may affect the manometric studies [93, 94]. However, knowledge of the function of the esophagus will greatly enhance care of the dysphagic postoperative patient.

pH testing has limited relevance in the diagnosis of a paraesophageal hernia, but is critical to identify the presence of increased esophageal acid exposure in patients with sliding hiatal hernias who might benefit from antireflux surgery. Confirmation of abnormal gastroesophageal reflux either by the identification of erosive esophagitis or Barrett's esophagus on upper endoscopy, or by demonstration of increased esophageal acid exposure on pH monitoring is necessary prior to consideration of operative intervention in patients with a sliding hiatal hernia.

Nuclear medicine studies, Nuclear medicine gastric emptying studies can be useful in assessing a reoperative patient where previous vagal injury is a possibility [95]. Care must be taken when interpreting these studies as simply considering the gastric emptying half-time can be misleading. Closer review of the scintigraphic images may demonstrate retention of radionucleotide in the distal esophagus or the part of the stomach proximal to a volvulus. In these cases, emptying time is not dependent on vagal activity but also on mechanical distortion of the stomach [95].

Echocardiogram [96] and endoscopic ultrasound can also demonstrate hiatal hernias but are not routinely used for diagnosis. Echocardiogram may demonstrate compression of the left atrium, inferior pulmonary vein and coronary sinus by a large hiatal hernia [97]. This may be useful in determining whether the symptom of dyspnea may be due to the hernia. By directing a patient to consume a volume of carbonated beverage, the stomach can be inflated while monitoring the effect on cardiac chamber compression.

The mainstays of evaluation for patients with a hiatal hernia, particularly prior to operative intervention, are upper endoscopy and barium swallow. Contrast studies are reported to be more sensitive than endoscopy in detecting sliding hiatal hernia [98]. The role of the various diagnostic techniques may depend on the clinical presentation of the patient. Incidentally detected hiatal hernias, or those hernias which are minimally symptomatic, may be assessed by endoscopy and contrast radiology. A CT scan can be performed if additional information is needed to aid in further clinical decision making [82]. Findings of a stomach in an unusually high position or with an abnormal axis in a patient with acute abdominal pain and vomiting should make one suspect gastric volvulus [99]. Emergency presentations of hiatal hernia, such as with gastric obstruction or ischemia, may first be decompressed with a nasogastric tube followed by a plain chest radiograph and endoscopy. Excessive investigation in emergency presentation may lead to delay in treatment and suboptimal outcomes [100]. CT scan may be especially useful in cases of diagnostic dilemma, though in retrospect, the diagnosis is frequently evident on prior imaging [101].

Summary of the preoperative diagnostic workup:

The evidence for various approaches to the preoperative workup for GERD and hiatal hernia has been provided above. However, this chapter also aims to include the personal approach and opinions of the author, who utilizes a standard approach to the assessment of these patients.

All patients being assessed by this author for this type of surgery will have:

1. Contrast video esophagram; to assess esophageal anatomy, length of the esophagus, the presence of any proximal pathology such as a proximal diverticulum and to assess contrast flow into the stomach
2. Esophagogastroduodenoscopy; to assess for mucosal disease, esophagitis, strictures, Barrett's metaplasia or alternative diagnosis
3. Esophageal physiology studies (high resolution esophageal manometry and ambulatory pH study); to confirm the diagnosis of reflux, to assess esophageal motility (which may aid in the postoperative treatment of dysphagia) and to estimate esophageal length (to allow for planning of intraoperative treatment for short-esophagus, if present).
4. Physiological assessment of fitness for surgery and anesthesia

What Is the Current Knowledge and What Future Direction Is Required

- GERD is a very common problem affecting up to 20% of the population of the Western World. Preoperative workup aims to provide objective evidence for reflux. If present, antireflux surgery is a well-proven and effective treatment, particularly for the management of 'typical' reflux symptoms. 'Atypical' symptoms are more difficult to treat and increasing importance is placed on impedance assessment and other alternative diagnostic tools. Prediction of response to antireflux surgery of atypical symptoms is currently difficult and remains an area of future investigation.
- Hiatal hernia treatment overlaps with that of the treatment of GERD. GERD is associated with many smaller Type I hiatal hernias; therapy is directed towards treatment of the GERD symptoms rather than the hernia per se. For larger hiatal hernias, often termed paraesophageal hernias, heartburn and regurgitation are only two of a common constellation of symptoms. Indications for surgery include treatment of these reflux symptoms but also of obstructive symptoms and to prevent emergent presentations. Preoperative assessment is directed to determining the presence of the hiatal hernia, confirming it as the cause of the patient's symptoms and assessing fitness for surgery. Where large asympatomatic hernias exist, particulary in the elderly, optimal management is less certain and controversy exists about whether suergery is indicated solely to prevent future complications.

References

1. Fedorak RN, Veldhuyzen van Zanten S, Bridges R. Canadian Digestive Health Foundation Public Impact Series: gastroesophageal reflux disease in Canada: incidence, prevalence, and direct and indirect economic impact. Can J Gastroenterol. 2010;24:431–4.
2. Locke GR III, Talley NJ, Fett SL, Zinsmeister AR, Melton LJ III. Prevalence and clinical spectrum of gastroesophageal reflux: a population-based study in Olmsted County, Minnesota. Gastroenterology. 1997;112:1448–56.
3. Mohammed I, Cherkas LF, Riley SA, Spector TD, Trudgill NJ. Genetic influences in gastro-oesophageal reflux disease: a twin study. Gut. 2003;52:1085–9.
4. Isolauri J, Laippala P. Prevalence of symptoms suggestive of gastro-oesophageal reflux disease in an adult population. Ann Med. 1995;27:67–70.
5. Knox SA, Harrison CM, Britt HC, Henderson JV. Estimating prevalence of common chronic morbidities in Australia. Med J Aust. 2008;189:66–70.
6. Kahrilas PJ, Shaheen NJ, Vaezi MF, et al. American Gastroenterological Association Medical Position Statement on the management of gastroesophageal reflux disease. Gastroenterology. 2008;135:1383–91. 91 e1-5.
7. Vakil N, van Zanten SV, Kahrilas P, Dent J, Jones R, Global Consensus G. The Montreal definition and classification of gastroesophageal reflux disease: a global evidence-based consensus. Am J Gastroenterol. 2006;101:1900–20. quiz 43.
8. Stefanidis D, Hope WW, Kohn GP, et al. Guidelines for surgical treatment of gastroesophageal reflux disease. Surg Endosc. 2010;24:2647–69.
9. Lundell LR, Dent J, Bennett JR, et al. Endoscopic assessment of oesophagitis: clinical and functional correlates and further validation of the Los Angeles classification. Gut. 1999;45:172–80.
10. Dent J. Endoscopic grading of reflux oesophagitis: the past, present and future. Best Pract Res Clin Gastroenterol. 2008;22:585–99.
11. Armstrong D, Bennett JR, Blum AL, et al. The endoscopic assessment of esophagitis: a progress report on observer agreement. Gastroenterology. 1996;111:85–92.
12. Lowes H, Somarathna T, Shepherd NA. Definition, derivation, and diagnosis of Barrett's esophagus: pathological perspectives. Adv Exp Med Biol. 2016;908:111–36.
13. Orlando RC. Pathogenesis of reflux esophagitis and Barrett's esophagus. Med Clin North Am. 2005;89:219–41. vii.
14. Bremner CG, Lynch VP, Ellis FH Jr. Barrett's esophagus: congenital or acquired? An experimental study of esophageal mucosal regeneration in the dog. Surgery. 1970;68:209–16.
15. Chen MY, Ott DJ, Sinclair JW, Wu WC, Gelfand DW. Gastroesophageal reflux disease: correlation of esophageal pH testing and radiographic findings. Radiology. 1992;185:483–6.
16. Thompson JK, Koehler RE, Richter JE. Detection of gastroesophageal reflux: value of barium studies compared with 24-hr pH monitoring. AJR Am J Roentgenol. 1994;162:621–6.
17. Bombeck CT, Helfrich GB, Nyhus LM. Planning surgery for reflux esophagitis and hiatus hernia. Surg Clin North Am. 1970;50:29–44.
18. Mattox HE III, Richter JE. Prolonged ambulatory esophageal pH monitoring in the evaluation of gastroesophageal reflux disease. Am J Med. 1990;89:345–56.
19. Pope CE II. Pathophysiology and diagnosis of reflux esophagitis. Gastroenterology. 1976;70:445–54.
20. Wiener GJ, Morgan TM, Copper JB, et al. Ambulatory 24-hour esophageal pH monitoring. Reproducibility and variability of pH parameters. Dig Dis Sci. 1988;33:1127–33.
21. Kohn GP. pH and impedance evaluation of the esophagus. In: Yeo CJ, editor. Shackelford's surgery of the alimentary tract. 8th ed. Philadelphia, PA: Elsevier; in press.
22. Hirano I, Richter JE, Practice Parameters Committee of the American College of G. ACG practice guidelines: esophageal reflux testing. Am J Gastroenterol. 2007;102:668–85.
23. Ter RB, Johnston BT, Castell DO. Exclusion of the meal period improves the clinical reliability of esophageal pH monitoring. J Clin Gastroenterol. 1997;25:314–6.

24. Arora AS, Murray JA. Streamlining 24-hour pH study for GERD: use of a 3-hour postprandial test. Dig Dis Sci. 2003;48:10–5.
25. Wong WM, Bautista J, Dekel R, et al. Feasibility and tolerability of transnasal/per-oral placement of the wireless pH capsule vs. traditional 24-h oesophageal pH monitoring--a randomized trial. Aliment Pharmacol Ther. 2005;21:155–63.
26. Pandolfino JE, Richter JE, Ours T, Guardino JM, Chapman J, Kahrilas PJ. Ambulatory esophageal pH monitoring using a wireless system. Am J Gastroenterol. 2003;98:740–9.
27. Wenner J, Johnsson F, Johansson J, Oberg S. Wireless esophageal pH monitoring is better tolerated than the catheter-based technique: results from a randomized cross-over trial. Am J Gastroenterol. 2007;102:239–45.
28. Prakash C, Clouse RE. Value of extended recording time with wireless pH monitoring in evaluating gastroesophageal reflux disease. Clin Gastroenterol Hepatol. 2005;3:329–34.
29. Ahlawat SK, Novak DJ, Williams DC, Maher KA, Barton F, Benjamin SB. Day-to-day variability in acid reflux patterns using the BRAVO pH monitoring system. J Clin Gastroenterol. 2006;40:20–4.
30. Bhat YM, McGrath KM, Bielefeldt K. Wireless esophageal pH monitoring: new technique means new questions. J Clin Gastroenterol. 2006;40:116–21.
31. Hirano I, Zhang Q, Pandolfino JE, Kahrilas PJ. Four-day Bravo pH capsule monitoring with and without proton pump inhibitor therapy. Clin Gastroenterol Hepatol. 2005;3:1083–8.
32. Anggiansah A, Sumboonnanonda K, Wang J, Linsell J, Hale P, Owen WJ. Significantly reduced acid detection at 10 centimeters compared to 5 centimeters above lower esophageal sphincter in patients with acid reflux. Am J Gastroenterol. 1993;88:842–6.
33. Wenner J, Johnsson F, Johansson J, Oberg S. Acid reflux immediately above the squamocolumnar junction and in the distal esophagus: simultaneous pH monitoring using the wireless capsule pH system. Am J Gastroenterol. 2006;101:1734–41.
34. Lee YY, Whiting JG, Robertson EV, et al. Kinetics of transient hiatus hernia during transient lower esophageal sphincter relaxations and swallows in healthy subjects. Neurogastroenterol Motil. 2012;24:990–e539.
35. Edmundowicz SA, Clouse RE. Shortening of the esophagus in response to swallowing. Am J Physiol. 1991;260:G512–6.
36. Kahrilas PJ, Quigley EM. Clinical esophageal pH recording: a technical review for practice guideline development. Gastroenterology 1996;110:1982–96.
37. Mattox HE III, Richter JE, Sinclair JW, Price JE, Case LD. Gastroesophageal pH step-up inaccurately locates proximal border of lower esophageal sphincter. Dig Dis Sci. 1992;37:1185–91.
38. Kahrilas PJ, Lin S, Chen J, Manka M. The effect of hiatus hernia on gastro-oesophageal junction pressure. Gut. 1999;44:476–82.
39. Ayazi S, Lipham JC, Portale G, et al. Bravo catheter-free pH monitoring: normal values, concordance, optimal diagnostic thresholds, and accuracy. Clin Gastroenterol Hepatol. 2009;7:60–7.
40. Tuttle SG, Rufin F, Bettarello A. The physiology of heartburn. Ann Intern Med. 1961;55:292–300.
41. Ouatu-Lascar R, Lin OS, Fitzgerald RC, Triadafilopoulos G. Upright versus supine reflux in gastroesophageal reflux disease. J Gastroenterol Hepatol. 2001;16:1184–90.
42. Campos GM, Peters JH, DeMeester TR, Oberg S, Crookes PF, Mason RJ. The pattern of esophageal acid exposure in gastroesophageal reflux disease influences the severity of the disease. Arch Surg. 1999;134:882–7. discussion 7–8.
43. Saraswat VA, Dhiman RK, Mishra A, Naik SR. Correlation of 24-hr esophageal pH patterns with clinical features and endoscopy in gastroesophageal reflux disease. Dig Dis Sci. 1994;39:199–205.
44. Johnson LF, Demeester TR. Twenty-four-hour pH monitoring of the distal esophagus. A quantitative measure of gastroesophageal reflux. Am J Gastroenterol. 1974;62:325–32.
45. Bredenoord AJ, Weusten BL, Smout AJ. Symptom association analysis in ambulatory gastro-oesophageal reflux monitoring. Gut. 2005;54:1810–7.

46. Öberg S. Esophageal pH monitoring. In: Yeo CJ, editor. Shackelford's surgery of the alimentary tract. 7th ed. Philadelphia, PA: Saunders; 2013. p. 147–53.
47. Tutuian R, Castell DO. Gastroesophageal reflux monitoring: pH and impedance. GI Motility Online. 2006.
48. Weusten BL, Roelofs JM, Akkermans LM, Van Berge-Henegouwen GP, Smout AJ. The symptom-association probability: an improved method for symptom analysis of 24-hour esophageal pH data. Gastroenterology. 1994;107:1741–5.
49. Fackler WK, Ours TM, Vaezi MF, Richter JE. Long-term effect of H2RA therapy on nocturnal gastric acid breakthrough. Gastroenterology. 2002;122:625–32.
50. Bell NJ, Burget D, Howden CW, Wilkinson J, Hunt RH. Appropriate acid suppression for the management of gastro-oesophageal reflux disease. Digestion. 1992;51(Suppl 1):59–67.
51. Johnsson F, Joelsson B, Isberg PE. Ambulatory 24 hour intraesophageal pH-monitoring in the diagnosis of gastroesophageal reflux disease. Gut. 1987;28:1145–50.
52. Jamieson JR, Stein HJ, DeMeester TR, et al. Ambulatory 24-h esophageal pH monitoring: normal values, optimal thresholds, specificity, sensitivity, and reproducibility. Am J Gastroenterol. 1992;87:1102–11.
53. Wenner J, Johansson J, Johnsson F, Oberg S. Optimal thresholds and discriminatory power of 48-h wireless esophageal pH monitoring in the diagnosisof GERD. Am J Gastroenterol. 2007;102:1862–9.
54. Venables TL, Newland RD, Patel AC, Hole J, Wilcock C, Turbitt ML. Omeprazole 10 milligrams once daily, omeprazole 20 milligrams once daily, or ranitidine 150 milligrams twice daily, evaluated as initial therapy for the relief of symptoms of gastro-oesophageal reflux disease in general practice. Scand J Gastroenterol. 1997;32:965–73.
55. Cherry J, Margulies SI. Contact ulcer of the larynx. Laryngoscope. 1968;78:1937–40.
56. Mahieu HF. Review article: the laryngological manifestations of reflux disease; why the scepticism? Aliment Pharmacol Ther. 2007;26(Suppl 2):17–24.
57. Ayazi S, Hagen JA, Zehetner J, et al. Proximal esophageal pH monitoring: improved definition of normal values and determination of a composite pH score. J Am Coll Surg. 2010;210:345–50.
58. Chen RY, Thomas RJ. Results of laparoscopic fundoplication where atypical symptoms coexist with oesophageal reflux. Aust N Z J Surg. 2000;70:840–2.
59. Swoger J, Ponsky J, Hicks DM, et al. Surgical fundoplication in laryngopharyngeal reflux unresponsive to aggressive acid suppression: a controlled study. Clin Gastroenterol Hepatol. 2006;4:433–41.
60. Ummarino D, Vandermeulen L, Roosens B, Urbain D, Hauser B, Vandenplas Y. Gastroesophageal reflux evaluation in patients affected by chronic cough: restech versus multichannel intraluminal impedance/pH metry. Laryngoscope. 2013;123:980–4.
61. Patel DA, Harb AH, Vaezi MF. Oropharyngeal reflux monitoring and atypical gastroesophageal reflux disease. Curr Gastroenterol Rep. 2016;18:12.
62. Tutuian R, Castell DO. Multichannel intraluminal impedance. In: Yeo CJ, editor. Shackelford's surgery of the alimentary tract. 7th ed. Philadelphia, PA: Saunders; 2013. p. 154–61.
63. Mainie I, Tutuian R, Agrawal A, Adams D, Castell DO. Combined multichannel intraluminal impedance-pH monitoring to select patients with persistent gastro-oesophageal reflux for laparoscopic Nissen fundoplication. Br J Surg. 2006;93:1483–7.
64. Sifrim D, Castell D, Dent J, Kahrilas PJ. Gastro-oesophageal reflux monitoring: review and consensus report on detection and definitions of acid, non-acid, and gas reflux. Gut. 2004;53:1024–31.
65. Shay S, Tutuian R, Sifrim D, et al. Twenty-four hour ambulatory simultaneous impedance and pH monitoring: a multicenter report of normal values from 60 healthy volunteers. Am J Gastroenterol. 2004;99:1037–43.
66. Ndebia EJ, Sammon AM, Umapathy E, Iputo JE. Normal values of 24-hour ambulatory esophageal impedance-pH monitoring in a rural South African cohort of healthy participants. Dis Esophagus. 2016;29:385.

67. Xiao YL, Lin JK, Cheung TK, et al. Normal values of 24-hour combined esophageal multichannel intraluminal impedance and pH monitoring in the Chinese population. Digestion. 2009;79:109–14.
68. Zerbib F, des Varannes SB, Roman S, et al. Normal values and day-to-day variability of 24-h ambulatory oesophageal impedance-pH monitoring in a Belgian-French cohort of healthy subjects. Aliment Pharmacol Ther. 2005;22:1011–21.
69. Ribolsi M, Savarino E, De Bortoli N, et al. Reflux pattern and role of impedance-pH variables in predicting PPI response in patients with suspected GERD-related chronic cough. Aliment Pharmacol Ther. 2014;40:966–73.
70. del Genio G, Tolone S, del Genio F, et al. Prospective assessment of patient selection for antireflux surgery by combined multichannel intraluminal impedance pH monitoring. J Gastrointest Surg. 2008;12:1491–6.
71. Malhotra A, Freston JW, Aziz K. Use of pH-impedance testing to evaluate patients with suspected extraesophageal manifestations of gastroesophageal reflux disease. J Clin Gastroenterol. 2008;42:271–8.
72. Bajbouj M, Becker V, Neuber M, Schmid RM, Meining A. Combined pH-metry/impedance monitoring increases the diagnostic yield in patients with atypical gastroesophageal reflux symptoms. Digestion. 2007;76:223–8.
73. Forootan M, Ardeshiri M, Etemadi N, Maghsoodi N, Poorsaadati S. Findings of impedance pH-monitoring in patients with atypical gastroesophageal reflux symptoms. Gastroenterol Hepatol Bed Bench. 2013;6:S117–21.
74. Chakravorty P, Bashah KF, Kohn GP. PS01.054 Correlation between pH studies and esophageal impedance in the evaluation of typical GERD symptoms (poster). 15th International Society for Diseases of the Esophagus World Congress. 2016.
75. Attwood SE, Lundell L, Hatlebakk JG, et al. Medical or surgical management of GERD patients with Barrett's esophagus: the LOTUS trial 3-year experience. J Gastrointest Surg. 2008;12:1646–54. discussion 54–5.
76. Pessaux P, Arnaud JP, Delattre JF, Meyer C, Baulieux J, Mosnier H. Laparoscopic antireflux surgery: five-year results and beyond in 1340 patients. Arch Surg. 2005;140:946–51.
77. O'Boyle CJ, Watson DI, Jamieson GG, Myers JC, Game PA, Devitt PG. Division of short gastric vessels at laparoscopic nissen fundoplication: a prospective double-blind randomized trial with 5-year follow-up. Ann Surg. 2002;235:165–70.
78. Triponez F, Dumonceau JM, Azagury D, et al. Reflux, dysphagia, and gas bloat after laparoscopic fundoplication in patients with incidentally discovered hiatal hernia and in a control group. Surgery. 2005;137:235–42.
79. Brehant O, Pessaux P, Arnaud JP, et al. Long-term outcome of laparoscopic antireflux surgery in the elderly. J Gastrointest Surg. 2006;10:439–44.
80. Anvari M, Allen C. Five-year comprehensive outcomes evaluation in 181 patients after laparoscopic Nissen fundoplication. J Am Coll Surg. 2003;196:51–7. discussion 7–8; author reply 8–9.
81. Wayman J, Myers JC, Jamieson GG. Preoperative gastric emptying and patterns of reflux as predictors of outcome after laparoscopic fundoplication. Br J Surg. 2007;94:592–8.
82. Kohn GP, Price RR, Demeester SR, et al. Guidelines for the management of hiatal hernia. Surg Endosc. 2013;27:4409–28.
83. Scheffer RC, Bredenoord AJ, Hebbard GS, Smout AJ, Samsom M. Effect of proximal gastric volume on hiatal hernia. Neurogastroenterol Motil. 2010;22:552–6. e120.
84. Fornari F, Madalosso CA, Farre R, Gurski RR, Thiesen V, Callegari-Jacques SM. The role of gastro-oesophageal pressure gradient and sliding hiatal hernia on pathological gastro-oesophageal reflux in severely obese patients. Eur J Gastroenterol Hepatol. 2010;22:404–11.
85. Franzen T, Tibbling L. Is the severity of gastroesophageal reflux dependent on hiatus hernia size? World J Gastroenterol. 2014;20:1582–4.
86. Ott DJ, Glauser SJ, Ledbetter MS, Chen MY, Koufman JA, Gelfand DW. Association of hiatal hernia and gastroesophageal reflux: correlation between presence and size of hiatal hernia and 24-hour pH monitoring of the esophagus. AJR Am J Roentgenol. 1995;165:557–9.

87. Mittal SK, Awad ZT, Tasset M, et al. The preoperative predictability of the short esophagus in patients with stricture or paraesophageal hernia. Surg Endosc. 2000;14:464–8.
88. Morcos SK. Review article: effects of radiographic contrast media on the lung. Br J Radiol. 2003;76:290–5.
89. Kahrilas PJ, Kim HC, Pandolfino JE. Approaches to the diagnosis and grading of hiatal hernia. Best Pract Res Clin Gastroenterol. 2008;22:601–16.
90. Swanstrom LL, Jobe BA, Kinzie LR, Horvath KD. Esophageal motility and outcomes following laparoscopic paraesophageal hernia repair and fundoplication. Am J Surg. 1999;177:359–63.
91. Boushey RP, Moloo H, Burpee S, et al. Laparoscopic repair of paraesophageal hernias: a Canadian experience. Can J Surg. 2008;51:355–60.
92. Nagpal AP, Soni H, Haribhakti S. Is oesophageal manometry a must before laparoscopic fundoplication? Analysis of 46 consecutive patients treated without preoperative manometry. J Minim Access Surg. 2010;6:66–9.
93. Roman S, Kahrilas PJ, Kia L, Luger D, Soper N, Pandolfino JE. Effects of large hiatal hernias on esophageal peristalsis. Arch Surg. 2012;147:352–7.
94. Ye P, Li ZS, Xu GM, Zou DW, Xu XR, Lu RH. Esophageal motility in patients with sliding hiatal hernia with reflux esophagitis. Chin Med J (Engl). 2008;121:898–903.
95. Shih WJ, Milan PP. Gastric-emptying scintigraphy of type III hiatal hernia: a case report. J Nucl Med Technol. 2005;33:83–5.
96. Khouzam RN, Akhtar A, Minderman D, Kaiser J, D'Cruz IA. Echocardiographic aspects of hiatal hernia: a review. J Clin Ultrasound. 2007;35:196–203.
97. Naoum C, Falk GL, Ng AC, et al. Left atrial compression and the mechanism of exercise impairment in patients with a large hiatal hernia. J Am Coll Cardiol. 2011;58:1624–34.
98. Fornari F, Gurski RR, Navarini D, Thiesen V, Mestriner LH, Madalosso CA. Clinical utility of endoscopy and barium swallow X-ray in the diagnosis of sliding hiatal hernia in morbidly obese patients: a study before and after gastric bypass. Obes Surg. 2010;20:702–8.
99. Gourgiotis S, Vougas V, Germanos S, Baratsis S. Acute gastric volvulus: diagnosis and management over 10 years. Dig Surg. 2006;23:169–72.
100. Shafii AE, Agle SC, Zervos EE. Perforated gastric corpus in a strangulated paraesophageal hernia: a case report. J Med Case Reports. 2009;3:6507.
101. Chang CC, Tseng CL, Chang YC. A surgical emergency due to an incarcerated paraesophageal hernia. Am J Emerg Med. 2009;27:134.e1–3.

Chapter 5
Indications and Procedures for Surgical Therapy of GERD with Hiatal Hernia

Monica T. Young and Brant K. Oelschlager

5.1 Introduction

Gastroesophageal reflux disease (GERD) is defined as a condition of symptoms or complications occurring secondary to reflux from the stomach into the distal esophagus. Hiatal hernias are frequently an incidental finding during work-up of symptomatic reflux. While asymptomatic hiatal hernias do not inherently require surgical repair, the exception is when this diagnosis is found in association with pathologic reflux. In this chapter we will review the work-up of symptomatic GERD, indications for laparoscopic antireflux surgery (LARS) with hiatal hernia repair, and fundoplication options.

5.2 Pathophysiology of GERD

Gastroesophageal reflux occurs during exposure of the esophageal epithelium to gastric secretions. A certain degree of esophageal acid exposure is considered physiologic, resulting from transient relaxation of the lower esophageal sphincter (LES) complex. GERD arises when the esophageal acid exposure exceeds the normal frequency and length of time seen in healthy individuals. This may result in typical and atypical symptoms of GERD as well as mucosal damage to the esophagus. The main anatomic barrier to GER is the LES, which is made up of several anatomic things including: intrinsic smooth muscle of the gastroesophageal (GE) junction, the intraabdominal segment of esophagus, the diaphragmatic crura, the phreno-esophageal membrane and the angle of His. Of these, the intrinsic muscle is the primary structure to prevent reflux of gastric contents into the esophagus. It is a

M.T. Young, M.D. • B.K. Oelschlager, M.D. (✉)
Division of General Surgery, Department of Surgery, UW Medical Center,
University of Washington, 1959 NE Pacific St., Box 356410, Seattle, WA 98195, USA
e-mail: Brant@uw.edu

M.A. Memon (ed.), *Hiatal Hernia Surgery*,
https://doi.org/10.1007/978-3-319-64003-7_5

3–4 cm zone of high pressure that separates two adjacent lower-pressure zones. The LES is constructed of smooth muscle which is tonically contracted except when it relaxes in response to a peristaltic wave. Resting LES tone ranges from 10 to 30 mmHg above intragastric pressure [1].

Pathologic reflux occurs when intragastric pressure rises above the high-pressure zone of the LES. This can develop from abnormal LES relaxation (spontaneous or nonfunctional) and when the baseline LES resting pressure is low, described as a hypotensive LES. Hiatal hernias are often associated with a hypotensive LES due to displacement of the sphincter above the crura of the diaphragm. This results in symptoms of GERD, which frequently prompts the initial workup leading to diagnosis of the hiatal hernia.

5.3 Clinical Presentation

Clinical manifestations of GERD can be categorized into typical or atypical symptoms (Table 5.1). The most common presenting symptoms are heartburn and regurgitation. Other typical symptoms include water brash, chest pain and dysphagia. Heartburn is described as an epigastric or retrosternal burning sensation and is considered specific to GERD. Regurgitation in the setting of reflux is described as digested food coming up from the stomach along with gastric secretions. The presence of gastric acid in the oropharynx can result in a sour or bile taste in the back of the throat, referred to as water brash.

5.3.1 Atypical Symptoms

Atypical or extraesophageal symptoms of GERD arise from the respiratory tract and are most commonly thought to be caused by microaspiration of gastric contents. They can be divided into laryngeal symptoms such as hoarseness, throat pain and Globus sensation; and pulmonary symptoms including cough, shortness of breath and asthma (either with or without associated chronic lung injury). Although aspiration is the most likely route of injury, distal esophageal acid exposure may activate the vagus nerve. Due to common innervation of the trachea and esophagus, this may

Table 5.1 Typical and atypical symptoms of GERD

Typical	Atypical
Heartburn	Hoarseness
Regurgitation	Throat pain
Chest pain	Globus sensation
Water brash	Cough
Dysphagia	Shortness of breath
Belching	Asthma
Bloating	

result in bronchospasm and cough. Atypical symptoms are much more difficult to elicit an etiology for as they can also occur from respiratory or pulmonary causes. Furthermore, extraesophageal GERD symptoms less commonly resolve with proton pump inhibitor (PPI) therapy. This is attributed to persistent microaspiration causing ongoing injury, even when acid production is suppressed by medical therapy [2]. When patients present with extraesophageal symptoms and GER, it is our practice to refer patients for evaluation by a laryngologist or pulmonologist. If a nongastrointestinal cause cannot be identified it is appropriate to proceed with LARS.

5.3.2 *Dysphagia*

Patients referred for surgical evaluation will occasionally experience dysphagia related to their GERD. In this patient population, the most common cause is esophageal mucosal inflammation and damage. The inflammatory changes can manifest as diffuse esophageal inflammation, a Schatzki ring or a peptic stricture. Although the incidence of peptic strictures has significantly decreased in the age of PPI therapy, they are considered pathognomonic for long-standing reflux. If found on upper endoscopy, peptic strictures should always be biopsied to rule out intestinal metaplasia, dysplasia or malignancy. Similarly to peptic strictures, Schatzki rings also arise in the distal esophagus. They can be differentiated on endoscopy by the appearance of submucosal fibrotic bands as opposed to the mucosal scarring seen in peptic stricture disease. Both should be dilated to relieve obstruction but Schatzki rings do not need to be biopsied unless there is a visible mucosal abnormality. Some patients with dysphagia in the setting of GERD have no identifiable anatomic etiology. In these cases the dysphagia usually resolves with control of reflux. Patients who present with sudden dysphagia to solids and liquids without anatomic abnormalities should be evaluated for neuromuscular or autoimmune disorders.

5.4 Preoperative Work-Up

Many patients present for surgical evaluation with a longstanding diagnosis of GERD based on typical symptoms and response to PPI therapy. However, there are four key diagnostic tests to help establish a diagnosis of GERD as well as evaluate gastroesophageal anatomy and function. These tests can help guide surgeon decision making and predict the success of an antireflux operation.

5.4.1 *pH Monitoring*

The gold standard test to diagnosis GERD is a 24-hour ambulatory pH study. This is performed using a thin nasoesophageal catheter. The catheter is positioned with the distal probe approximately 5 cm above the LES, whose location is determined using

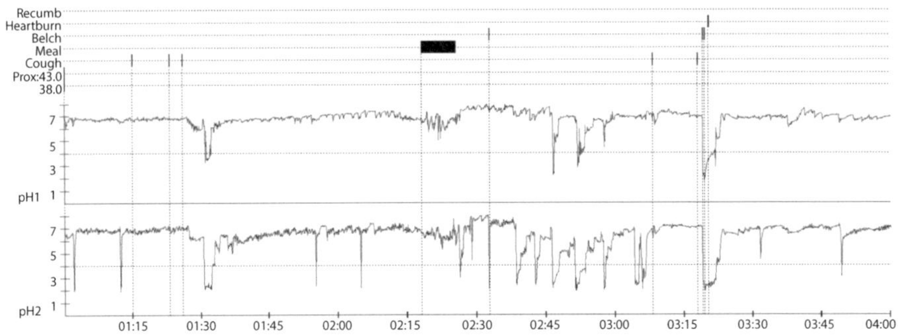

Fig. 5.1 Sample pH study tracing demonstrating episodes of reflux when pH drops below 4, indicated by *dotted line*

esophageal manometry. Another option for assessment is ambulatory pH monitoring performed using an endoscopically placed wireless pH sensor. Both studies record data on the duration and number of acid episodes (defined as pH < 4), including the number of episodes lasting longer than 5 min and the percentage of time spent in reflux during upright and supine position (Fig. 5.1). Based on these results a composite DeMeester score may be calculated. Abnormal distal esophageal acid exposure is defined as >4–5% of time spent with pH < 4 or a DeMeester score of 14.7 or higher. Symptom correlation is also recorded by having the patient press a button to track reflux-related symptoms. If >50% of episodes correlate with patient symptoms then drops in pH are considered positive. A strong correlation with symptoms can occasionally be helpful in equivocal cases. It is important to note that patients sometimes modify their behavior and eating patterns when the catheter is in place. Therefore, a comprehensive interpretation of the study is necessary to help predict the effectiveness of LARS.

5.4.2 *Esophageal Manometry*

Esophageal manometry should be performed on all patients being evaluated for LARS. High resolution esophageal manometry has become increasingly prevalent and has improved the sensitivity and specificity of testing. A transnasal catheter with pressure-sensing devices is passed down the esophagus and into the stomach. The patient performs 10 swallows which are displayed as a color-contour plot based on pressure recordings (Fig. 5.2). This study assesses function of the esophageal body by measuring amplitude and efficacy of swallow-induced peristalsis. The length, location and pressure of the LES is evaluated along with sphincter relaxation during swallowing. Manometry can identify esophageal motility disorders and therefore identify patients who may be at higher risk for postoperative dysphagia. It can also help screen patients with atypical symptoms who may have an underlying primary motility abnormality, such as achalasia or scleroderma.

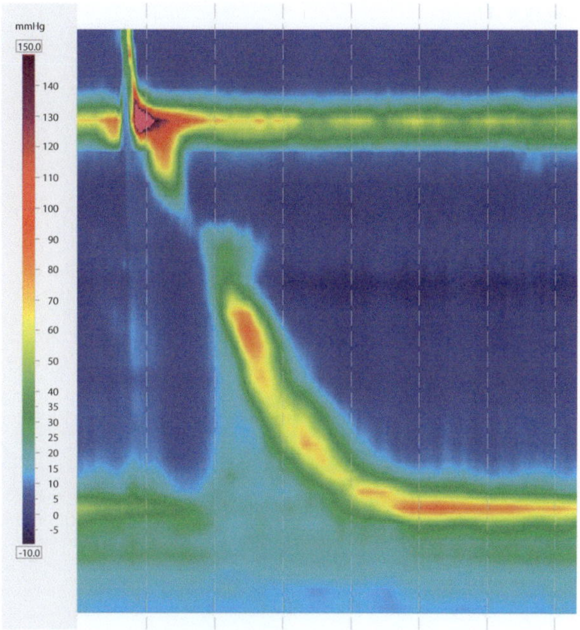

Fig. 5.2 High-resolution manometry tracing demonstrating normal swallow, peristalsis and lower esophageal sphincter relaxation

5.4.3 Esophagogastroduodenoscopy

Preoperative endoscopy is necessary to evaluate the esophageal mucosa, the GE junction flap valve and check for the presence of a hiatal hernia. If the patient has esophageal complications of GERD (e.g. esophagitis, ulcerations, peptic stricture or Barrett's esophagus), ambulatory pH testing might not be required. Patients with atypical symptoms such as dysphagia should be evaluated for additional anatomic abnormalities. Depending on the findings, biopsies can be taken or strictures can be dilated, making upper endoscopy diagnostic as well as therapeutic.

5.4.4 Barium Esophagram

Contrast radiographs of the upper gastrointestinal tract help delineate anatomy and identify the presence of a hiatal hernia or paraesophageal hernia (PEH) (Fig. 5.3). A large PEH or shortened esophagus can add to the complexity of the operation and should be identified preoperatively. Although sometimes the radiologist will comment on reflux of contrast into the distal esophagus, barium esophagram is not a reliable way to diagnose GERD. If the anatomy and function of the esophagus is clear with EGD, manometry and pH monitoring, then one can consider dropping the UGI. However, many other pathologies can be identified such as esophageal diverticula, peptic strictures, achalasia, esophageal dysmotility, gastroparesis and malignancy.

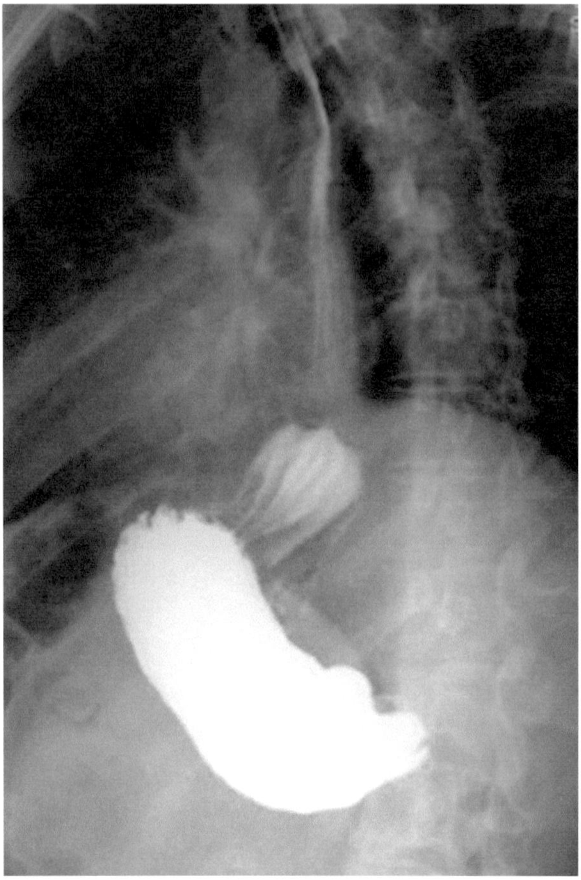

Fig. 5.3 Upper gastrointestinal series X-ray showing hiatal hernia with stomach above the level of the diaphragm

5.4.5 Impedance Testing

Esophageal impedance testing is a technique for assessing episodes of nonacid reflux. Similarly to pH monitoring, this outpatient study is performed using a thin, flexible catheter placed through the nares into the esophagus. Impedance catheters detect changes in resistance based on the flow of an electrical current. By recording different levels of impedance the catheter can help analyze movement of gas and liquid in the esophagus [3]. Combined impedance-pH testing has been reported to be more sensitive than pH testing alone. However, these tests require a lot of education and human oversight, and often contradict the gold standard pH monitoring. Therefore, a normal impedance study portion and normal pH portion should be treated with caution. As such, more research is needed to determine the role of impedance in guiding surgical therapies for GERD [4, 5].

5.5 Additional Preoperative Considerations

5.5.1 Obesity

There are several additional factors which should be considered prior to LARS. Obese patients have been shown to have a high failure rate with hiatal hernia repair and fundoplication [6–8]. For morbidly obese patients (Body mass index >40) we typically consider Roux-en-Y gastric bypass as an alternative antireflux operation [9]. Gastric bypass can aid in weight loss and reverse medical comorbidities while also eliminating acid exposure in the distal esophagus. Other preoperative considerations include patients with severe cardiopulmonary disease who may not tolerate general anesthesia or pneumoperitoneum. Previous operations on the stomach may make dissection at the hiatus more difficult or preclude construction of the fundoplication.

5.5.2 Partial Versus Complete Fundoplication

There has been a long history of controversy over the optimal fundoplication to provide superior treatment of reflux while mitigating postoperative side effects of dysphagia and gas-bloat. The most commonly seen options include 180-degree anterior (Dor fundoplication), 270-degree posterior (Toupet fundoplication) and 360-degree esophagogastric fundoplication (Nissen fundoplication).

The anterior Dor fundoplication has generally been found to be less effective for reflux control, with more patients requiring reoperations for symptomatic GERD [10–13]. However, debate remains on differences in outcomes between Toupet and Nissen fundoplications. Short-term data appears to favor partial fundoplication with fewer side effects and similar control of reflux compared to complete fundoplication [10, 14–21]. In 2010 Shan and colleagues reviewed 32 studies, including nine randomized controlled trials, comparing laparoscopic Nissen fundoplication with laparoscopic Toupet fundoplication. In patients with normal esophageal motility, no difference in postoperative dysphagia was found between groups. In patients with abnormal esophageal motility, laparoscopic Nissen fundoplication was found to be associated with higher rates of dysphagia. The study also found increased rates of postoperative gas-bloat and inability to belch in patients who underwent Nissen fundoplication. The authors concluded that laparoscopic Toupet fundoplication offers equivalent symptom relief with reduced adverse results compared to laparoscopic Nissen fundoplication [22].

However, long-term outcomes have trended in favor of the Nissen, with similar rates of dysphagia and some studies showing re-emergence of symptoms after partial fundoplication [23–25]. A very recent meta-analysis published by Du et al. reviewed eight randomized controlled trials comparing laparoscopic Nissen fundoplication and laparoscopic Toupet fundoplication [26]. There were no significant differences found with regard to hospital length of stay, perioperative complications, patient satisfaction or control of reflux symptoms. Although postoperative dysphagia was noted to be more prevalent after Nissen fundoplication, subgroup analysis showed that the difference between groups disappeared over time. A comparative outcome study of 161 patients undergoing partial and complete fundoplications showed a significantly increased prevalence of heartburn after laparoscopic Toupet fundoplication [25]. Quality of life results were collected using patient questionnaire with a mean follow-up of 88 months.

Multiple studies have also attempted to determine whether the type of fundoplication constructed should be tailored based on the patient's preoperative esophageal motility [27–29]. In patients with GERD and esophageal dysmotility it has been reasoned that a complete fundoplication will lead to greater postoperative dysphagia. Booth et al. performed a randomized controlled trial comparing outcomes of Nissen and Toupet fundoplication based on preoperative esophageal manometry [30]. Patients were stratified based on effective and ineffective esophageal motility. While there were no differences between groups for heartburn and regurgitation, dysphagia was more frequent after Nissen fundoplication at 1 year follow-up. However there was no difference seen in postoperative symptoms between the effective and ineffective motility groups. Based on these findings, the authors did not recommend tailoring the type of fundoplication based on preoperative manometry results. In our experience, performing a complete fundoplication in patients with esophageal dysmotility provides effective control of GERD symptoms without an increase in the development of dysphagia [31]. We utilize a partial fundoplication only in those patients with aperistalsis or severe ineffective esophageal motility.

Despite a large volume of literature, there is still no consensus regarding the fundoplication which provides maximal reflux control with the least side-effects. This is attributed to highly variable patient characteristics, patient selection and operative technique between studies. Based on current evidence, the Society of American Gastrointestinal and Endoscopic Surgeons guidelines for treatment of GERD do not currently recommend a modified approach based on esophageal motility [32]. Surgeons should perform the fundoplication that they are most comfortable with until further consensus has been achieved.

5.5.3 Barrett's Esophagus

Chronic distal esophageal exposure to acid reflux can lead to histologic change of the distal esophageal mucosa from stratified squamous epithelium to intestinal columnar epithelium. Biopsy results will show intestinal metaplasia, known as Barrett's esophagus. Endoscopically Barrett's is described as red "tongues" of mucosa extending proximally from the GE junction. If Barrett's esophagus is suspected, biopsies should be taken to establish the diagnosis as well as evaluation for the presence of dysplasia or malignancy. The incidence of esophageal adenocarcinoma is increased by about 40-fold in these patients compared to the general population. Although intestinal metaplasia in the distal esophagus is a complication of long term GERD, the presence of Barrett's itself is not an indication for surgery. Some evidence suggests that LARS may cause regression of intestinal metaplasia, however current studies are not conclusive [33–35]. For patients with Barrett's esophagus without GER symptoms there is no evidence that anti-reflux surgery will decrease patient risk of esophageal adenocarcinoma [36, 37].

5.6 Surgical Management

Surgical therapy should be considered in patients who have an objective diagnosis of GERD based on preoperative testing and inadequate symptom and disease control despite maximal medical therapy. Other indications include patients with extra-esophageal manifestations or complications of GERD such as peptic stricture, esophageal ulcerations, or recurrent aspiration [38–42]. Occasionally patients will have adequate symptoms control with medical management but request surgery to avoid prescriptions or medication side effects.

5.7 Operative Technique

We routinely administer preoperative antibiotics to reduce the risk of surgical site infection and preoperative subcutaneous heparin to reduce risk of venous thromboembolic events. Sequential compression devices are placed prior to induction. After initiation of general anesthesia, a Foley is inserted and the patient is placed in a modified low lithotomy position with all extremities well padded. The surgeon stands between the patient legs to obtain optimal ergonomics and the assistant stands at the patient's left. Steep reverse Trendelenburg is utilized to facilitate exposure of the hiatus and displace the abdominal viscera inferiorly. An 11 mm incision is made at the left costal margin lateral to the mid-clavicular line. A Veress needle is inserted and used to establish pneumoperitoneum. The abdomen is entered under visualization with a bladed optical access port. Three additional 5 mm ports are then placed (Fig. 5.4). The camera port is placed 2 cm to the left of the midline and 10 cm below the costal margin. The assistant drives camera and operates through the left inferior port. The primary surgeon operates through the left upper quadrant and left subcostal port. A Nathanson liver retractor is placed through a small subxyphoid incision.

Our dissection is first begun at the left crus by dividing the phrenogastric membrane. The lesser sac is entered at the inferior edge of the spleen and the short gastric vessels are ligated and divided to mobilize the gastric fundus. This is carried superiorly until the previously dissected left crus is encountered. After the fundus is mobilized to expose the left crus, the phrenoesophageal membrane is incised. The mediastinum is carefully entered through the phrenoesophageal membrane between the left crus and

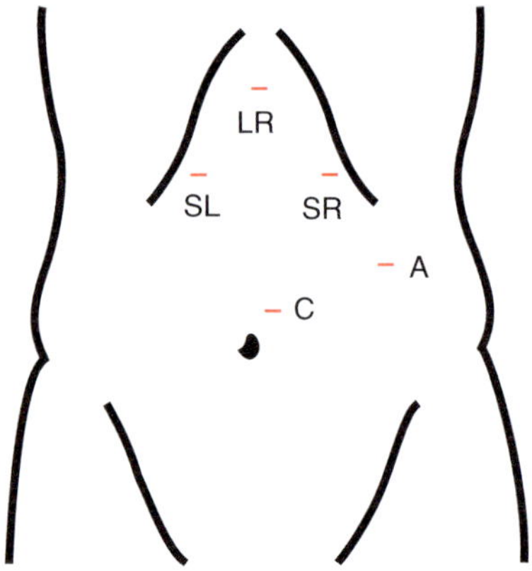

Fig. 5.4 Port placement for laparoscopic foregut surgery with patient in split-leg position. *C* camera port, *A* assistant port, *SR* surgeon right hand, *SL* surgeon left hand, *LR* liver retractor

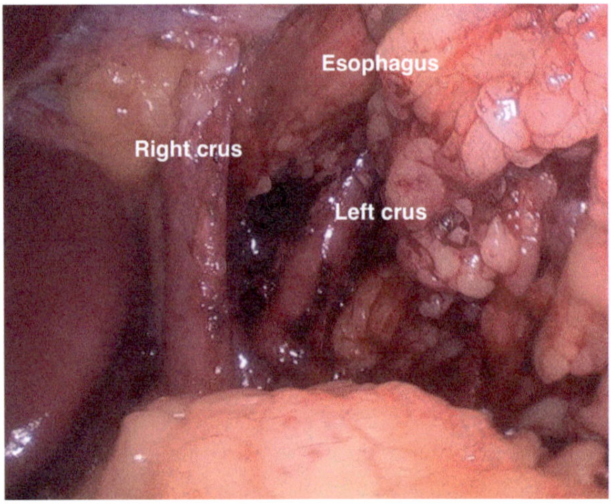

Fig. 5.5 Intraoperative anatomy visualizing the hiatus, esophagus, right and left crus

esophagus. The dissection is continued superiorly as well as anteriorly by dividing the peritoneum overlying the anterior crus. The gastrohepatic ligament is then divided to the level of the right crus. The right phrenoesophageal membrane is divided and right crural dissection is performed in a similar fashion to the left side (Fig. 5.5). A retroesophageal window is created and a penrose drain is placed around the esophagus. This is used to safely retract the esophagus during the mediastinal dissection and creation of the fundoplication. The esophagus is mobilized until at least 3 cm of intra-abdominal esophagus is achieved. During this dissection, care must be taken to preserve the anterior and posterior vagal nerves. The hiatus is closed posteriorly using permanent interrupted sutures and approximated to allow a 52-French bougie (Fig. 5.6). The crural fascia is incorporated into the closure rather than the muscle fibers alone. Closure begins posteriorly where the left and right crura join and then proceeds anteriorly. The esophagus should maintain straight orientation without excessive angulation and the bougie should pass easily. The repaired hiatus should allow passage of a closed laparoscopic instrument between the esophagus and crura.

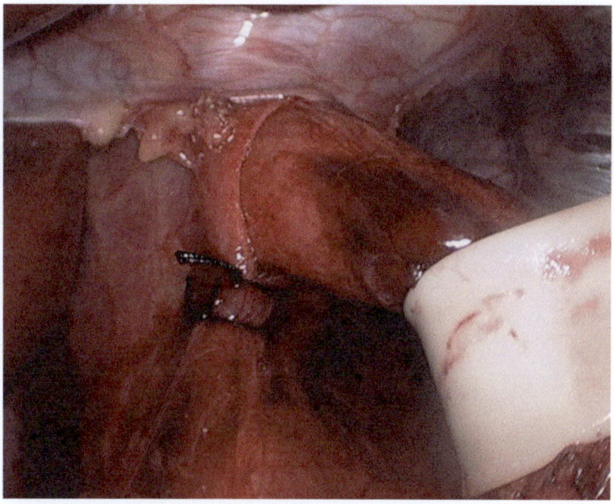

Fig. 5.6 Closure of the diaphragmatic hiatus with interrupted sutures

5.7.1 Creation of a Nissen Fundoplication

The Nissen fundoplication is the most commonly performed fundoplication worldwide [43]. It augments the intrinsic function of the LES by increasing resting pressure and decreasing transient relaxation, as well as by recreating the angle of His. The most common technical failure when constructing a Nissen fundoplication is incorrect fundoplication anatomy. It is critical for proper construction of the fundoplication that the two gastric fundus flaps are symmetrically wrapped around the distal esophagus. To maintain appropriate orientation, it is our practice to place a marking suture 3 cm distal to the GE junction and 2 cm from the greater curvature on the posterior fundus. The posterior fundus is then passed through the retroesophageal window from the patients left to right side. The marking suture is used to identify the correct site. The anterior fundus to the left of the esophagus is similarly grasped 2 cm from the greater curvature and 3 cm from the GE junction. By identifying two points equidistant from the greater curvature and GE junction we decrease the chance of constructing a fundoplication using the body of the stomach. This error creates a redundant portion in the posterior wrap which can compress the esophagus and result in dysphagia. Anterior and posterior portions of the fundus are positioned on the anterior aspect of the esophagus and secured together using three or four interrupted permanent sutures (Fig. 5.7). Care is taken to avoid entrapment of the anterior vagal nerve. The fundoplication is constructed to a length of approximately 2.5–3 cm. Similar to the hiatal repair, it should allow easy passage of a 52-French bougie. To prevent herniation through the hiatus we anchor the wrap to the esophagus and diaphragm. Two coronal sutures are placed to secure the right and left gastric flaps and a single caudal suture to secure the posterior wrap. We prefer these coronal sutures to incorporating the esophagus with the fundoplication in order to reduce the chance of including the vagus nerve with the closure.

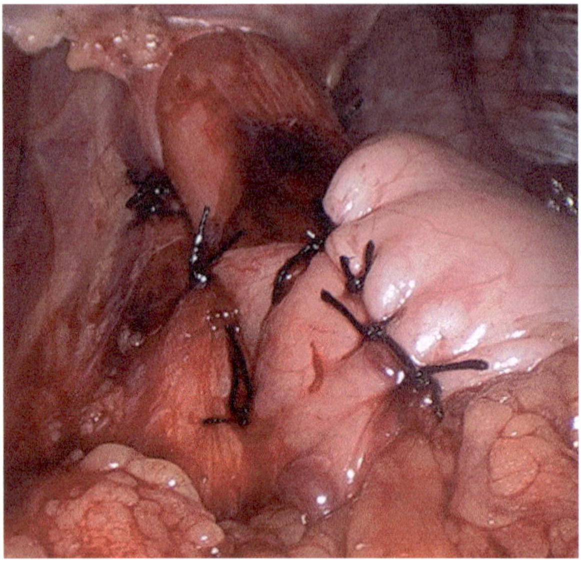

Fig. 5.7 Intraoperative view of 360-degree fundoplication

5.7.2 Creation of a Partial Fundoplication

The initial gastric and esophageal dissection is the same prior to the construction of a Nissen and Toupet however in a 270-degree fundoplication the gastric flaps are sutured to the anterior esophagus rather than to each other. To construct an anterior 180-degree Dor fundoplication the fundus is folded over the anterior aspect of the esophagus and anchored to the hiatus and esophagus. Anatomically the Dor fundoplication does not augment the LES or angle of His to the same degree and therefore is rarely used as a primary anti-reflux procedure. The Hill fundoplication has been traditionally referred to as a "cardioplasty" and involves suturing the GE junction intraabdominally at the level of the hiatus [43, 44].

5.7.3 Assessment of Esophageal Length

If a hiatal hernia is present, adequate mobilization of the hernia contents is essential to prevent recurrence and achieve a successful repair. This topic will be addressed more extensively in other chapters on PEH repair, however it is important to reiterate the importance of adequate intra-abdominal esophageal length prior to fundoplication. As the GE junction is displaced superiorly above the hiatus, the thoracic distance traversed by the esophagus shortens. Intrinsic shortening of the esophagus is also believed to occur from the chronic inflammation associated with GERD. Longitudinal as well as circumferential fibrosis manifested as stricture formation may potentiate this decreasing length [45]. While the incidence of a truly shortened esophagus is unknown, in the literature it has been reported to occur in 0–60% of patients [46–48]. A recent study published last year by Magaczewski et al. found no cases of shortened esophagus in their review of 202 patients undergoing laparoscopic Nissen fundoplication, 30 of which were reported to have a concurrent hiatal hernia [49]. Similarly, Madel et al. reported his outcomes of 628 fundoplications, with 351 requiring hiatal hernia repair and no esophageal lengthening procedures [50]. At our institution we have found that with adequate mobilization of the mediastinal esophagus the required 3 cm of intra-abdominal esophagus can almost always been obtained. In rare cases when esophageal length still is not adequate a vagotomy can yield an additional 2–3 cm of intra-abdominal esophagus. While vagotomy has been associated with delayed gastric emptying, diarrhea and dumping syndrome, we have not found this to be true in most cases. In our review of 102 patients undergoing reoperative antireflux surgery or PEH repair, 30 patients (29%) required a vagotomy to gain additional esophageal length. There was no difference found in severity of abdominal pain, bloating, diarrhea or early satiety between patients requiring vagotomy and those with vagi left intact [51, 52]. If intra-abdominal length cannot be obtained with these techniques a Collis gastroplasty or wedge gastroplasty is usually performed.

5.8 Postoperative Care

After the operation patients are admitted to the general surgical ward, unless their comorbidities require a higher level of care. Patients are given a clear liquid diet in the evening on postoperative day 0 and advanced to a full liquid diet on postoperative day 1. They are discharged home once tolerating a liquid diet and ambulating with good pain control on oral analgesics. Patients are given instructions on how to slowly introduce soft foods into their diet and generally have no dietary restrictions by 4–6 weeks.

5.9 Operative Complications and Side Effects

LARS has been found to have very low rates of perioperative morbidity and mortality [53]. According to a review of over 7500 laparoscopic fundoplication patients using the American College of Surgeons National Surgical Quality Improvement Program database 30-day mortality was found to be 0.19% and 30-day morbidity was 3.8% [53]. Minor causes of morbidity include ileus, urinary retention and wound infection. Although major complications are rare, it is important to mention pneumothorax, gastric or esophageal injuries and splenic injuries as intraoperative pitfalls specific to LARS. Perioperative complications requiring reoperation occur in <1% of patients. Common postoperative complaints include dysphagia, bloating, increased flatulence and inability to belch.

5.9.1 Pneumothorax

Intraoperative pneumothorax is one of the most common complications to occur during LARS. Violation of the pleura is usually identified by visualization of the thoracic cavity. Incidence has been described in up to 10% of patients [52]. Occasionally the pneumothorax will be discovered after a change in hemodynamics such as increased peak pressures on the ventilator or decreased blood pressure. Once identified, the pleura should be sutured closed. The carbon dioxide insufflation will then absorb rapidly in the pleural cavity, allowing the lung to re-expand. Since a small residual pneumothorax should be self-limiting, we do not routinely order a postoperative radiograph unless the patient is symptomatic. Tube thoracostomy placement is very rarely required.

5.9.2 Gastric and Esophageal Injuries

Gastric and esophageal injuries typically occur from traction injury or overaggressive manipulation during mediastinal dissection [54, 55]. Occasionally they can also be caused during advancement of the Bougie into the stomach. Reported incidence varies in the literature but in a retrospective study of 1340 patients undergoing laparoscopic fundoplication, Pessax and colleagues found 0.4% of patients had a gastric or esophageal perforation [56]. Risk of this complication is increased in reoperative cases when the anatomy is difficult to delineate and scar tissue is adherent to the esophageal wall. Utilization of a Penrose drain for retraction can decrease excessive manipulation of the distal esophagus. When an injury is identified early it can be repaired with suture or stapler, depending on the location. If a leak is discovered postoperatively the patient may require drain placement or possible reoperation.

5.9.3 Splenic Injury or Bleeding

Splenic injury or bleeding most often occurs during mobilization of the fundus and ligation of the short gastric vessels. By utilizing the "left crus approach" and first dividing the phrenogastric ligament we have found that the superior dissection can be completed with good visualization of the short gastric vessels. Care must be taken to avoid excessive traction on the splenogastric ligament which can result in tearing of the splenic capsule. Partial splenic infarction can occur when ligating short gastric vessels that are the primary blood supply to the superior pole of the spleen. This is occasionally unavoidable but rarely has any clinical significance.

5.9.4 *Bloating*

Aerophagia while eating or simply swallowing can lead to gastric distension. Transient LES relaxation mediated by the vagus nerve normally allows belching to relieve this pressure. Patients who have undergone fundoplication may find that they are unable to belch due to the reconstruction of the GE junction flap valve. This can lead to increased bloating and flatulence when patients are unable to release air from the proximal gastrointestinal tract. If significant gastric distension is identified in the immediate postoperative period a nasogastric tube can be placed for temporary decompression. No other intervention is generally required and many patients find symptoms improve over time.

5.9.5 *Dysphagia*

It is common for patients to experience mild symptoms of dysphagia during the first 2–4 weeks after LARS. These symptoms generally decrease over time and early dysphagia is attributed to postoperative edema at the fundoplication and hiatus. A minority of patients will have persistent symptoms and only 1–2% should require intervention such as esophageal dilation or reoperation. If a patient cannot tolerate liquids an upper gastrointestinal series should be obtained to ensure there is no significant anatomical obstruction. If no recurrent hernia or other cause is found watchful waiting can be initiated for 3 months postoperatively. For patients with severe symptoms, or persisting symptoms of dysphagia beyond 3 months, upper endoscopy can be used for evaluation and potential dilation of the GE junction.

5.10 Conclusion

GERD is frequently associated with hiatal hernias due to displacement of the GE junction and compromise of the LES resting pressure. Patients with symptomatic reflux can benefit from LARS, with approximately 90% reporting resolution of reflux symptoms at 5 and 10-year follow-up [41, 57]. However, they should first undergo preoperative testing to confirm the diagnosis and optimize surgical therapy. It is our preference to construct a laparoscopic Nissen fundoplication as it offers optimal reflux control with minimal side effects as well as very low morbidity and mortality. With appropriate selection and surgical experience, laparoscopic antireflux surgery can provide an effective treatment for the management of GERD.

What Is the Current Knowledge and What Future Direction Is Required

- Presentation of GERD can range from typical symptoms of heartburn or regurgitation to atypical respiratory symptoms and dysphagia.
- The four key diagnostic tests to help establish a diagnosis of GERD are pH monitoring, esophageal manometry, esophagogastroduodenoscopy and barium esophagram.
- Surgical therapy should be considered in patients with an objective diagnosis of GERD and inadequate disease control despite maximal medical therapy, or complications such as esophageal stricture, ulceration or recurrent aspiration.
- When a hiatal hernia is present, adequate mobilization of the hernia contents is essential to obtain 3 cm of intra-abdominal esophageal length and prevent recurrence.
- During construction of the fundoplication, the two gastric fundus flaps must be symmetrically wrapped around the distal esophagus. Identifying two points equidistant from the greater curvature and GE junction will decrease the chance of constructing a redundant fundoplication using the body of the stomach.
- Patients should be counseled on postoperative side effects of dysphagia, bloating, increased flatulence and inability to belch.
- With appropriate patient selection and experience, laparoscopic antireflux surgery has been shown to provide effective control of reflux symptoms.
- There is still controversy regarding tailoring the fundoplication based on esophageal motility. Current guidelines do not recommend a modified approach but further research could be helpful to determine which patients may benefit from partial versus complete fundoplication.

References

1. Sabiston DC, Townsend CM. Sabiston textbook of surgery: the biological basis of modern surgical practice. 19th ed. Philadelphia, PA: Elsevier Saunders; 2012. p. xxv. 2124 p.
2. Mainie I, Tutuian R, Shay S, Vela M, Zhang X, Sifrim D, et al. Acid and non-acid reflux in patients with persistent symptoms despite acid suppressive therapy: a multicentre study using combined ambulatory impedance-pH monitoring. Gut. 2006;55(10):1398–402.
3. Bredenoord AJ, Tutuian R, Smout AJ, Castell DO. Technology review: esophageal impedance monitoring. Am J Gastroenterol. 2007;102(1):187–94.
4. Bredenoord AJ, Weusten BL, Timmer R, Conchillo JM, Smout AJ. Addition of esophageal impedance monitoring to pH monitoring increases the yield of symptom association analysis in patients off PPI therapy. Am J Gastroenterol. 2006;101(3):453–9.
5. Patel A, Sayuk GS, Gyawali CP. Parameters on esophageal pH-impedance monitoring that predict outcomes of patients with gastroesophageal reflux disease. Clin Gastroenterol Hepatol. 2015;13(5):884–91.
6. Perez AR, Moncure AC, Rattner DW. Obesity adversely affects the outcome of antireflux operations. Surg Endosc. 2001;15(9):986–9.

7. Morgenthal CB, Lin E, Shane MD, Hunter JG, Smith CD. Who will fail laparoscopic Nissen fundoplication? Preoperative prediction of long-term outcomes. Surg Endosc. 2007;21(11):1978–84.
8. Andolfi C, Vigneswaran Y, Kavitt RT, Herbella FA, Patti MG. Laparoscopic antireflux surgery: importance of patient's selection and preoperative workup. J Laparoendosc Adv Surg Tech A. 2016;27:101.
9. Duke MC, Farrell TM. Surgery for gastroesophageal reflux disease in the morbidly obese patient. J Laparoendosc Adv Surg Tech A. 2017;27:12.
10. Spence GM, Watson DI, Jamiesion GG, Lally CJ, Devitt PG. Single center prospective randomized trial of laparoscopic Nissen versus anterior 90 degrees fundoplication. J Gastrointest Surg. 2006;10(5):698–705.
11. Cai W, Watson DI, Lally CJ, Devitt PG, Game PA, Jamieson GG. Ten-year clinical outcome of a prospective randomized clinical trial of laparoscopic Nissen versus anterior 180(degrees) partial fundoplication. Br J Surg. 2008;95(12):1501–5.
12. Woodcock SA, Watson DI, Lally C, Archer S, Bessell JR, Booth M, et al. Quality of life following laparoscopic anterior 90 degrees versus Nissen fundoplication: results from a multicenter randomized trial. World J Surg. 2006;30(10):1856–63.
13. Ludemann R, Watson DI, Jamieson GG, Game PA, Devitt PG. Five-year follow-up of a randomized clinical trial of laparoscopic total versus anterior 180 degrees fundoplication. Br J Surg. 2005;92(2):240–3.
14. Varin O, Velstra B, De Sutter S, Ceelen W. Total vs partial fundoplication in the treatment of gastroesophageal reflux disease: a meta-analysis. Arch Surg. 2009;144(3):273–8.
15. Catarci M, Gentileschi P, Papi C, Carrara A, Marrese R, Gaspari AL, et al. Evidence-based appraisal of antireflux fundoplication. Ann Surg. 2004;239(3):325–37.
16. Salminen PT, Hiekkanen HI, Rantala AP, Ovaska JT. Comparison of long-term outcome of laparoscopic and conventional nissen fundoplication: a prospective randomized study with an 11-year follow-up. Ann Surg. 2007;246(2):201–6.
17. Baigrie RJ, Cullis SN, Ndhluni AJ, Cariem A. Randomized double-blind trial of laparoscopic Nissen fundoplication versus anterior partial fundoplication. Br J Surg. 2005;92(7):819–23.
18. Chrysos E, Tsiaoussis J, Zoras OJ, Athanasakis E, Mantides A, Katsamouris A, et al. Laparoscopic surgery for gastroesophageal reflux disease patients with impaired esophageal peristalsis: total or partial fundoplication? J Am Coll Surg. 2003;197(1):8–15.
19. Laws HL, Clements RH, Swillie CM. A randomized, prospective comparison of the Nissen fundoplication versus the Toupet fundoplication for gastroesophageal reflux disease. Ann Surg. 1997;225(6):647–53. discussion 54.
20. Watson DI, Jamieson GG, Lally C, Archer S, Bessell JR, Booth M, et al. Multicenter, prospective, double-blind, randomized trial of laparoscopic nissen vs anterior 90 degrees partial fundoplication. Arch Surg. 2004;139(11):1160–7.
21. Strate U, Emmermann A, Fibbe C, Layer P, Zornig C. Laparoscopic fundoplication: Nissen versus Toupet two-year outcome of a prospective randomized study of 200 patients regarding preoperative esophageal motility. Surg Endosc. 2008;22(1):21–30.
22. Shan CX, Zhang W, Zheng XM, Jiang DZ, Liu S, Qiu M. Evidence-based appraisal in laparoscopic Nissen and Toupet fundoplications for gastroesophageal reflux disease. World J Gastroenterol. 2010;16(24):3063–71.
23. Limpert PA, Naunheim KS. Partial versus complete fundoplication: is there a correct answer? Surg Clin North Am. 2005;85(3):399–410.
24. Su F, Zhang C, Ke L, Wang Z, Li Y, Li H, et al. Efficacy comparison of laparoscopic Nissen, Toupet and Dor fundoplication in the treatment of hiatal hernia complicated with gastroesophageal reflux disease. Chin J Gastrointes Surg. 2016;19(9):1014–20.
25. Sgromo B, Irvine LA, Cuschieri A, Shimi SM. Long-term comparative outcome between laparoscopic total Nissen and Toupet fundoplication: symptomatic relief, patient satisfaction and quality of life. Surg Endosc. 2008;22(4):1048–53.
26. Du X, Hu Z, Yan C, Zhang C, Wang Z, Wu J. A meta-analysis of long follow-up outcomes of laparoscopic Nissen (total) versus Toupet (270 degrees) fundoplication for gastro-esophageal reflux disease based on randomized controlled trials in adults. BMC Gastroenterol. 2016;16(1):88.

27. Hunter JG, Trus TL, Branum GD, Waring JP, Wood WC. A physiologic approach to laparoscopic fundoplication for gastroesophageal reflux disease. Ann Surg. 1996;223(6):673–85. discussion 85–7.
28. Patti MG, Arcerito M, Feo CV, De Pinto M, Tong J, Gantert W, et al. An analysis of operations for gastroesophageal reflux disease: identifying the important technical elements. Arch Surg. 1998;133(6):600–6. discussion 6–7.
29. Zornig C, Strate U, Fibbe C, Emmermann A, Layer P. Nissen vs Toupet laparoscopic fundoplication. Surg Endosc. 2002;16(5):758–66.
30. Booth MI, Stratford J, Jones L, Dehn TC. Randomized clinical trial of laparoscopic total (Nissen) versus posterior partial (Toupet) fundoplication for gastro-oesophageal reflux disease based on preoperative oesophageal manometry. Br J Surg. 2008;95(1):57–63.
31. Oleynikov D, Eubanks TR, Oelschlager BK, Pellegrini CA. Total fundoplication is the operation of choice for patients with gastroesophageal reflux and defective peristalsis. Surg Endosc. 2002;16(6):909–13.
32. Stefanidis D, Hope WW, Kohn GP, Reardon PR, Richardson WS, Fanelli RD, et al. Guidelines for surgical treatment of gastroesophageal reflux disease. Surg Endosc. 2010;24(11):2647–69.
33. Kaufman JA, Houghland JE, Quiroga E, Cahill M, Pellegrini CA, Oelschlager BK. Long-term outcomes of laparoscopic antireflux surgery for gastroesophageal reflux disease (GERD)-related airway disorder. Surg Endosc. 2006;20(12):1824–30.
34. Hofstetter WL, Peters JH, DeMeester TR, Hagen JA, DeMeester SR, Crookes PF, et al. Long-term outcome of antireflux surgery in patients with Barrett's esophagus. Ann Surg. 2001;234(4):532–8. discussion 8–9.
35. Bowers SP, Mattar SG, Smith CD, Waring JP, Hunter JG. Clinical and histologic follow-up after antireflux surgery for Barrett's esophagus. J Gastrointest Surg. 2002;6(4):532–8. discussion 9.
36. Rossi M, Barreca M, de Bortoli N, Renzi C, Santi S, Gennai A, et al. Efficacy of Nissen fundoplication versus medical therapy in the regression of low-grade dysplasia in patients with Barrett esophagus: a prospective study. Ann Surg. 2006;243(1):58–63.
37. Chang EY, Morris CD, Seltman AK, O'Rourke RW, Chan BK, Hunter JG, et al. The effect of antireflux surgery on esophageal carcinogenesis in patients with barrett esophagus: a systematic review. Ann Surg. 2007;246(1):11–21.
38. Lagergren J, Bergstrom R, Lindgren A, Nyren O. Symptomatic gastroesophageal reflux as a risk factor for esophageal adenocarcinoma. N Engl J Med. 1999;340(11):825–31.
39. Spechler SJ, Goyal RK. The columnar-lined esophagus, intestinal metaplasia, and Norman Barrett. Gastroenterology. 1996;110(2):614–21.
40. Rakita S, Villadolid D, Thomas A, Bloomston M, Albrink M, Goldin S, et al. Laparoscopic Nissen fundoplication offers high patient satisfaction with relief of extraesophageal symptoms of gastroesophageal reflux disease. Am Surg. 2006;72(3):207–12.
41. Oelschlager BK, Eubanks TR, Oleynikov D, Pope C, Pellegrini CA. Symptomatic and physiologic outcomes after operative treatment for extraesophageal reflux. Surg Endosc. 2002;16(7):1032–6.
42. Lindstrom DR, Wallace J, Loehrl TA, Merati AL, Toohill RJ. Nissen fundoplication surgery for extraesophageal manifestations of gastroesophageal reflux (EER). Laryngoscope. 2002;112(10):1762–5.
43. Ferguson MK, Fennerty MB. Managing failed anti-reflux therapy. London: Springer; 2006. p. x. 196 p.
44. Lawrence PF, Bell RM, Dayton MT. Essentials of general surgery. 4th ed. Philadelphia, PA: Lippincott Williams & Wilkins; 2006. p. xiv. 613 p.
45. Horvath KD, Swanstrom LL, Jobe BA. The short esophagus: pathophysiology, incidence, presentation, and treatment in the era of laparoscopic antireflux surgery. Ann Surg. 2000;232(5):630–40.
46. Coster DD, Bower WH, Wilson VT, Brebrick RT, Richardson GL. Laparoscopic partial fundoplication vs laparoscopic Nissen-Rosetti fundoplication. Short-term results of 231 cases. Surg Endosc. 1997;11(6):625–31.

47. Hill LD, Gelfand M, Bauermeister D. Simplified management of reflux esophagitis with stricture. Ann Surg. 1970;172(4):638–51.
48. Pearson FG, Cooper JD, Patterson GA, Ramirez J, Todd TR. Gastroplasty and fundoplication for complex reflux problems. Long-term results. Ann Surg. 1987;206(4):473–81.
49. Migaczewski M, Zub-Pokrowiecka A, Grzesiak-Kuik A, Pedziwiatr M, Major P, Rubinkiewicz M, et al. Incidence of true short esophagus among patients submitted to laparoscopic Nissen fundoplication. Wideochir Inne Tech Maloinwazyjne. 2015;10(1):10–4.
50. Madan AK, Frantzides CT, Patsavas KL. The myth of the short esophagus. Surg Endosc. 2004;18(1):31–4.
51. Oelschlager BK, Yamamoto K, Woltman T, Pellegrini C. Vagotomy during hiatal hernia repair: a benign esophageal lengthening procedure. J Gastrointest Surg. 2008;12(7):1155–62.
52. Soper NJ, Swanström LL, Eubanks S. Mastery of endoscopic and laparoscopic surgery. 3rd ed. Philadelphia, PA: Lippincott Williams & Wilkins; 2009. p. xvii. 670 p.
53. Niebisch S, Fleming FJ, Galey KM, Wilshire CL, Jones CE, Litle VR, et al. Perioperative risk of laparoscopic fundoplication: safer than previously reported-analysis of the American College of Surgeons National Surgical Quality Improvement Program 2005 to 2009. J Am Coll Surg. 2012;215(1):61–8. discussion 8–9.
54. Bizekis C, Kent M, Luketich J. Complications after surgery for gastroesophageal reflux disease. Thorac Surg Clin. 2006;16(1):99–108.
55. Champault G. Gastroesophageal reflux. Treatment by laparoscopy. 940 cases--French experience. Ann Chir. 1994;48(2):159–64.
56. Pessaux P, Arnaud JP, Delattre JF, Meyer C, Baulieux J, Mosnier H. Laparoscopic antireflux surgery: five-year results and beyond in 1340 patients. Arch Surg. 2005;140(10):946–51.
57. Dallemagne B, Weerts J, Markiewicz S, Dewandre JM, Wahlen C, Monami B, et al. Clinical results of laparoscopic fundoplication at ten years after surgery. Surg Endosc. 2006;20(1):159–65.

Chapter 6
Anterior Versus Posterior Fundoplication, Are They Equal?

Courtney Olmsted and Peter Nau

6.1 Introduction

Gastroesophageal reflux disease (GERD) is a common condition in western societies with as many 40% experiencing symptoms monthly [1]. It can affect one's health related quality of life and is associated with a number of complications including an increased risk for esophageal adenocarcinoma [2]. The Nissen fundoplication has been the most widely used procedure for the surgical management of GERD and hiatal hernias for six decades. It was first described by Rudolf Nissen in 1956 for the treatment of GERD [3] and then later in 1961 for hiatal hernias [4]. With the advent of laparoscopic surgery it is primarily performed via a minimally invasive approach as it reduces the morbidity associated with an open procedure [5]. The long-term efficacy of anti-reflux surgery had been validated in numerous studies [6–10]. A prospective, randomized control trial with 10-year follow-up definitively establishes the safety and efficacy of both laparoscopic partial and Nissen fundoplications [9, 10]. After 10 years, a minority of patients had return of reflux symptoms, and when surveyed, nearly all were satisfied with their outcome and decision to have undergone the surgery [9, 10].

Notwithstanding the efficacy of the operation, the utilization of antireflux surgery has declined substantially in recent years [11]. This is likely secondary to a myriad of unwanted side effects including dysphagia and what have been called "wind-related" complications. These complaints have led to several technical modifications aimed at reducing postoperative morbidity. The procedures are

C. Olmsted, M.D., M.S.C.I. • P. Nau, M.D., M.S. (✉)
Department of Surgery, Carver College of Medicine, University of Iowa,
200 Hawkins Drive, Primary Office 4626 JCP, Iowa City, IA 52242, USA
e-mail: peter-nau@uiowa.edu

M.A. Memon (ed.), *Hiatal Hernia Surgery*,
https://doi.org/10.1007/978-3-319-64003-7_6

similar to the laparoscopic Nissen fundoplication (LNF) in that they augment the lower esophageal sphincter (LES) pressure, but to a lesser degree than that which is accomplished with a 360° wrap. Given the improved side effect profile, partial fundoplications have gained popularity over the past several years. This increase in the utilization of a partial wrap has been associated with a debate on the competence of the LES and the associated reflux control. Further, there has been some contestation as to if anterior or posterior partial fundoplication is superior. Several meta-analyses and systematic reviews have examined the topic [6–8]. This chapter aims to describe the current procedures being used in addition to comparing and contrasting the procedures so they may be selected in the appropriate patient.

6.2 Preoperative Evaluation

GERD is characterized by the pathologic reflux of gastric contents into the esophagus. Classic symptoms of GERD include acid regurgitation, heartburn and dysphagia. Atypical or extraesophageal symptoms include chest pain, chronic cough, voice changes and globus sensation. Medical management is the first line approach to GERD. Unfortunately, up to 44% will report inadequate resolution of symptoms with proton pump inhibitors (PPI's) [12]. It is this population who responds to PPI's, but has persistent or refractory symptoms that is best suited for surgical intervention [13].

Prior to proceeding with definitive surgical treatment for GERD, all patients need a complete evaluation including a thorough history and physical. Lifestyle changes including weight loss and elevating the head of the bed [14] should be made in addition to initiation of acid-suppressing medications [15]. PPI's display superior efficacy in the treatment of GERD-related esophagitis and are the standard of care for the medical management of GERD [16]. In those whose symptoms are refractory to medical management or suffer from untoward medication side effects, it is appropriate to move forward with evaluation for surgical intervention.

The surgical work-up for GERD consists of an objective evaluation for acidic effluent in the esophagus as well as an overall assessment of esophageal anatomy and function. Acid reflux is best evaluated through the use of a pH monitor placed within the lumen of the esophagus (Fig. 6.1). The addition of multichannel intraluminal impedance has improved the sensitivity of the test via the ability to test for both acidic and non-acidic reflux [17]. All patients should undergo an endoscopy to screen for mucosal changes or other anatomic pathology prior to any antireflux surgery. While not exceedingly specific for pathologic levels of GERD, an esophagram is an important test of esophageal function and anatomy prior to antireflux surgery (Fig. 6.2). Last, in the setting of dysphagia it is reasonable to complete a high resolution esophageal manometry (HREM) (Fig. 6.3). With objective evidence of impaired esophageal peristalsis, one may consider catering the wrap to the patient's esophageal function.

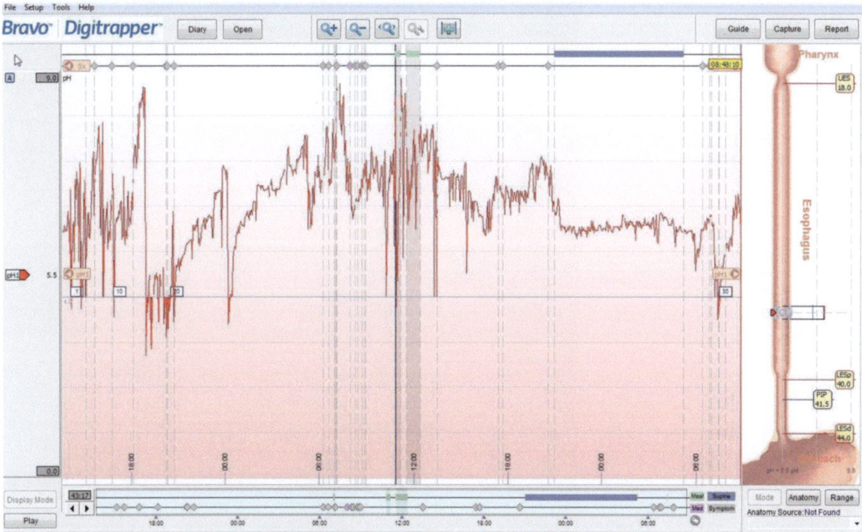

Fig. 6.1 Sample tracing from Bravo pH evaluation

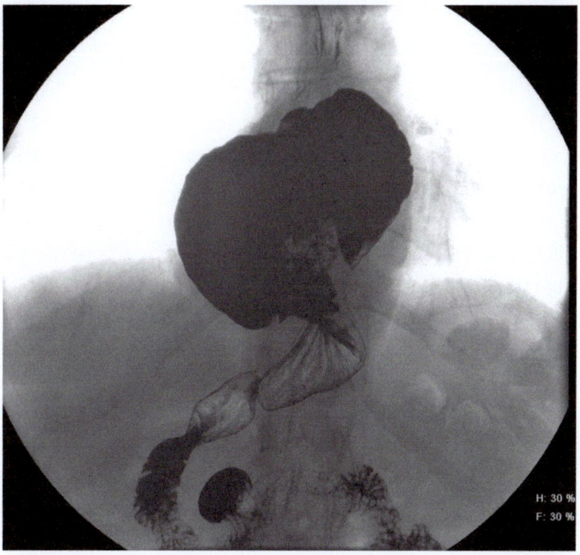

Fig. 6.2 Sample esophagram with evidence of large hiatal hernia with element of organoaxial volvulus

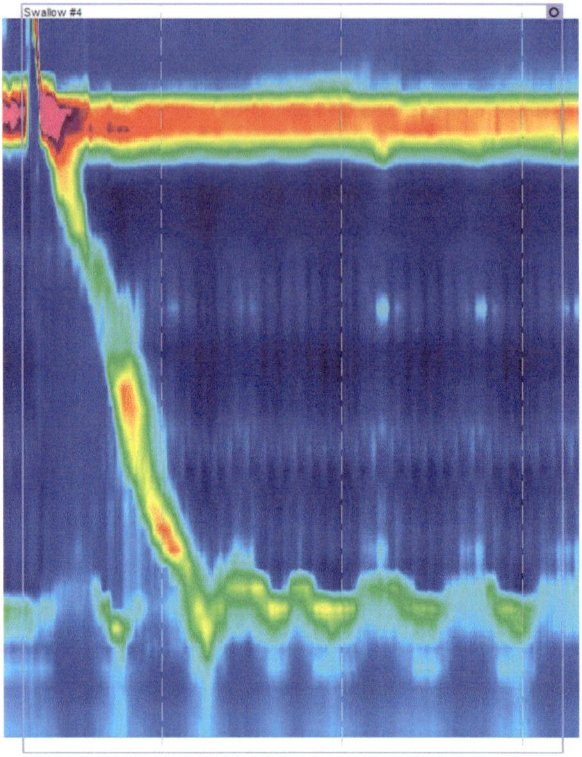

Fig. 6.3 Representative sample of high resolution esophageal manometry

6.3 Partial Anterior Fundoplication Technique

The laparoscopic partial anterior fundoplications (LAF) have been described as 90°, 180° (Dor Fundoplication) [18], or 120° (Watson Fundoplication) [19]. Anterior wraps have three main components: mobilize sufficient abdominal esophagus, secure distal esophagus to crural repair, and close the angle of His via a partial fundoplication. The 90° fundoplication detailed by Krysztopik et al. [20] is described here. The patient positioning and port placement are the same as that described for the laparoscopic Nissen [5]. Briefly, the patient is placed in a modified Lloyd Davies position in reverse Trendelenburg with the operating surgeon standing between the patient's legs and the assistant at the patient's left side. A five-port technique is utilized for the operation (Fig. 6.4). The camera port is placed cephalad of the umbilicus and to the left of midline to provide for visualization of the structures within the hiatus. One must be able to extend the laparoscope all the way to the hiatus in order to visualize mediastinal mobilization of the esophagus. Next, 5 mm trocars are placed bilaterally in the anterior axillary lines for retraction of the liver and the surgeon's assistant. A 12 mm trocar is beneath the costal margin in the left midclavicular line. It is important to place this port lateral so as to maintain appropriate triangulation at the hiatus. Lastly, with the liver retracted through the right lateral

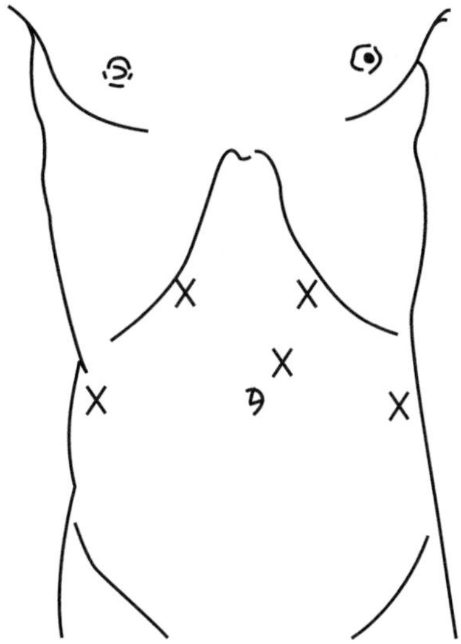

Fig. 6.4 Illustration of the abdomen with "*X*'s" marking the trochar placement utilized for laparoscopic antireflux surgery

port, the final 5 mm trocar is placed in the right midclavicular line. Placement of this port prior to liver retraction can result in obstructed access to the hiatus.

The operation is begun with dissection and isolation of the esophagus from the surrounding structures. This is started by transection of the pars flaccida, moving cephalad so as to identify the right crus. The phrenoesophageal ligament is transected moving anteriorly from right to left. This dissection is carried laterally and posteriorly as far as possible until visualization is limited by the gastric fundus. Next, the short gastric vessels are divided moving cephalad until the left crus can be completely identified and all posterior short gastric vessels are sacrificed. A Penrose drain is then passed posterior to the esophagus to facilitate retraction. The hiatus is restored posteriorly with nonabsorbable suture. The fundoplication begins with an esophagopexy between the right posterolateral side of the esophagus (proximal to the gastroesophageal (GE) junction) to either the right or both crura. Next, the fat pad overlying the cardia is retracted inferiorly to reconstruct the angle of His, and an additional suture is placed between the left lateral esophagus and the neighboring gastric fundus. Another suture is placed more cranially to close the angle of His. This suture brings the left portion of the intra-abdominal esophagus to the gastric body in juxtaposition to the left crura. The left crura can be included in this suture to gain additional length of the intraabdominal esophagus. Next, the gastric fundus is directed midline to sit loosely over the anterior portion of the esophagus. An apical suture, the highest extent of the fundoplication, is placed from the fundus to the anterior esophagus including the apex of the hiatus. The inferior portion of the fundal fold is secured midline to the anterior esophagus at the EG junction. In this 90° wrap, the short gastric vessels are left intact and no bougie is needed [20]. The Watson fundoplication is similar to the above yet the fundus is brought over as a 120° wrap. In the Dor fundoplication the short gastric vessels are ligated and the fundus is secured in place as a 180° wrap.

6.4 Posterior Partial Fundoplication Technique

The laparoscopic posterior partial fundoplication (LPF) that has been described for the treatment of GERD is the Toupet (270° wrap) [21] although according to Nissen, a 360° fundoplication is a type of posterior fundoplication [7]. The laparoscopic Toupet fundoplication described by Wenck is discussed here. Somewhat similar to the LAF, the posterior consists of three main steps: mobilizing the abdominal esophagus, mobilizing the posterior portion of the fundus, and esophogastroplasty with phrenogastroplasty. The patient positioning and port placement mirrors that of the aforementioned LAF. Essential operative steps including esophageal isolation and mobilization as well as the crural repair are also the same. To complete the fundoplication, a portion of the superior fundus is drawn posterior to the esophagus to the right side. Following this, a shoeshine maneuver is performed to verify that the fundus is appropriately oriented and that there is not undue tension due to persistent caudal or posterior short gastric vessels. The right portion of the fundus is secured to right lateral aspect of the esophagus with three distinct stitches. The most cephalad stitch also incorporates the right crura to anchor the wrap within the abdomen. This is then completed on the left side in a mirror image of the right. Finally, the posterior wrap is affixed to the crural closure with two interrupted stitches to deter from cephalad migration of the wrap postoperatively [22].

6.5 Posterior Complete Fundoplication Technique

As stated previously, the 360° fundoplication is a type of a posterior fundoplication [7] and is briefly narrated herein. Much like the partial wraps, there are three essential steps to the 360° fundoplication including mobilization of the esophagus in order to achieve appropriate abdominal length, transection of the short gastric vessels to afford for a tension-free wrap, and esophogastroplasty with phrenogastroplasty. The patient positioning and port placement mirrors that of the aforementioned procedures. Essential operative steps including esophageal isolation and mobilization as well as the crural repair are also the same. To complete the fundoplication, a portion of the superior fundus is drawn posterior to the esophagus towards the right. A shoeshine maneuver is performed to verify that the fundus is appropriately oriented and that there is not undue tension. A 2.0–2.5 cm complete fundoplication is then created with permanent stitches. The most cephalad stitch often incorporates the muscular esophagus to help prevent slippage of the wrap down onto the stomach. Further, many will anchor the wrap to the crura pillars bilaterally to deter cephalad herniation into the thoracic cavity. Finally, the posterior wrap is affixed to the crural closure with two interrupted stitches to complete intra-abdominal fixation [22].

6.6 Medical Management Versus Surgery

Medical management remains the first line treatment for GERD. Recent publications have identified associations between PPI usage and dementia [23], chronic kidney disease [24], and even risk of infections [25, 26]. These findings have produced consternation amongst millions of chronic PPI users and have led to uncertainty as to the superiority of medical management of GERD. It is with this ambiguity in mind that investigators have assessed the efficacy of the two treatment options. A randomized study by Mahon et al. noted that anti-reflux surgery objectively improved the acid exposure within the esophagus while also significantly benefiting patient gastrointestinal and general well-being [27]. In another randomized controlled study by Goeree et al., surgery produced fewer heartburn days and improved overall quality of life when compared with medical management alone [28]. Perhaps more importantly, the long-term cost-effectiveness of surgery has been validated in two distinct trials out to at least 5 years post-operatively [2, 28]. While these studies have lacked standardized patient-oriented outcomes and are limited in length of follow-up, there is compelling evidence that the surgical management of GERD is successful and with an acceptable side effect profile.

6.7 Durability of Fundoplication Long-Term

Many reviews have been published with over 10 years of follow up data for the LPF versus LAF. These studies demonstrate that the posterior partial fundoplication is a durable surgical treatment for GERD with better reflux control than an anterior wrap at the expense of mild increase in dysphagia [8–10, 29]. Patients with anterior fundoplication have been found to need significantly more antisecretory drugs post-operatively and reoperative surgery for their recurrent GERD. This is evidence that an anterior fundoplication is overall less durable than a posterior wrap [30]. Of note, the anterior partial fundoplication is technically simpler its counterpart [30] which may continue to make it a popular procedure despite the evidence suggesting it to be an inferior operation in the long-term.

6.8 Dysphagia Side Effects

The incidence of post-operative dysphagia is up to 70% following a 360° fundoplication [31]. The vast majority of these cases are transient and related to post-operative edema. Advocates for a Toupet fundoplication assert that reflux control is comparable, but the incidence of post-operative dysphagia is lower than that of the LNF [32]. Specifically, those patients with preoperative esophageal dysmotility are thought to be better served with the looser partial fundoplication [33]. To date, the literature has been inconsistent its support of this assertion. Zornig et al. noted that, while the Toupet was a superior operation for prevention of dysphagia, the outcome was independent of preoperative motility. Conversely, others have noted that the presence of dysphagia is similar between the two operations [29]. Perhaps most importantly, a meta-analysis of over 400 patients found that the LNF was significantly more likely to require dilation for persistent dysphagia [34]. Few have investigated the differences between LAF and the LNF. While limited by a follow-up of only 6 months, one group noted fewer side effects following the LAF [35]. Another paper reported improved outcomes following LAF out to 10 years. It is notable that their investigations into improved reflux control and side effect profiles were based strictly on subjective evaluation by the patient.

The issue of post-operative dysphagia has also been investigated for the LAF and LPF. A randomized, controlled trial of 95 patients noted no difference in the compliant of dysphagia post-operatively based on type of fundoplication [36]. Others have observed a higher incidence of early dysphagia with the LPF, but that this resolved by 6 months post procedure [37]. Of note, the LPF performed in setting of a Heller myotomy for achalasia has been found to be associated with improved postoperative dysphagia with nearly identical reflux control in comparison to partial anterior fundoplication [38]. While it is not as intensely debated when considering the anterior versus partial wrap, there is evidence to support that neither is superior in prevention of post-operative dysphagia.

6.9 Bloating and Wind-Related Side Effects

For many prospective patients one of the principal deterrents to anti-reflux surgery is anxiety at the prospects of an inability to belch or vomit, excess flatulence and abdominal bloating. These so called wind-related side effects can be identified in up to 60% of patients depending on the complaint [8, 39]. When compared to the Nissen, the LAF has been shown to have less flatus, abdominal bloating, inability to belch and vomit, and other gas-related symptoms [7]. Those with a LPF also noted less flatulence and postprandial fullness compared to those undergoing a 360° fundoplication [29]. When comparing the LAF and LPF, the results have been less uniform. Well-designed studies with a follow-up up to 5 years found no difference in the complaints of flatulence or inability to belch between the LAF and LPF cohorts. Conversely, other investigations have noted that those who underwent LAF were significantly more likely to be able to vomit [28, 32]. Hagedorn et al. observed an improved ability to vomit as well as fewer complaints of flatulence in those undergoing an LAF [36]. While the literature is more conclusive when comparing a partial to a full wrap, there is more ambiguity with the LAF and LPF. Perhaps the only area where there is a more explicit difference is the improved ability to vomit following LAF.

6.10 Control of Reflux Symptoms

There have been several comparisons via randomized controlled trials and meta-analyses of the Nissen to both the LAF and LPF [7, 8, 10, 29, 30, 36, 37, 40–43]. While thoughtfully designed, many of these investigations have been limited by short-term follow-up. For instance, using 24-h pH testing Zornig et al. identified no difference in reflux control up to 4 months post-operatively [32]. This result was replicated in a randomized study with 1 year follow-up using impedance pH testing [33]. A meta-analysis of the available studies showed that the ability to heal esophagitis was not significantly different between the two operations (LNF vs. LPF was 6.28% vs. 8.63% respectively, P = 0.42). Certainly the durability of a partial wrap remains a concern in that any degree of unwrapping would negatively affect the increased LES pressures. With that said, the available data speaks to the equivalence of the LPF to the LNF for reflux control.

The LAF has also been compared to Nissen for the long-term control of reflux symptoms. One group reported equivalent outcomes with regard to reflux symptoms out to 10 years for a 180° LAF. Of note, this was a subjective evaluation only and had a relatively small sample size [10]. This same collaborative showed that a 90° LAF was inferior to a LNF for control of reflux symptoms at 5 years [44]. While not powered to evaluate for differences in reflux, Djerf showed that there was a higher incidence of heartburn and acid regurgitation in those that had undergone a LAF versus LNF [45]. While there are investigations into the equivalence of the LAF to the LNF, most of the studies are underpowered or lack objective evaluations for reflux control.

Investigators have also contrasted the efficacy of the LAF and LPF to control acid reflux. Engstrom compared a 120° anterior fundoplication to a Toupet and found the anterior had inferior control of reflux related symptoms (heartburn and acid regurgitation) with patients who had been randomized to the LAF [30]. Another randomized, controlled trial identified better objective reflux control as well as fewer complaints of heartburn and acid regurgitation after posterior fundoplication [36]. It should be noted that, while the results were inferior for reflux control, patients who underwent 90° LAF had similar overall satisfaction [42, 43]. Certainly the LAF and LPF both reduce acid exposure to the esophagus; however, the majority with a posterior fundoplication are able to achieve normal pH levels postoperatively as opposed to those receiving a partial anterior fundoplication [36]. Given these findings, there is compelling evidence that the effectiveness and durability of the LPF for control of GERD-related symptoms is superior to that of the LAF.

6.11 Conclusions

Both anterior and posterior partial fundoplication procedures are safe operative treatments for GERD. Among partial fundoplications, the LPF has been shown to offer superior symptom control. Furthermore, the side effect profile of the two operations remains comparable. Given this, in the hands of a competent surgeon, a posterior partial fundoplication is recommended over anterior partial fundoplication. The debate between a LPF and Nissen fundoplication is less well-defined. Certainly, the evidence supports the stance that the reflux control of the LPF is comparable, but with improved morbidity, when compared with the Nissen. With that said, there is a dearth of long-term evidence for the durability of the LPF. This is particularly important when considering a younger population and the decreased efficacy of a revisional operation should the index procedure fail. While a compelling argument can be made for the universal application of the toupet, it is not unreasonable to consider a full wrap in a very young population as it is only with the Nissen that there is long-term data at this time.

What is the current knowledge?	What questions need answering?
The anterior fundoplication provides inferior long-term reflux control	Is tailoring the fundoplication to esophageal function appropriate?
There is an improved side effect profile when comparing a toupet vs. nissen fundoplication	What is the long-term durability of a toupet fundoplication?
Pre-op evaluation for anti-reflux surgery includes objective evaluation for reflux, esophageal function and anatomic variants	Is there an absolute contraction vigor below which a 360° fundoplication is contraindicated?
All fundoplications share the necessity of achieving adequate intra-abdominal esophagus prior to wrap creation	Is there an indication for an anterior wrap outside of an operation for achalasia?

References

1. Locke GR III, et al. Prevalence and clinical spectrum of gastroesophageal reflux: a population-based study in Olmsted County, Minnesota. Gastroenterology. 1997;112(5):1448–56.
2. Faria R, et al. Cost-effectiveness of laparoscopic fundoplication versus continued medical management for the treatment of gastro-oesophageal reflux disease based on long-term follow-up of the REFLUX trial. Br J Surg. 2013;100(9):1205–13.
3. Nissen R. A simple operation for control of reflux esophagitis. Schweiz Med Wochenschr. 1956;86(Suppl 20):590–2.
4. Nissen R. Gastropexy and "fundoplication" in surgical treatment of hiatal hernia. Am J Dig Dis. 1961;6:954–61.
5. Peters MJ, Mukhtar A, Yunus RM, Khan S, Pappalardo J, Memon B, Memon MA. Meta-analysis of randomized clinical trials comparing open and laparoscopic anti-reflux surgery. Am J Gastroenterol. 2009;104(6):1548–61. quiz 1547, 1562.
6. Broeders JA, et al. Laparoscopic anterior versus posterior fundoplication for gastroesophageal reflux disease: systematic review and meta-analysis of randomized clinical trials. Ann Surg. 2011;254(1):39–47.
7. Broeders JA, et al. Laparoscopic anterior 180-degree versus nissen fundoplication for gastroesophageal reflux disease: systematic review and meta-analysis of randomized clinical trials. Ann Surg. 2013;257(5):850–9.

8. Memon MA, et al. Laparoscopic anterior versus posterior fundoplication for gastro-esophageal reflux disease: a meta-analysis and systematic review. World J Surg. 2015;39(4):981–96.
9. Chew CR, et al. Prospective randomized trial of laparoscopic Nissen fundoplication with anterior versus posterior hiatal repair: late outcomes. World J Surg. 2011;35(9):2038–44.
10. Cai W, et al. Ten-year clinical outcome of a prospective randomized clinical trial of laparoscopic Nissen versus anterior 180(degrees) partial fundoplication. Br J Surg. 2008;95(12):1501–5.
11. Finks JF, Wei Y, Birkmeyer JD. The rise and fall of antireflux surgery in the United States. Surg Endosc. 2006;20(11):1698–701.
12. Dickman R, et al. Comparison of clinical characteristics of patients with gastroesophageal reflux disease who failed proton pump inhibitor therapy versus those who fully responded. J Neurogastroenterol Motil. 2011;17(4):387–94.
13. Hamdy E, et al. Outcome of laparoscopic Nissen fundoplication for gastroesophageal reflux disease in non-responders to proton pump inhibitors. J Gastrointest Surg. 2014;18(9):1557–62.
14. Kaltenbach T, Crockett S, Gerson LB. Are lifestyle measures effective in patients with gastroesophageal reflux disease? An evidence-based approach. Arch Intern Med. 2006;166(9):965–71.
15. Badillo R, Francis D. Diagnosis and treatment of gastroesophageal reflux disease. World J Gastrointest Pharmacol Ther. 2014;5(3):105–12.
16. Khan M, et al. Medical treatments in the short term management of reflux oesophagitis. Cochrane Database Syst Rev. 2007;2:CD003244.
17. Hong SK, Vaezi MF. Gastroesophageal reflux monitoring: pH (catheter and capsule) and impedance. Gastrointest Endosc Clin N Am. 2009;19(1):1–22. v.
18. Dor J, et al. Treatment of reflux by the so-called modified Heller-Nissen technic. Presse Med. 1967;75(50):2563–5.
19. Watson A, et al. A more physiological alternative to total fundoplication for the surgical correction of resistant gastro-oesophageal reflux. Br J Surg. 1991;78(9):1088–94.
20. Krysztopik RJ, et al. A further modification of fundoplication. 90 degrees anterior fundoplication. Surg Endosc. 2002;16(10):1446–51.
21. Toupet A. Technic of esophago-gastroplasty with phrenogastropexy used in radical treatment of hiatal hernias as a supplement to Heller's operation in cardiospasms. Mem Acad Chir (Paris). 1963;89:384–9.
22. Wenck C, Zornig C. Laparoscopic Toupet fundoplication. Langenbecks Arch Surg. 2010; 395(4):459–61.
23. Gomm W, et al. Association of proton pump inhibitors with risk of dementia: a pharmacoepidemiological claims data analysis. JAMA Neurol. 2016;73(4):410–6.
24. Lazarus B, et al. Proton pump inhibitor use and the risk of chronic kidney disease. JAMA Intern Med. 2016;176(2):238–46.
25. McDonald EG, et al. Continuous proton pump inhibitor therapy and the associated risk of recurrent clostridium difficile infection. JAMA Intern Med. 2015;175(5):784–91.
26. Lambert AA, et al. Risk of community-acquired pneumonia with outpatient proton-pump inhibitor therapy: a systematic review and meta-analysis. PLoS One. 2015;10(6):e0128004.
27. Mahon D, et al. Randomized clinical trial of laparoscopic Nissen fundoplication compared with proton-pump inhibitors for treatment of chronic gastro-oesophageal reflux. Br J Surg. 2005;92(6):695–9.
28. Goeree R, et al. Cost-utility of laparoscopic Nissen fundoplication versus proton pump inhibitors for chronic and controlled gastroesophageal reflux disease: a 3-year prospective randomized controlled trial and economic evaluation. Value Health. 2011;14(2):263–73.
29. Hagedorn C, et al. Long-term efficacy of total (Nissen-Rossetti) and posterior partial (Toupet) fundoplication: results of a randomized clinical trial. J Gastrointest Surg. 2002;6(4):540–5.
30. Engstrom C, et al. An anterior or posterior approach to partial fundoplication? Long-term results of a randomized trial. World J Surg. 2007;31(6):1221–5. discussion 1226–7.
31. Sato K, et al. Causes of long-term dysphagia after laparoscopic Nissen fundoplication. JSLS. 2002;6(1):35–40.

32. Zornig C, et al. Nissen vs Toupet laparoscopic fundoplication. Surg Endosc. 2002;16(5):758–66.
33. Koch OO, et al. Comparison of results from a randomized trial 1 year after laparoscopic Nissen and Toupet fundoplications. Surg Endosc. 2013;27(7):2383–90.
34. Broeders JA, et al. Systematic review and meta-analysis of laparoscopic Nissen (posterior total) versus Toupet (posterior partial) fundoplication for gastro-oesophageal reflux disease. Br J Surg. 2010;97(9):1318–30.
35. Watson DI, et al. Prospective randomized double-blind trial between laparoscopic Nissen fundoplication and anterior partial fundoplication. Br J Surg. 1999;86(1):123–30.
36. Hagedorn C, et al. Efficacy of an anterior as compared with a posterior laparoscopic partial fundoplication: results of a randomized, controlled clinical trial. Ann Surg. 2003;238(2):189–96.
37. Khan M, et al. Randomized controlled trial of laparoscopic anterior versus posterior fundoplication for gastro-oesophageal reflux disease. ANZ J Surg. 2010;80(7-8):500–5.
38. Kurian AA, et al. Partial anterior vs partial posterior fundoplication following transabdominal esophagocardiomyotomy for achalasia of the esophagus: meta-regression of objective postoperative gastroesophageal reflux and dysphagia. JAMA Surg. 2013;148(1):85–90.
39. Luostarinen M, et al. Fate of Nissen fundoplication after 20 years. A clinical, endoscopical, and functional analysis. Gut. 1993;34(8):1015–20.
40. Engstrom C, et al. Manometric characteristics of the gastroesophageal junction after anterior versus posterior partial fundoplication. Dis Esophagus. 2005;18(1):31–6.
41. Chrysos E, et al. The effect of total and anterior partial fundoplication on antireflux mechanisms of the gastroesophageal junction. Am J Surg. 2004;188(1):39–44.
42. Watson DI, et al. Anterior 90 degrees partial vs Nissen fundoplication--5 year follow-up of a single-centre randomised trial. J Gastrointest Surg. 2012;16(9):1653–8.
43. Spence GM, et al. Single center prospective randomized trial of laparoscopic Nissen versus anterior 90 degrees fundoplication. J Gastrointest Surg. 2006;10(5):698–705.
44. Nijjar RS, et al. Five-year follow-up of a multicenter, double-blind randomized clinical trial of laparoscopic Nissen vs anterior 90 degrees partial fundoplication. Arch Surg. 2010;145(6):552–7.
45. Djerf P, et al. One- and ten-year outcome of laparoscopic anterior 120 degrees versus total fundoplication: a double-blind, randomized multicenter study. Surg Endosc. 2016;30(1):168–77.

Chapter 7
Novel Endoscopic Antireflux Procedures: Do They Have a Role in Patients with Hiatus Hernia?

George Triadafilopoulos

Abbreviations

ARMS	Anti-reflux mucosectomy
EART	Endoscopic anti-reflux therapy
GEJ	Gastro-esophageal junction
GERD	Gastroesophageal reflux disease
GERD-HRQL	GERD health related quality of life
LARS	Laparoscopic antireflux surgery
LESP	Lower esophageal sphincter pressure
PPI	Proton pump inhibitors
TF	Transoral fundoplication

7.1 Introduction

Endoscopic anti-reflux therapy (EART) is a relatively novel concept in the management of gastro-esophageal reflux disease (GERD) that intends to address three key issues: First, the need to treat refractory GERD, that is, to eliminate symptoms that are not completely controlled by proton pump inhibitor (PPI) use; second to eliminate long-term PPI use in those patients who, although well-controlled pharmacologically, are concerned about drug-related adverse events; and third to minimize the need for laparoscopic anti-reflux surgery (LARS) and its peri-operative and long-term sequelae [1]. Over the past 15 years, these clinical issues have

G. Triadafilopoulos, M.D.
Stanford Multidimensional Program for Innovation and Research in the Esophagus (S-MPIRE), Division of Gastroenterology and Hepatology, Stanford University School of Medicine, Stanford, CA 94305, USA
e-mail: vagt@stanford.edu

M.A. Memon (ed.), *Hiatal Hernia Surgery*,
https://doi.org/10.1007/978-3-319-64003-7_7

become increasingly prevalent and clinically significant, thereby expanding the potential applicability and clinical value of EART. It has also become clear that not all patients with GERD are suitable candidates for such an option and that a careful, objective evaluation is needed in order to phenotypically characterize the disease and tailor therapy, aiming at producing the best long-term efficacy and safety.

7.2 Precision GERD Management

Prior to considering any therapy for GERD, one needs to address several key questions (Table 7.1): Addressing these questions using various tools is essential in decision-making as to what options are available to the particular patient and which among them is the best.

7.2.1 GERD Validation

Although the symptoms of heartburn and acid regurgitation are highly specific for GERD, they are imperfect and other non-GERD diagnoses need to be considered. A significant number of symptomatic patients without erosive disease are found not have excessive reflux suggestive that their esophagus is hypersensitive. The best way to validate the diagnosis in a patient with a negative endoscopic examination is ambulatory esophageal pH monitoring, that is performed either using a trans-nasal catheter (impedance/pH), or wirelessly, by placing the Bravo pH probe (Fig. 7.1) [2]. These tools quantify esophageal acid exposure and are invaluable in establishing the diagnosis of GERD and, further, assessing its magnitude, occurrence in the

Table 7.1 Ten key questions for precision GERD management

1. Is GERD truly present and validated by endoscopy and/or pH monitoring?
2. Does GERD affect the patient's quality of life?
3. Is there a confounding illness that makes GERD worse?
4. Has pharmacologic therapy been optimized?
5. Is there a sliding hiatal hernia that would require repair?
6. Are GERD complications (i.e. strictures, Barrett's esophagus) present?
7.Is the esophageal structure and function adequate to undertake an endoscopic or surgical intervention?
8. Is the patient treatment-naïve or has failed or inadequately responded to previous therapies?
9. Is there significant obesity present that would be amenable to endoscopic or surgical therapy?
10. Are there extra-esophageal manifestations present, either alone or together with typical GER symptoms?

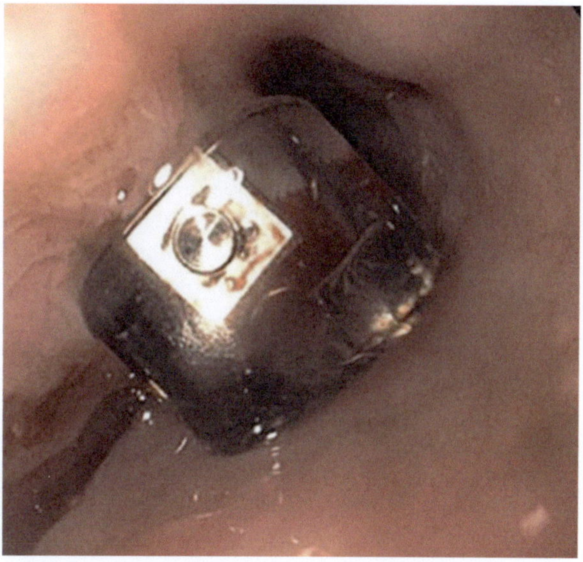

Fig. 7.1 Antegrade endoscopic view of Bravo pH capsule that was placed in order to confirm pathologic acid exposure in a patient with endoscopy-negative GERD

upright or supine position, and relating acid reflux events to symptoms. If the pH/impedance study is negative, other possibilities, particularly achalasia, esophageal spasm, or gastroparesis, need to be considered. Yet, even if the pH/impedance study is positive, overlap syndromes may occur. For example, in a recent study, pathologic acid reflux was found in 44% of patients with esophageal dysmotility/achalasia and 73% of patients with gastroparesis [3].

It is also useful to examine the impact of GERD on the patients' quality of life (GERD-HRQL) by asking the patient to fill out standardized, disease-specific questionnaires. This way, the decision to proceed with potentially beneficial yet invasive interventions, endoscopic or surgical, can be adequately balanced against their respective risks [4]. Ideally, these GERD-HRQL assessments should be done at baseline as well as during a trial of PPI therapy. In a patient using PPIs, it is useful to ask what happens if these drugs are transiently discontinued. Under such circumstances, *bone fide* patients with GERD quickly develop heartburn and acid regurgitation (or other more atypical symptoms) while patients with other diagnoses tend to tolerate PPI abstinence for quite some time. The latter group of patients should not be considered as good candidates for invasive procedures but instead be evaluated further to define the underlying reason for their symptoms.

Another important question to be addressed is the presence of regurgitation, or "volume" reflux, particularly while patients are on PPI therapy. Its presence suggests more severe, mostly supine GERD, but also a higher likelihood of underlying hiatal hernia, complicated disease (i.e. Barrett's esophagus) and respiratory manifestations. Regurgitation is a key point in the discussion of pursuing endoscopic and surgical therapies for GERD [5].

7.2.2 *Hiatal Hernia Assessment*

The presence, type and dimensions of hiatal herniation play a pivotal role in further decision-making (Fig. 7.2). Classic para-esophageal hernias readily disqualify from endoscopic intervention. The same is true for mixed hernias that are typically large enough and fixed to lend themselves to a successful endoscopic repair. On the other hand properly assessed sliding hernias that are <3 cm in length could be amenable to transoral fundoplication (TF). Available evidence thus far has questioned the feasibility and efficacy of the other endoscopic modalities if the hiatal length exceeds 2 cm.

There are several ways to assess for hiatal hernia. Traditionally, barium esophagography has been used, but it has a sensitivity of only 34% and cannot be definitively diagnostic for GERD. If a hiatal hernia is found, it is likely to be contributing to the symptoms and should be repaired surgically. CT scanning is increasingly used, since it provides important information on the structures surrounding the hernia, a better definition of the diaphragmatic defect size and esophageal wall thickening and rigidity, all elements that are important in tissue mobilization. Novel methods for *in vivo* measurement of esophageal hiatal surface area using MDCT multi-planar reconstruction have been introduced [6]. The presence of fluid levels within the esophagus or the hiatal hernia on CT imaging implies more severe disease with impaired motility and esophageal clearance and should raise suspicion for achalasia. High-resolution esophageal manometry (HRM) provides a reliable assessment of the length of the hiatal hernia under physiologic conditions and highlights the relationship between the lower esophageal sphincter (LES) and the crural diaphragm and the spatial dynamics of the esophago-gastric junction (EGJ) at rest and upon swallowing (Fig. 7.3) [7].

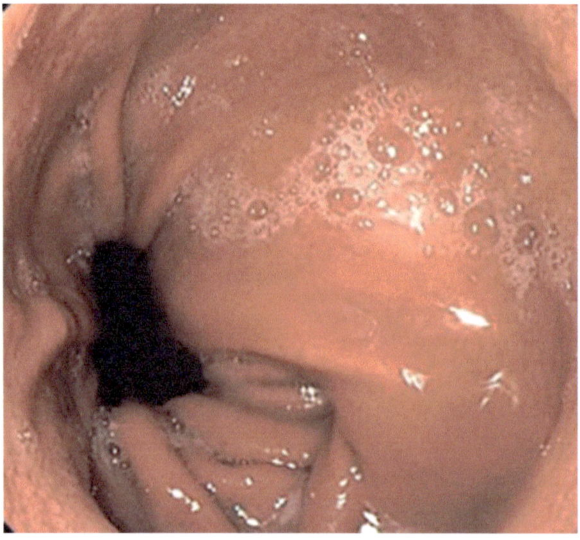

Fig. 7.2 Antegrade endoscopic view of a 4 cm sliding hiatal hernia in a patient after fundoplication

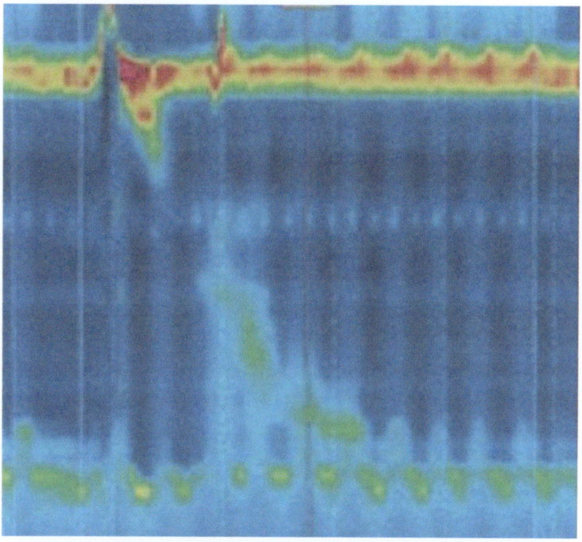

Fig. 7.3 HRM revealing significant impairment of esophageal peristalsis that would negate the performance of a 360° (Nissen) fundoplication

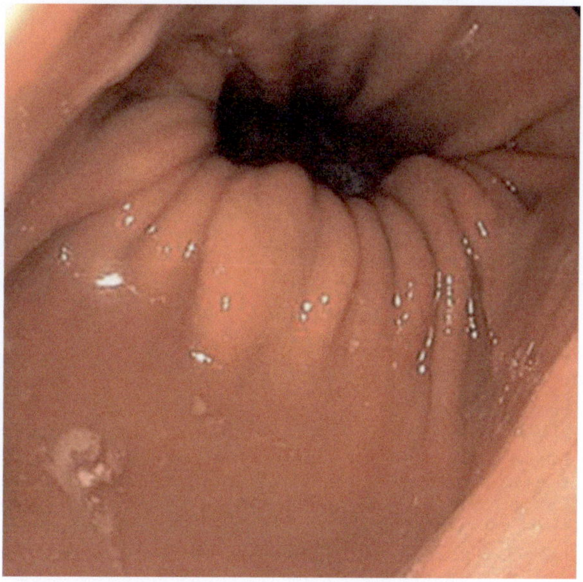

Fig. 7.4 Antegrade endoscopic view of a 5 cm sliding hiatal hernia. Note the accumulation of clear fluid on the left bottom at the time of endoscopy. Such a sizable hernia cannot be corrected with EART

In order to provide useful information, endoscopy requires attention to the GEJ at various levels of air distention, forward and retrograde viewing and a meticulous detailing of the mucosa. If the distance of the GEJ from the incisors does not vary significantly with insufflation one can expect wall fibrosis and esophageal foreshortening both messengers of a challenging surgical repair. Fluid pooling, stricture formation or tissue nodularity imply atony and complicated disease and are expected to be associated with suboptimal endoscopic or surgical outcomes (Fig. 7.4).

Retroflexed views of the cardia during endoscopy are essential not only to confirm the type and size of the hernia but also to assess the GEJ using the Hill classification, a grading system that is easy to learn and has been used and validated for over 20 years (Fig. 7.5) [8]. In controls without GERD, there is a prominent tissue fold of tissue along the lesser curvature of the stomach that closely apposes to the endoscope (Hill Grade I). Less commonly, in Hill Grade II, the fold is present but there are times of opening and closing around the endoscope. In contrast, in patients with GERD the fold is not prominent and there is inadequate grip of the endoscope by the GEJ tissues (Hill Grade III) and a sliding hiatal hernia may be present (Fig. 7.6). Patients with GERD and hiatal hernia have essentially no fold and the lumen of the esophagus remains open, allowing the squamous esophageal epithelium, proximal to the GEJ, to be seen from below (Hill Grade IV). In the original study of this classification, the sensitivity and specificity of an abnormal cardia (Hill Grades III and IV) in predicting reflux was 91%, with a positive predictive value of 95%, and a negative predictive value of 87%.

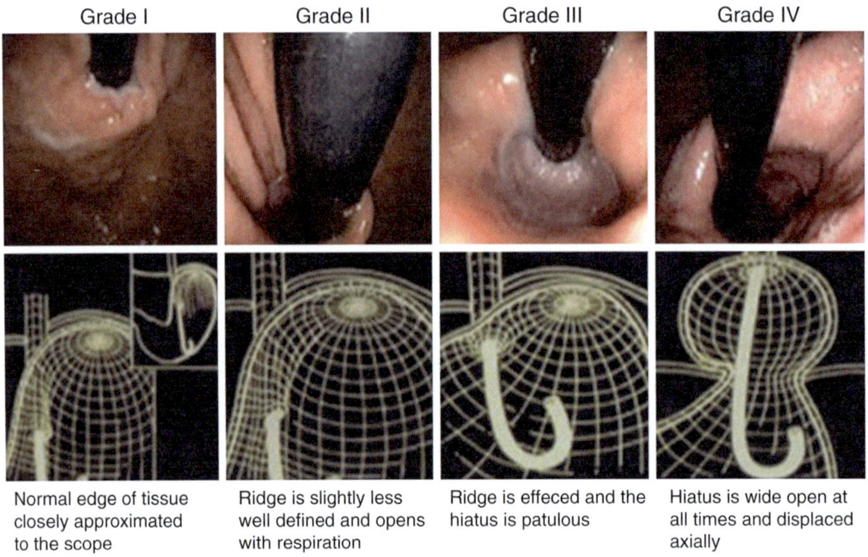

Fig. 7.5 Hill's endoscopic classification. Grade I flap valve appearance showing the ridge of tissue to be closely approximated to the shaft of the retroflexed endoscope. It extends 3–4 cm along the lesser curve. Grade II flap valve appearance. The ridge is slightly less well defined opening rarely with respiration and closing promptly. Grade III flap valve appearance. The ridge is barely present, and there is often failure to close around the endoscope. This is nearly always accompanied by a hiatal hernia. Grade IV flap valve appearance. There is no muscular ridge, the gastroesophageal area stays open all the time and squamous epithelium can often be seen from the retroflexed position. A hiatus hernia is always present (*Reproduced from ref.* [8])

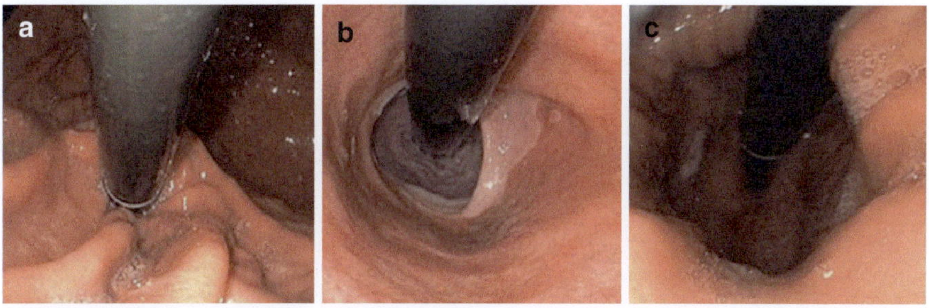

Fig. 7.6 (**a**) Retrograde appearance of the cardia, revealing a Hill grade I appearance. The white marking on the endoscope surface is fully encircled by the tissues of the cardia, suggestive of an anti-reflux effect. In a symptomatic patient with pH-confirmed GERD, EART can be performed. (**b**) Retrograde appearance of a Hill grade IV cardia. The endoscope can be advanced into the distal esophagus and easily visualize the squamous epithelium. (**c**) Retrograde view of a large sliding hiatal hernia in a patient with GERD and Barrett's esophagus. Neither (**b**) nor (**c**) are amenable to EART and surgery is required

7.2.3 Esophageal Structure and Function

Both these elements need to be examined in every patient with GERD. Esophageal structure is best assessed by endoscopy, first to exclude other conditions (i.e. other forms of esophagitis or cancer), and to carefully define mucosal integrity, ruling out dysplastic Barrett's esophagus that will require attention prior to any endoscopic or surgical therapy for GERD being applied (Fig. 7.7) [9]. Most EART studies have excluded patients with Barrett's esophagus, hence the efficacy of these procedures in such patients is not well established. In contrast, we have better efficacy data on Barrett's esophagus patients undergoing anti-reflux surgery. Moreover, patients with long segment Barrett's esophagus tend to have large sliding hiatal hernias in need for operative hernia repair and anti-reflux surgery.

Functional assessment mainly aims to exclude achalasia or other forms of severe peristaltic failure that would impede the placement of a magnetic sphincter (LINX) or a 360° fundoplication and may favor instead a partial 270° (Toupet) fundoplication or a Collis gastroplasty. It is debatable to what degree ineffective esophageal peristalsis and other lesser disorders of function detected by HRM serve as contraindications to surgery or endoscopic management. As a general rule, the creation of a tight anti-reflux barrier may aggravate dysphagia and difficulties with throat clearance and any invasive option needs to be carefully examined and individualized.

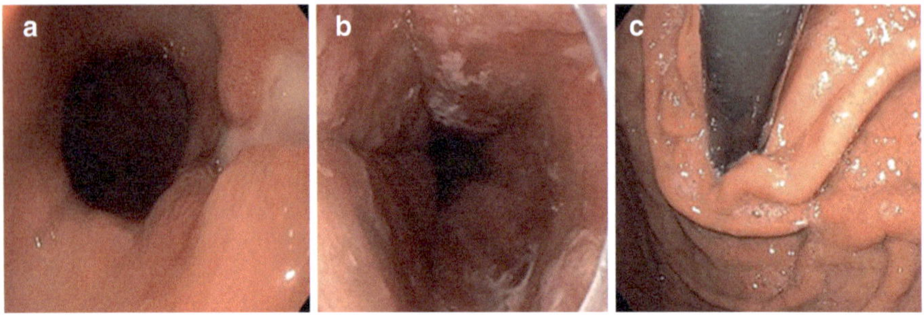

Fig. 7.7 (**a**) Antegrade view of a >1 cm esophageal ulcer on the substrate of Barrett's esophagus. Healing of the ulcer using PPI therapy and reassessment of the Barrett's epithelium 2 months later revealed high-grade dysplasia. (**b**) Antegrade endoscopic appearance of Barrett's esophagus immediately after HALO-360° ablation. This patient was first treated using HALO ablation for his dysplastic Barrett's esophagus and then, upon resolution of both the dysplasia and metaplasia underwent a 270° laparoscopic fundoplication for GERD symptom control. (**c**) Retrograde appearance of the cardia 3 months postoperatively, showing the desired anti-reflux effect

7.2.4 Prior Therapies

Complete non-response to PPI therapy is a warning against either endoscopic or surgical intervention for GERD. This is different than PPI-refractory disease, where patients exhibit some (partial) response to pharmacologic therapy. This latter group of patients constitutes the majority of patients referred for invasive therapies. Perception modulators, such as the SSRI citalopram, can reduce esophageal hypersensitivity not limited to acid, as well as other add-on therapies, such as prokinetics, inhibitors of transient lower sphincter relaxations or alginates also play an important therapeutic role. Another group of patients, those who respond well to PPI therapy but do not wish to continue them long-term fearful of adverse events. Such patients may have lesser endoscopic burden of disease that makes them better candidates for any invasive therapies. There are very limited data in patients who have previously undergone either endoscopic or surgical therapies for GERD and present with refractory symptoms. Radiofrequency therapy of GEJ (Stretta) can be performed repeatedly or in a patient post anti-reflux surgery but not after magnetic sphincter implantation, but there is no published data on its efficacy. In a patient presenting with recurrent GERD after anti-reflux surgery, the degree of wrap displacement, if any, plays an essential role in decision-making (Fig. 7.8). If present, there is no role for EART and surgical repair is the only option [10]. Revisional anti-reflux surgery is always more challenging to perform and its outcomes are considered less robust than those of the initial intervention. The use of mesh to close large hiatal defects that contributed to prior failure remains controversial and needs to be individualized. Finally, patients with prior esophageal injury or those with complicated disease (i.e., long peptic strictures) that are resistant to medical therapy lone or in combination with temporary endoscopic stenting, may require esophagectomy instead of EART or anti-reflux surgery.

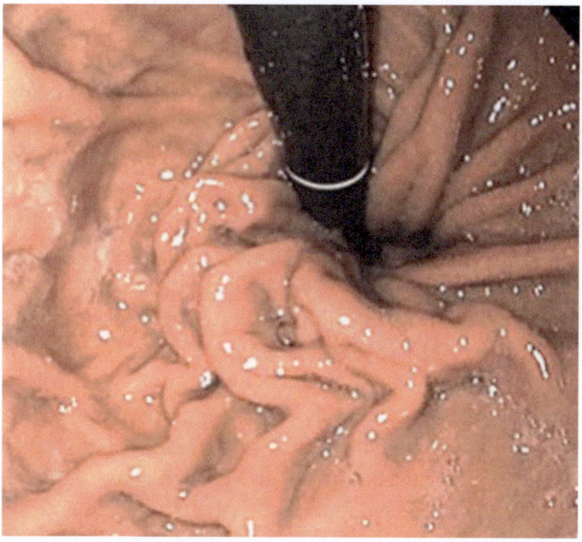

Fig. 7.8 Retrograde view of the displaced fundoplication, revealing laxity around the shaft of the endoscope. This is not amenable to endoscopic repair and a revisional surgery is needed

7.2.5 Obesity

Patients with morbid obesity have been excluded from EART trials and data on efficacy and safety are scant. In general, if a patient with GERD is a candidate for anti-obesity surgery, the performance of Roux-en-Y bypass is the best surgical option. Sleeve gastrectomy is less likely to be associated with complete control of GERD symptoms, but if such symptoms occur postoperatively, radiofrequency therapy of EGJ is feasible and effective [11]. Regardless of the choice of invasive therapy, endoscopic or surgical, peri-operative morbidity is high in obese patients and needs to be considered and balanced against the anticipated gains.

7.2.6 Extra-Esophageal Symptoms

The efficacy of EART in controlling extra-esophageal symptoms—particularly if such symptoms occur in the absence of typical GERD—has not been adequately explored and more data is needed. Non-cardiac chest pain, cough, asthma, recurrent hoarseness and dental erosions, are less responsive to pharmacologic, endoscopic or surgical interventions. Prior proof that GERD is inducing such symptoms is generally advised in order to maximize gains.

7.3 Endoscopic Anti-Reflux Therapies (EART)

Currently, there are four EART options available for patients with GERD. Radiofrequency therapy of GEJ (Stretta) used for over 15 years has the best long-term data [12]. The transoral fundoplication (TF) device creates molding of the GEJ through endoscopic placement of polypropylene suture material; its short-term efficacy and safety have been recently demonstrated in controlled clinical trials. The MUSE™ endoscopic stapling system is a recent technique that creates an endoscopic partial fundoplication under ultrasound guidance, but clinical data is still scant. More recently, the use of conventional endoscopic dissection tools to perform anti-reflux mucosectomy (ARMS) has been reported from Japan [13].

The presence of a sliding hiatal hernia plays an important role when selecting EART. Since Stretta treats the intrinsic LES muscle without interfering with the crural diaphragm element of the anti-reflux mechanism, the dissociation of the two in the setting of a hernia longer than 2 cm serves as a contraindication for the procedure since the treated area will remain above the diaphragm, possibly creating an acid pocket effect (Fig. 7.9). Radiofrequency therapy may be most helpful in those with TLESR as the cause of their reflux. The same is probably true for ARMS, although we do not have enough information on this issue. Since they create a partial valvular structure at the GEJ, both TF and MUSE may be feasible and effective in patients with <3 cm hernias that, during the procedure, can be stretched and mobilized aborally, but more data will be needed on their durability in such patients.

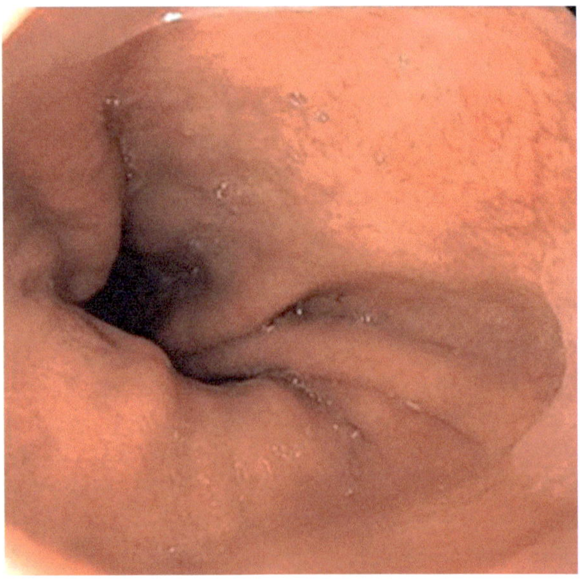

Fig. 7.9 Antegrade view of a <2 cm sliding hiatal hernia that could be treated with EART

Since many open and controlled studies and recent reviews have addressed the safety, efficacy and durability of EART, the discussion below focuses on the specifics of these procedures in patients with Hill grades I and II and sliding hiatal hernias <3 cm. It is with such understanding that a balanced decision towards endoscopic or surgical therapy can be made, aiming at optimizing clinical outcomes, particularly in the long-term.

7.3.1 Radiofrequency Treatment of the EGJ (Stretta)

Radiofrequency energy delivery to the EGJ muscle (Stretta) has been used extensively and has long-term data (10 years) (Fig. 7.10) [14]. In general, Stretta is most effective in patients without hiatal hernia; its mechanism of action is mostly driven by enhancement of the lower esophageal sphincter (LES) tone and reduction of transient LES relaxations [15]. The presence of a hiatal hernia >2 cm is a contraindication to the performance of Stretta, hence feasibility and efficacy studies on patients with significant (>3 cm) hiatal hernia are lacking. In the first randomized, sham-controlled trial, patients (40% with hiatal hernia <2 cm) who were treated with Stretta had significantly improved symptoms and quality of life scores without improvement seen in the sham group. Stretta reduced PPI usage by 46% compared to 29% in the sham group [16]. In another prospective, randomized, double-blinded, sham-controlled trial, patients with hiatal hernia <2 cm were treated with either

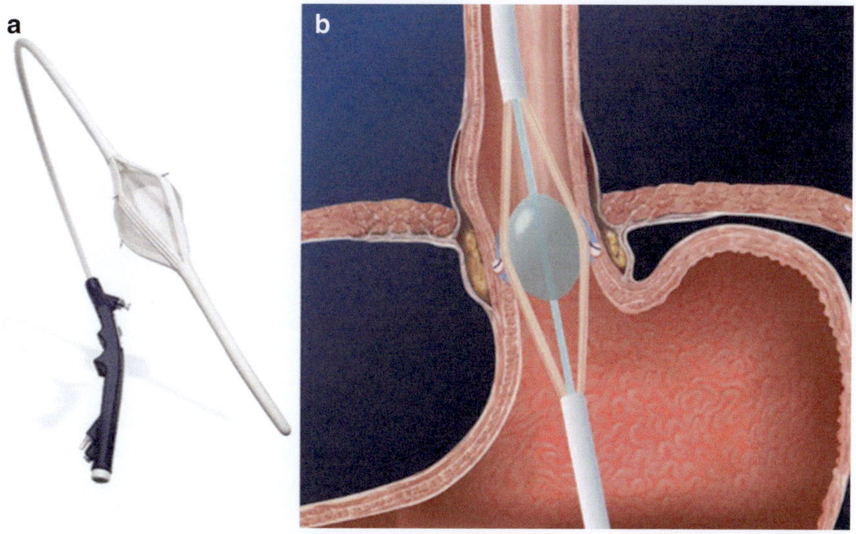

Fig. 7.10 (**a**) Stretta catheter. Upon inflation of the balloon, the four needles are impregnated into the muscle of the EGJ prior to radiofrequency application

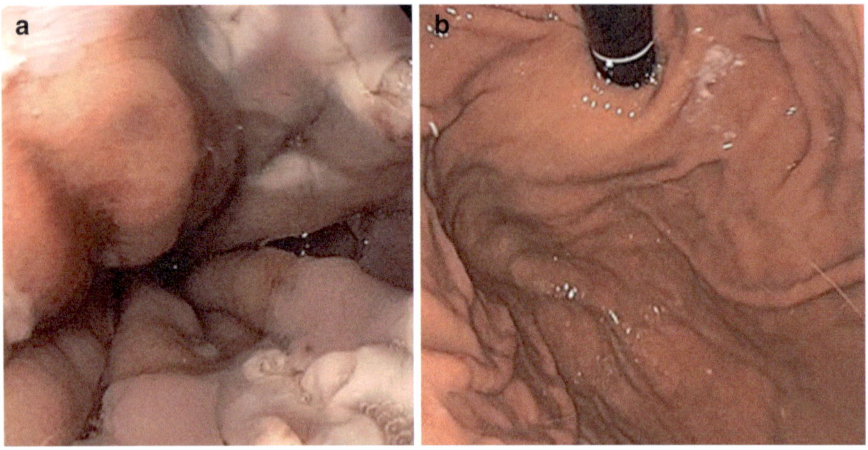

Fig. 7.11 (**a**) Endoscopic view of the EGJ immediately after Stretta, revealing the white mucosal markings where the radiofrequency treatment was administered at the level of the EGJ and cardia. (**b**) Retrograde view of the cardia in the same patient 2 months afterwards revealing a Hill grade I appearance. The endoscope is snug around the tissues of the cardia

Stretta once, Stretta twice, or with a sham procedure. At 12 months there was a significant symptom improvement in both active treatments, but not the sham group. LES pressures and pH improved in both the single- and double-treatment groups, with non-significant changes seen in the sham group [17] (Fig. 7.11).

7.3.2 Transoral Fundoplication (TF)

Trans-oral, incisionless fundoplication (TF) treats GERD by creating a full-thickness esophago-gastric plication using trans-mural fasteners (Fig. 7.12) and a large number of studies over the past several years have validated its safety and effectiveness. TF can fill the "therapeutic gap" that exists between PPI and laparoscopic fundoplication but TF cannot effectively close a significant hiatal hernia. In the earliest TF study [18], upper endoscopy was performed before and after the procedure in order to grade esophagitis and to exclude Barrett's esophagus. A hiatal hernia was diagnosed when the Z-line was above the diaphragmatic pinch caused by external compression by the crus or when a herniation was visible on the retroflexed endoscopic view. Hiatal hernias (<3 cm) were present in 13 patients (76%) and they were all reduced and remained reduced in 62% of cases.

The recent randomized study of 44 patients (22 TF and 22 sham) excluded patients with body mass index (BMI) >35, Hill grade IV, and hiatal hernia >3 cm [19]. Based on their data, the authors concluded that ideal TF candidates would be patients with persistent GERD symptoms and with the following anatomic

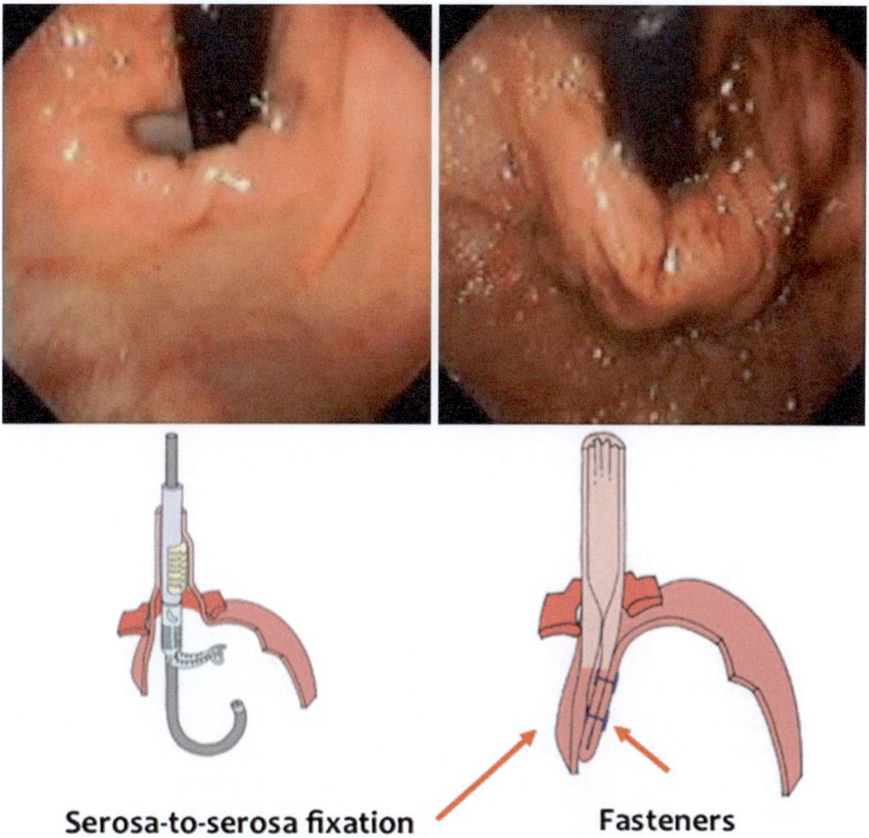

Fig. 7.12 (*Top*) Retrograde endoscopic appearance of the cardia before and after TF. (*Bottom*). Diagrammatic representation of the transmural fasteners, creating the partial fundoplication affect

characteristics: (i) hiatal hernia <2 cm without an enlarged hiatus; (ii) normal esophageal motility; (iii) abnormal ambulatory pH or evidence of reflux esophagitis on endoscopy or biopsy; (iv) Hill grade II–III at the GEJ.

In a prospective randomized trial, of patients poorly responsive to PPI therapy, high-resolution esophageal manometry confirmed the absence of esophageal motor dysfunction, endoscopy was performed to grade the appearance of the anti-reflux barrier (Hill grade), to confirm the absence of long segment Barrett's esophagus, and to grade esophagitis, if present. Cine-esophagography was performed to confirm the absence of hiatal hernia or a hiatal hernia ≤2 cm in length. There were no patients with larger hernias [5].

Similarly, another controlled study of TF included only highly selected GERD patients with a small (≤2 cm) hiatal hernia [20]. The authors of another study with TF considered preoperative endoscopy as mandatory to determine the diaphragmatic hiatus, and the greatest transverse dimension of the hiatus under full gastric distension [21]. They claimed that only a hiatal hernia <2.5 cm long can be fully reduced below the diaphragm, while a plication performed in a hiatus with a transverse dimension >3.0 cm can end up in the thorax, which reduces the efficacy of the newly created valve. In that series, hiatal hernia, even <2.5 cm and ineffective esophageal motility increased the risk of symptomatic recurrence. In another study, patients were required to have Hill grades II, III, or IV, while patients with a hiatal hernia >3 cm, esophageal motility disorders, diverticula, strictures, previous gastroesophageal surgery, or Barrett's esophagus were excluded. Fifteen patients (55%) had hernia <2 cm [22].

7.3.3 MUSE

The MUSE™ endoscopic stapling system creates an endoscopic partial fundoplication (Fig. 7.13). The MUSE endoscope is inserted and advanced into the stomach and retroflexed, pulling it back to the correct stapling level above the GEJ. Tissue is then stapled under ultrasonographic gap finder. The procedure is repeated circumferentially to form a 180° fundoplication.

A multi-center, prospective study evaluated 69 patients; no patients with sliding hiatal hernia >3 cm were enrolled. During general anesthesia all patients were ventilated with a PEEP setting of 5 mmHg; if a hernia was still evident, PEEP was gradually increased to 10 mmHg until the hernia was reduced and the procedure was performed. Of the 66 patients who completed follow-up 6 months after the procedure, the GERD-HRQL score improved by >50% off PPI in 73% of patients and 64.6% were no longer using daily PPIs. The proportions of patients with an unacceptable Hill Grade (>2) dropped dramatically after the procedure. There were two severe adverse events (empyema and gastrointestinal bleeding) requiring intervention [23]. Larger randomized studies and registry trials with longer periods of follow up will be required.

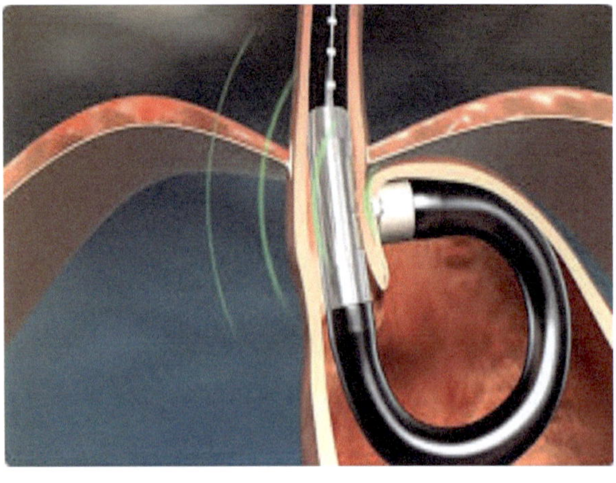

Fig. 7.13 Diagrammatic representation of the MUSE device, creating the partial fundoplication affect

7.3.4 Anti-Reflux Mucosectomy (ARMS)

ARMS is performed using endoscopic mucosal resection (EMR) and endoscopic submucosal dissection (ESD) of the distal 1 cm of the esophagus and proximal 2 cm of the stomach, with the resection length at the cardia measured in retroflexion (Fig. 7.14). The presence of a sliding hiatal hernia is a contraindication for ARMS. The procedure is preferably performed along the lesser curve of the stomach, thus preserving a sharp mucosal valve at gastric cardia. In one study, GERD symptoms, pH as well as bile reflux scores improved significantly after the procedure. In two cases of total circumferential resection, repeat balloon dilation was necessary to control distal esophageal stricture. In all cases, PPI therapy was stopped. Larger studies with long-term follow up will be needed [24].

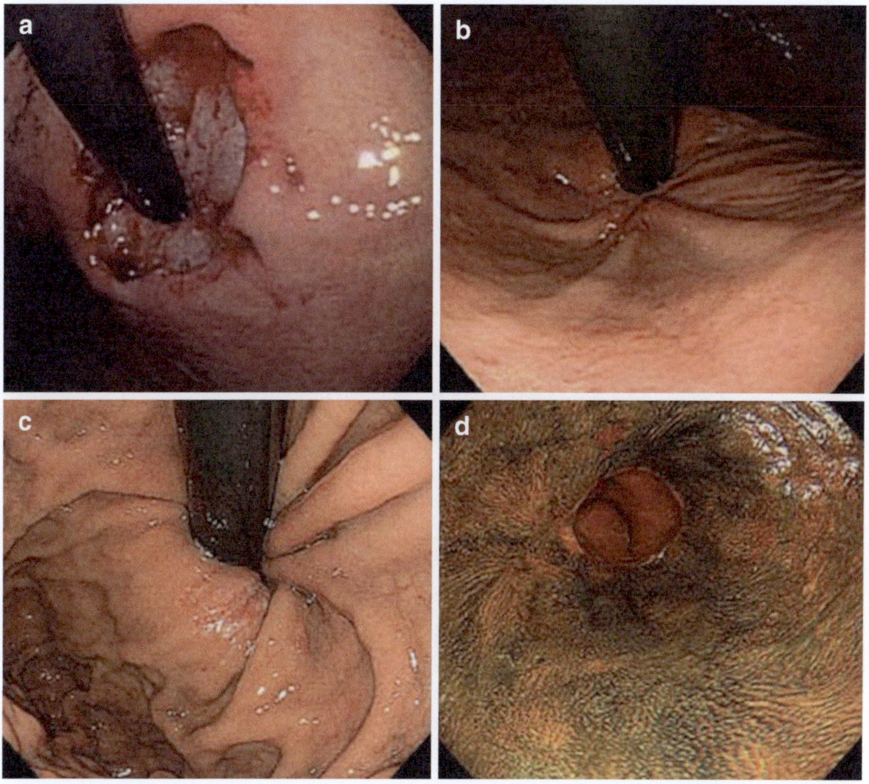

Fig. 7.14 Endoscopic follow up of circumferential anti-reflux mucosectomy (ARMS) (retroflexed views). (**a**) Immediately after ARMS showing a 2 cm-wide gastric cardia mucosa that was circumferentially resected by cap-endoscopic mucosal resection. (**b**) Appearance at 3 years, a tight gastroesophageal junction revealing convergence of three gastric folds along the gastric lesser curve. (**c**) More than 10 years after circumferential ARMS shows an appearance that is similar to (**b**). (**d**) Forward view of the EGJ >10 years after circumferential ARMS. Chromoendoscopy with Lugol's solution demonstrates well-stained squamous epithelium, with neither recurrence of esophagitis nor Barrett's esophagus (*Reproduced from ref.* [24])

7.4 Conclusions

The clinical and phenotypic complexity of GERD requires that a detailed, multimodality diagnostic evaluation prior to decision-making for EART or surgical therapies. Each of the four currently available endoscopic modalities has unique features and limitations, particularly in regards to hiatal hernia size. A tailored and individualized selection has to be based on symptoms, clinical presentation, proper disease definition, therapeutic objectives, and available local endoscopic and surgical expertise. As these novel endoscopic and laparoscopic technologies evolve and mature and long-term data becomes available, decision-making will remain in flux but best done at multi-disciplinary esophageal centers of excellence.

What Is the Current Knowledge and What Future Direction Is Required

- GERD is a more complex and multifactorial disease than previously thought and results from imbalance between several offensive and protective factors
- Reflux hypersensitivity is increasingly recognized and add-on therapies may be required
- Precision GERD management requires several key questions to be addressed
- Although gastric acid hypersecretion is not a pathogenetic factor in GERD, acid inhibition is the mainstay of GERD therapy.
- When acid inhibition fails, laparoscopic anti-reflux surgery with or without hernia repair is the best-validated option.
- Not all patients with GERD are suitable candidates for endoscopic anti-reflux therapy
- The effectiveness and adverse effects of all new endoscopic treatment modalities must be investigated in randomized controlled and comparative efficacy trials

Compliance with Ethical Standards *Conflict of Interest*: The author has equity position with Mederi Therapeutics, C2 Therapeutics and EndoStim.
Human and Animal Rights and Informed Consent: This article does not contain any studies with human or animal subjects performed by the author.

References

1. Triadafilopoulos G. Endoscopic options for gastroesophageal reflux: where are we now and what does the future hold? Curr Gastroenterol Rep. 2016;18(9):47. https://doi.org/10.1007/s11894-016-0521-1.
2. de Bortoli N, Martinucci I, Bertani L, Russo S, Franchi R, Furnari M, Tolone S, Bodini G, Bolognesi V, Bellini M, Savarino V, Marchi S, Savarino EV. Esophageal testing: what we have so far. World J Gastrointest Pathophysiol. 2016;7(1):72–85. https://doi.org/10.4291/wjgp.v7.i1.72.

3. Galindo G, Vassalle J, Marcus SN, Triadafilopoulos G. Multimodality evaluation of patients with gastroesophageal reflux disease symptoms who have failed empiric proton pump inhibitor therapy. Dis Esophagus. 2013;26(5):443–50. https://doi.org/10.1111/j.1442-2050.2012.01381.x.
4. Bedell A, Taft TH, Keefer L, Pandolfino J. Development of the northwestern esophageal quality of life scale: a hybrid measure for use across esophageal conditions. Am J Gastroenterol. 2016;111(4):493–9. https://doi.org/10.1038/ajg.2016.20.
5. Hunter JG, Kahrilas PJ, Bell RC, Wilson EB, Trad KS, Dolan JP, Perry KA, Oelschlager BK, Soper NJ, Snyder BE, Burch MA, Melvin WS, Reavis KM, Turgeon DG, Hungness ES, Diggs BS. Efficacy of transoral fundoplication vs omeprazole for treatment of regurgitation in a randomized controlled trial. Gastroenterology. 2015;148(2):324–333.e5. https://doi.org/10.1053/j.gastro.2014.10.009.
6. Ouyang W, Dass C, Zhao H, Kim C, Criner G. COPDGene Investigators. Multiplanar MDCT measurement of esophageal hiatus surface area: association with hiatal hernia and GERD. Surg Endosc. 2016;30(6):2465–72. https://doi.org/10.1007/s00464-015-4499-9.
7. Kahrilas PJ, Bredenoord AJ, Fox M, Gyawali CP, Roman S, Smout AJ, Pandolfino JE. International High Resolution Manometry Working Group. The Chicago Classification of esophageal motility disorders, v3.0. Neurogastroenterol Motil. 2015;27(2):160–74. https://doi.org/10.1111/nmo.12477.
8. Hill LD, Kozarek RA, Kraemer SJ, Aye RW, Mercer CD, Low DE, Pope CE II. The gastroesophageal flap valve: in vitro and in vivo observations. Gastrointest Endosc. 1996;44(5):541–7.
9. Singhal V, Khaitan L. Preoperative evaluation of gastroesophageal reflux disease. Surg Clin North Am. 2015;95(3):615–27. https://doi.org/10.1016/j.suc.2015.02.013.
10. Lin DC, Chun CL, Triadafilopoulos G. Evaluation and management of patients with symptoms after anti-reflux surgery. Dis Esophagus. 2015;28(1):1–10. https://doi.org/10.1111/dote.12103.
11. Iannelli A, Sans A, Martini F, Santonicola A, Iovino P, Angrisani L. Hiatal hernia, GERD, and sleeve gastrectomy: a complex interplay. Obes Surg. 2016;26(10):2485–7. https://doi.org/10.1007/s11695-016-2291-0.
12. Triadafilopoulos G. Stretta: a valuable endoscopic treatment modality for gastroesophageal reflux disease. World J Gastroenterol. 2014;20:7730–8. https://doi.org/10.3748/wjg.v20.i24.7730.
13. Triadafilopoulos G, Azagury D. How can we deal with the GERD treatment gap? Ann N Y Acad Sci. 2016;1381(1):14–20. https://doi.org/10.1111/nyas.13104.
14. Noar M, Squires P, Noar E, Lee M. Long-term maintenance effect of radiofrequency energy delivery for refractory GERD: a decade later. Surg Endosc. 2014;28:2323–33.
15. Arts J, Bisschops R, Blondeau K, Farré R, Vos R, Holvoet L, Caenepeel P, Lerut A, Tack J. A double-blind sham-controlled study of the effect of radiofrequency energy on symptoms and distensibility of the gastro-esophageal junction in GERD. Am J Gastroenterol. 2012;107:222–30.
16. Corley DA, Katz P, Wo JM, Stefan A, Patti M, Rothstein R, Edmundowicz S, Kline M, Mason R, Wolfe MM. Improvement of gastroesophageal reflux symptoms after radiofrequency energy: a randomized, sham-controlled trial. Gastroenterology. 2003;125:668–76.
17. Aziz AM, El-Khayat HR, Sadek A, Mattar SG, McNulty G, Kongkam P, Guda MF, Lehman GA. A prospective randomized trial of sham, single-dose Stretta, and double-dose Stretta for the treatment of gastroesophageal reflux disease. Surg Endosc. 2010;24:818–25.
18. Cadière GB, Rajan A, Germay O, Himpens J. Endoluminal fundoplication by a transoral device for the treatment of GERD: a feasibility study. Surg Endosc. 2008;22:333–42. https://doi.org/10.1007/s00464-007-9618-9.
19. Håkansson B, Montgomery M, Cadiere GB, Rajan A, Bruley des Varannes S, Lerhun M, Coron E, Tack J, Bischops R, Thorell A, Arnelo U, Lundell L. Randomised clinical trial: transoral incisionless fundoplication vs. sham intervention to control chronic GERD. Aliment Pharmacol Ther. 2015;42:1261–70. https://doi.org/10.1111/apt.13427.
20. Witteman BPL, Conchillo JM, Rinsma NF, Betzel B, Peeters A, Koek GH, Stassen LPS, Bouvy ND. Randomized controlled trial of transoral incisionless fundoplication vs. proton pump inhibitors for treatment of gastroesophageal reflux disease. Am J Gastroenterol. 2015;110:531–42. https://doi.org/10.1038/ajg.2015.28.

21. Testoni PA, Vailati C. Transoral incisionless fundoplication with EsophyX® for treatment of gastro-oesphageal reflux disease. Dig Liver Dis. 2012;44:631–5. https://doi.org/10.1016/j.dld.2012.03.019.
22. Repici A, Fumagalli U, Malesci A, Barbera R, Gambaro C, Rosati R. Endoluminal fundoplication (ELF) for GERD using EsophyX: a 12-month follow-up in a single-center experience. J Gastrointest Surg. 2010;14:1–6. https://doi.org/10.1007/s11605-009-1077-2.
23. Zacherl J, Roy-Shapira A, Bonavina L, Bapaye A, Kiesslich R, Schoppmann SF, Kessler WR, Selzer DJ, Broderick RC, Lehman GA, Horgan S. Endoscopic anterior fundoplication with the Medigus Ultrasonic Surgical Endostapler (MUSE™) for gastroesophageal reflux disease: 6-month results from a multi-center prospective trial. Surg Endosc. 2015;29:220–9.
24. Inoue H, Ito H, Ikeda H, Sato C, Sato H, Phalanusitthepha C, Hayee B, Eleftheriadis N, Kudo SE. Anti-reflux mucosectomy for gastroesophageal reflux disease in the absence of hiatus hernia: a pilot study. Ann Gastroenterol. 2014;27:346–51.

Chapter 8
Magnetic Sphincter Augmentation for Symptomatic Small Hiatus Hernia

Luigi Bonavina, Andrea Sironi, and Emanuele Asti

Therapy for gastroesophageal reflux disease and hiatus hernia remains unsatisfactory. About 40% of patients are partial responders to proton-pump inhibitors, and even high dose escalation may be inadequate to maintain in a symptom-free state individuals with a mechanically defective lower esophageal sphincter and volume regurgitation [1]. Furthermore, there are growing concerns over the long-term impact of chronic acid suppression on multiple metabolic and physiologic pathways, and there is evidence that patients suffering from uncontrolled esophageal acid exposure may progress to serious complications of the disease, such as pulmonary aspiration and fibrosis, esophagitis and peptic stricture, and Barrett's metaplasia, the leading risk factor for esophageal adenocarcinoma [2].

The laparoscopic Nissen fundoplication is the current surgical gold standard for the treatment of gastroesophageal reflux disease. This procedure is safe, effective and durable if performed in specialized centers with appropriate technique and correct indications. A multicenter European trial comparing medical therapy with fundoplication performed by expert surgeons showed that 92% of medical patients and 85% of surgical patients remained in remission at 5 years of follow-up [3]. Despite a remarkably low morbidity and mortality rates, the Nissen fundoplication, is underused due to the perceived side effects and fear of failure in the long-term. As a consequence, only patients with severe symptoms/complications and partial response to pharmacological therapy are usually referred for fundoplication [4].

The most common side effects of the Nissen fundoplication are bloating, inability to belch and vomit, and persistent dysphagia that may occasionally require revisional surgery. These are the main reasons why gastroenterologists tend to limit their referrals for fundoplication only to patients with long-lasting severe disease

L. Bonavina (✉) • A. Sironi • E. Asti
Division of General Surgery, Department of Biomedical Sciences for Health, IRCCS Policlinico San Donato, University of Milano School of Medicine,
Via Morandi 30, 20097, San Donato Milanese, Milano, Italy
e-mail: luigi.bonavina@unimi.it

M.A. Memon (ed.), *Hiatal Hernia Surgery*,
https://doi.org/10.1007/978-3-319-64003-7_8

and large hiatal hernias, and a reduced utilization of surgical fundoplication has been noted in the United States over the past decade [5].

The limitations of both drug therapy and fundoplication have left many patients and clinicians in the ambiguous position to either tolerate a life-time drug dependence with incomplete symptom relief, or to undertake the risk of a surgical procedure that alters gastric anatomy, may have substantial side-effects, and may deteriorate over time. The Linx™ Reflux Management System is an FDA approved method aimed to provide a permanent solution to gastroesophageal reflux disease by augmenting the sphincter barrier with a standardized laparoscopic procedure.

8.1 Biomechanics of Magnetic Sphincter Augmentation

The Linx is a mechanical device that consists of a series of biocompatible titanium beads with magnetic cores hermetically sealed inside. The beads are interlinked with independent titanium wires to form an expandable ring. The beads can move independent of the adjacent beads, creating a dynamic implant that does not compress the esophagus and does not limit its range of motion upon swallowing, belching, and vomiting. The Linx is designed to augment the physiologic barrier to reflux by magnetic force and is manufactured in different sizes: for reflux to occur, the intragastric pressure must overcome the resistance to opening of both the patient's native LES pressure and the magnetic bonds of the device. The device, while augmenting the LES, allows for expansion to accommodate a swallowed bolus or the escape of elevated gastric pressure associated with belching or vomiting. Following the implant, the Linx is encapsulated in a fibrous tissue reaction outside the esophageal wall, making possible its surgical removal without damaging the esophagus. The device has recently received magnetic resonance imaging approval for scanning in systems up 1.5 T.

8.2 Operative Technique and Perioperative Management

The device is implanted under general anesthesia using a typical 5-port laparoscopic access. The Linx procedure requires a few standardized steps and dissection should be minimized with preservation of the phreno-esophageal ligament (Fig. 8.1). The operation starts by dividing the peritoneum on the anterior surface of the gastroesophageal junction below the insertion of the inferior leaf of the phreno-esophageal ligament and above the hepatic branch of the anterior vagus nerve. The lateral surface of the left crus is freed from the posterior fundic wall without dividing any short gastric vessel. The gastro-hepatic ligament is opened above and below the hepatic branch to facilitate the preparation of the retro-esophageal window. Gentle dissection from the right side is made towards the left crus just above the crural decussation to identify the posterior vagus nerve. A tunnel is then created between the vagus and the posterior esophageal wall, and a penrose drain is passed in a left

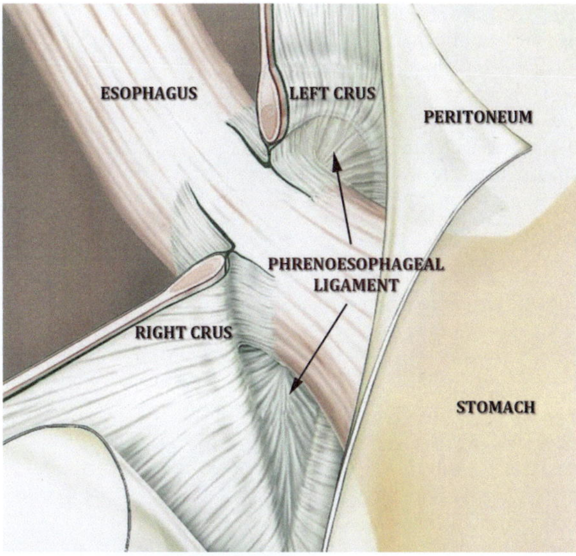

Fig. 8.1 Anatomy of the gastroesophageal junction. Minimal dissection with possible preservation of phreno-esophageal ligament is required to implant the magnetic sphincter augmentation device

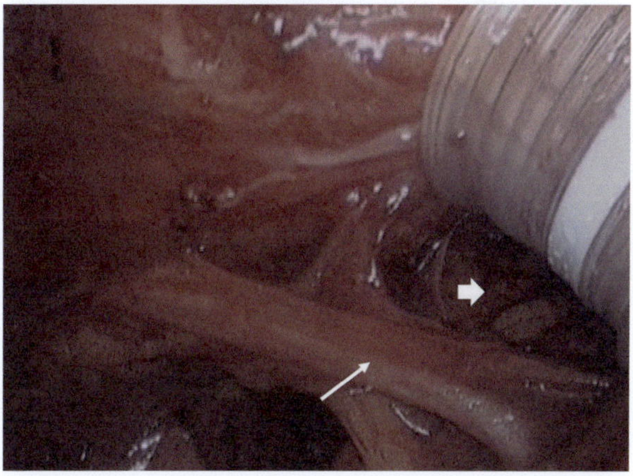

Fig. 8.2 Laparoscopic view of the retro-esophageal dissection. A tunnel between esophagus and posterior esophageal is made to insert the Linx device in the proper position

to right direction (Fig. 8.2). The circumference of the esophagus is measured to determine the proper size of the Linx device to be implanted. The sizing tool is a laparoscopic instrument with a soft, circular curved tip actuated through a handset with a numerical indicator that corresponds to the size range of the Linx device. The gauge is placed around the esophagus in the tunnel made between the esophageal wall and the posterior vagus nerve bundle. The appropriate size of Linx device is introduced through the tunnel and its opposing ends/clasps are brought to the anterior surface of the esophagus and engaged together. The decision to proceed with a posterior crural repair depends on the size of the hernia found intra-operatively: in most patients with a small and reducible hernia, a formal hiatus repair is usually not necessary if the lower mediastinum has not been entered (Fig. 8.3).

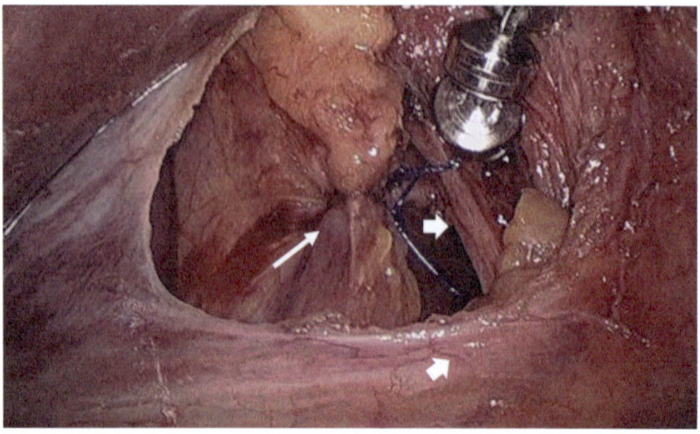

Fig. 8.3 Linx procedure and posterior hiatoplasty: crura repair (*arrow*), posterior vagus (*upper arrowhead*), preserved hepatic branch of the anterior vagus (*lower arrowhead*)

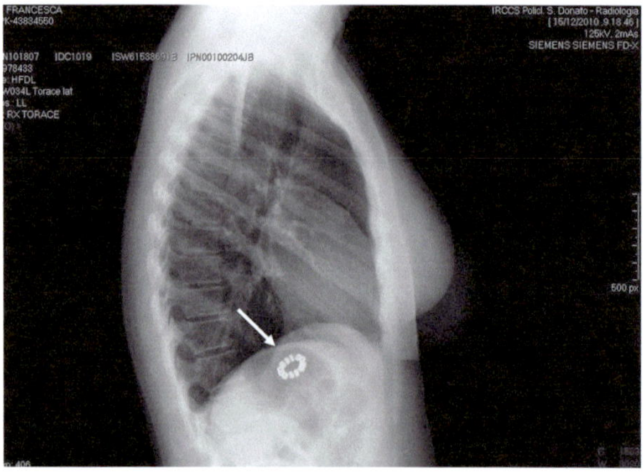

Fig. 8.4 Chest film lateral view showing the Linx device in the sub-diaphragmatic position with typical inclination angle

A chest film is performed after surgery to check the correct placement of the device (Fig. 8.4), and patients are discharged the same day or on the first post-operative day. They are counselled to progressively return to a normal diet, chew well and take small volume meals, and discontinue the use of proton pump inhibitors.

8.3 Synopsis of Clinical Experience

The first clinical implant of Linx device was performed a decade ago. Since then, all reported studies have consistently confirmed a high rate of symptom relief and discontinuation of PPI therapy, an objective reduction of esophageal acid exposure, and an improved quality of life.

The *feasibility study* included 44 patients implanted with the Linx at four study centers in USA and in Europe between February 2007 and October 2008. The short-term, mid-term, 4-year, and final results of this study have been previously published [6–9]. In the feasibility study patients served as their own control to assess the effect of treatment on esophageal acid exposure, symptoms, and use of proton pump inhibitors. The primary criteria for inclusion in the trial were age >18 and <85 years, typical reflux symptoms at least partially responsive to proton pump inhibitors, abnormal esophageal acid exposure, and normal contractile amplitude and wave form in the esophageal body. The primary criteria for exclusion were history of dysphagia, previous upper abdominal surgery, previous endoluminal antireflux procedures, sliding hiatal hernia >3 cm, esophagitis >grade A, and/or the presence of histologically documented Barrett's esophagus. Patients with abnormal manometric findings (distal esophageal contraction amplitude of <35 mmHg on wet swallows or <70% propulsive peristaltic sequences) were also excluded. Preoperative evaluation consisted of symptom questionnaire and Gastro-Esophageal Reflux Disease-Health Related Quality of Life (GERD-HRQL) questionnaire, upper gastrointestinal endoscopy, barium swallow, standard esophageal manometry, and 24–48 h esophageal pH monitoring. All Linx devices were successfully implanted via a standard laparoscopic approach. The median operative time was 40 min. No intraoperative complications occurred. Patients were instructed to resume a regular diet after a chest film and radiological assessment of the esophageal transit were performed. All patients except one were discharged within 48 h. Thirty-three patients (75%) were followed at 5 years. The mean total GERD-HRQL score off PPI decreased from 25.7 at baseline to 2.9 at year 5 ($p < 0.001$), and 94% (31/33) patients had a >50% reduction in the total score compared to baseline; 91% of patients reported of being satisfied with their current condition. Esophageal pH testing was completed in 20 patients at 5 years: 85% of patients achieved either normal esophageal acid exposure or had at least a 50% reduction from baseline. Normalization of esophageal pH was achieved in 70% of patients. Complete cessation of drug therapy or a reduction of 50% or more of the daily dose at 5 years was achieved by 88% and 94% of patients, respectively. Forty-three percent of patients complained of mild dysphagia during the postoperative period which resolved by 3 months without treatment. Laparoscopic device explant was necessary because of persistent dysphagia in one patient, the need to undergo magnetic resonance imaging in another, and the persisting reflux symptoms in a third individual.

A *randomized single-arm trial* was performed in a cohort of 100 patients at 13 centers in the United States and one in the Netherlands [10]. The criteria of inclusion and perioperative subjective and objective evaluations were similar to the feasibility study. Significant improvements were seen in GERD related quality of life, regurgitation, and esophageal acid exposure. Use of PPI dropped to 13% at 3 years and patient satisfaction with reflux control increased to 94% after implantation. Importantly, these positive results were stable showing no degradation over the study time period. Although 14% of patients reported non severe bloating after implantation, all study patients retained their ability to belch and vomit. Dysphagia was present to some extent in 68% of patients but decreased to 4% by 3 years. Five percent of patients rated the dysphagia as severe and required endoscopic balloon dilation or surgical removal of device with complete resolution.

Two *single-center studies* have further validated the efficacy of the Linx procedure. In Milan, Italy, 100 consecutive patients underwent Linx implantation between 2007 and 2012. The median implant duration was 3 years, ranging from 378 days to 6 years. There was a significant reduction of acid exposure time and improvement of GERD-HRQL score, and freedom from daily dependence on PPI was achieved in 85% of the patients [11]. Another study from USA, including 66 patients with an average follow-up of 5.8 months, showed similar satisfactory results [12].

Three *case-control studies* found comparable control of reflux symptoms after surgical fundoplication or Linx implant up to 1 year follow up. However, the fundoplication group showed a higher rate of patients with inability to belch and vomit, along with more severe gas-bloat symptoms [13–15].

A *safety profile analysis study* of the first 1000 implants in 82 hospitals worldwide showed 1.3% hospital readmission rate, 5.6% need of postoperative endoscopic dilations, and 3.4% reoperation rate [16]. All reoperations were performed non-emergently for device removal. Among the 36 patients who had the device removed, the most commons symptoms were dysphagia and recurrence of reflux symptoms. In addition, 7% of patients enrolled in the randomized multicenter single-arm trial had the device removed due to persistent dysphagia in four, vomiting in one, chest pain in one, and reflux in one [17].

A *single-center cohort study* focused on reoperations for Linx removal and reported the long-term results of one-stage laparoscopic removal and fundoplication [18]. Eleven (6.7%) out of 164 patients who underwent a laparoscopic Linx implant with a median follow-up of 48 months were explanted at a later date. The main presenting symptom requiring device removal was recurrence of heartburn or regurgitation in 46%, dysphagia in 37%, and chest pain in 18%. In two patients (1.2%) full-thickness erosion of the esophageal wall with partial endoluminal penetration of the device occurred. Although the course of this complication appeared to be benign and easy to treat, it is possible that the long-term erosion rate of the Linx device will be higher than it has been reported so far. The median implant duration was 20 months, with 82% of the patients being explanted between 12 and 24 months after the implant. Device removal was combined with partial fundoplication, most commonly Toupet or Dor, in 11 patients and with reconstruction of the angle of His in one. There were no conversions to laparotomy and the postoperative course was uneventful in all patients. At the latest follow-up after reoperation (1–5 years), the GERD-HRQL score was within normal limits in all patients.

8.4 Role of Magnetic Sphincter Augmentation in Hiatus Hernia

The Linx procedure was developed as a less invasive and more standardized surgical option for patients who are partially responders to proton pump inhibitors, have troublesome regurgitation or develop progressive symptoms despite continuous medical therapy. Minimal dissection is required to create the space where the device would encircle the lower esophageal sphincter area when implanted. Proper surgical dissection with preservation of the phreno-esophageal ligament allows objective sizing of the distal esophagus and placement of the magnetic device at the esophago-gastric junction without altering gastric anatomy and without entering the mediastinum. A more extensive dissection is needed only when the distal esophagus does not easily reduce into the abdomen or when there is intraoperative evidence of sliding hiatus hernia. In such circumstances, a posterior crural repair can be added to the Linx procedure. In a single center series, a hiatoplasty was performed in 44% of patients with 1–2 non-resorbable stitches; however, a formal mediastinal dissection was required only in three patients with type I or III hernia. The presence of a hiatus hernia and the concurrent crura repair were not predictive of subsequent removal of the device [11]. On the other hand, a more recent study has concluded that the Linx procedure can be safely offered to patients with hiatal hernia larger than 3 cm [19]. A total of 192 implanted patients were reviewed, and 52 (27%) had a large hernia. Compared to patients with smaller hernias, postoperative requirement of proton pump inhibitors was less and mean GERD-HRQL scores were lower. Also, the rate of postoperative intervention for dysphagia and the incidence of symptom resolution or improvement were similar.

8.5 Conclusions

The Linx procedure provides a simple and physiologic solution to gastroesophageal reflux with a favorable side-effect profile. Magnetic sphincter augmentation is highly effective in decreasing esophageal acid exposure, reducing typical reflux symptoms, reducing daily drug dependence, and improving patients' quality of life. Safety issues such as device erosions or migrations have been rare and not associated with mortality. The device can be easily removed if necessary, thereby preserving the option of fundoplication or other therapies in the future. The potential limitations of this innovative procedure are the current contraindication to undergo scanning in MRI systems >1.5 T, and the potential long-term consequences of a permanent foreign body implant. The efficacy of the Linx in the presence of large hiatal hernia and Barrett's esophagus remains to be tested in further comparative studies.

What Is the Current Knowledge and What Future Direction Is Required

- Magnetic sphincter augmentation provides a minimally invasive and standardized antireflux repair in patients with small hiatus hernia.
- It is effective in decreasing esophageal acid exposure, reducing typical reflux symptoms and drug dependence, and improving patients' quality of life.
- Device erosions have been rare and not associated with mortality.
- The device can be removed, if necessary, without side-effects.
- Scanning with magnetic resonance systems >1.5 T is currently contraindicated.

References

1. Kahrilas PJ, Howden CW, Hughes N. Response of regurgitation to proton pump inhibitor therapy in clinical trials of gastroesophageal reflux disease. Am J Gastroenterol. 2011;106:1419–25.
2. Malfertheiner P, Nocon M, Vieth M, et al. Evolution of gastro-oesophageal reflux disease over 5 years under routine medical care – the ProGERD study. Aliment Pharmacol Ther. 2012;35:154–64.
3. Galmiche JP, Hatlebakk J, Attwood S, et al. Laparoscopic antireflux surgery vs esomeprazole treatment for chronic GERD: the LOTUS randomized clinical trial. JAMA. 2011;305(19):1969–77.
4. Richter JE, Dempsey DT. Laparoscopic antireflux surgery: key to success in the community setting. Am J Gastroenterol. 2008;103:289–91.
5. Khan F, Maradey-Romero C, Ganocy S, Frazier R, Fass R. Utilisation of surgical fundoplication for patients with gastro-oesophageal reflux disease in the USA has declined rapidly between 2009 and 2013. Aliment Pharmacol Ther. 2016;43:1124–31.
6. Bonavina L, Saino G, Bona D, et al. Magnetic augmentation of the lower esophageal sphincter: results of a feasibility clinical trial. J Gastrointest Surg. 2008;12:2133–40.
7. Bonavina L, DeMeester TR, Fockens P, et al. Laparoscopic sphincter augmentation device eliminates reflux symptoms and normalizes esophageal acid exposure. Ann Surg. 2010;252:857–62.
8. Lipham JC, DeMeester TR, Ganz RA, et al. The Linx reflux management system: confirmed safety and efficacy now at 4 years. Surg Endosc. 2012;26:2944–9.
9. Saino G, Bonavina L, Lipham J, Dunn D, Ganz RA. Magnetic sphincter augmentation for gastroesophageal reflux at 5 years: final results of a pilot study show long-term acid reduction and symptom improvement. J Laparoendosc Adv Surg Tech A. 2015;25:787–92.
10. Ganz RA, Peters JH, Horgan S, et al. Esophageal sphincter device for gastroesophageal reflux disease. N Engl J Med. 2013;368:719–27.
11. Bonavina L, Saino G, Bona D, et al. One hundred consecutive patients treated with magnetic sphincter augmentation for gastroesophageal reflux disease: 6 years of clinical experience from a single center. J Am Coll Surg. 2013;217:577–85.
12. Smith CD, Devault KR, Buchanan M. Introduction of mechanical sphincter augmentation for gastroesophageal reflux disease into practice: early clinical outcomes and keys to successful adoption. J Am Coll Surg. 2014;218:776–81.
13. Louie BE, Farivar AS, Schultz D, et al. Short-term outcomes using magnetic sphincter augmentation versus Nissen fundoplication for medically resistant gastroesophageal reflux disease. Ann Thorac Surg. 2014;98:498–504.
14. Riegler M, Schoppman SF, Bonavina L, et al. Magnetic sphincter augmentation and fundoplication for GERD in clinical practice: one-year results of a multicenter, prospective observational study. Surg Endosc. 2015;29:1123–9.
15. Reynolds J, Zehetner J, Wu P, et al. Laparoscopic magnetic sphincter augmentation vs laparoscopic Nissen fundoplication; a matched-pair analysis of 100 patients. Ann Surg. 2015;221:123–8.
16. Lipham JC, Taiganides PA, Louie BE, et al. Safety analysis of first 1000 patients treated with magnetic sphincter augmentation for gastroesophageal reflux disease. Dis Esophagus. 2015;28:305–11.
17. Ganz RA, Edmundowicz SA, Taiganides PA, et al. Long-term outcomes of patients receiving a magnetic sphincter augmentation device for gastroesophageal reflux. Clin Gastroenterol Hepatol. 2016;14:671–7.
18. Asti E, Siboni S, Lazzari V, et al. Removal of the magnetic sphincter device. Surgical technique and results of a single-center cohort study. Ann Surg. 2017;265(5):941–5. PMID:27163959.
19. Rona KA, Reynolds J, Schwameis K, et al. Efficacy of magnetic sphincter augmentation in patients with large hiatal hernias. Surg Endosc. 2017;31(5):2096–102. PMID:27553803.

Chapter 9
Laparoscopic Repair of Paraesophageal Hiatus Hernia: Suture Cruroplasty or Prosthetic Repair

Manjunath Siddaiah-Subramanya, Breda Memon, and Muhammed Ashraf Memon

9.1 Introduction

Large paraesophageal hiatus hernias (PHH) account for almost 50% of the cases encountered during contemporary laparoscopic hiatal hernia repair [1] (Fig. 9.1). PHH, using upper gastrointestinal contrast study, was first reported in 1926 [2]. Since the introduction of laparoscopic hiatal hernia repair in 1991 [3], there has been contentious debate as to which surgical method of repair offers the best outcome in these large PHH in the chronic setting. The four available methods i.e., conventional laparoscopic, robotic, transthoracic and open transabdominal, have shown more or less equivalent results [4]. Furthermore, there also remains discussion regarding the technical aspects of surgical repair which requires two critical

M. Siddaiah-Subramanya, M.B.B.S., M.R.C.S., F.R.A.C.S.
Department of General Surgery, Logan Hospital, Meadowbrook, Brisbane, QLD, Australia
e-mail: manjunathbss9@yahoo.com

B. Memon, R.N., L.L.B., P.G.C.Ed.
South East Queensland Surgery (SEQS) and Sunnybank Obesity Centre,
Suite 9, McCullough Centre, 259 McCullough Street, Sunnybank, QLD, Australia
e-mail: bmemon@yahoo.com

M.A. Memon, M.B.B.S., F.A.C.S., F.R.A.C.S. (✉)
South East Queensland Surgery (SEQS) and Sunnybank Obesity Centre,
Suite 9, McCullough Centre, 259 McCullough Street, Sunnybank, QLD, Australia

Mayne Medical School, School of Medicine, University of Queensland,
Brisbane, QLD, Australia

Faculty of Health Sciences and Medicine, Bond University, Gold Coast, QLD, Australia

Faculty of Health and Social Science, Bolton University, Bolton, Lancashire, UK

School of Agricultural, Computing and Environmental Sciences, International Centre for Applied Climate Sciences and Centre for Health Sciences Research, University of Southern Queensland, Toowoomba, QLD, Australia
e-mail: mmemon@yahoo.com

M.A. Memon (ed.), *Hiatal Hernia Surgery*,
https://doi.org/10.1007/978-3-319-64003-7_9

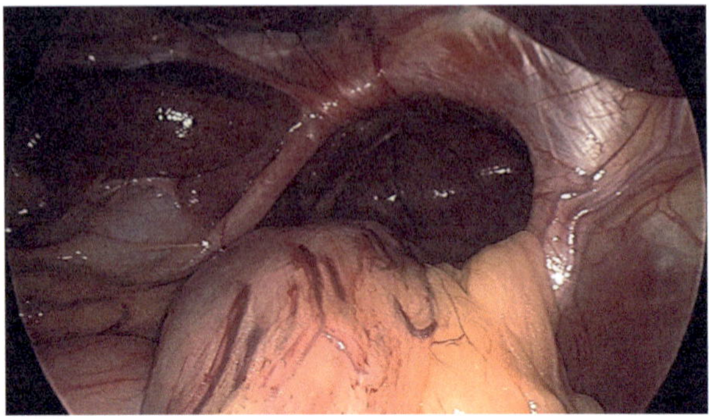

Fig. 9.1 Large PHH

steps in the repair of these large PHH; (1) aggressive mobilization of the esophagus to restore intra-abdominal length to minimize axial tension; and (2) selecting the best way to close the crural pillars of these large PHH. Crural closure can be achieved either by using suture or mesh because the dehiscence of ineffective crural repair due to radial tension may lead to intrathoracic migration of the wrap. This may result in either acute hiatal hernia requiring emergency surgery or recurrence of reflux and/or dysphagia over a period of time requiring difficult revisional surgery. These issues will have significant impact on the patient's short and long term outcome and quality of life (QOL). Several studies analyzing laparoscopic repair of very large PHH by X-ray or endoscopy reveal between 11% and 67% failure rate due to disruption of the hiatal hernia repair suggesting significant room for improvement [5–9]. It has also been suggested that the inherent actions of the diaphragm during both respiratory (breathing, sneezing and coughing) and non-respiratory (vomiting, straining at stools and laughing) movements exerts repetitive stress upon the repair of the crura, which if closed under tension using suture technique may lead to the disruption of such a repair. However, it has been proposed that the addition of mesh in a tension free manner as an alternative to reinforce the crural pillars may decrease hiatal disruption and reduce the recurrence rate by minimizing radial tension. Nevertheless, non-absorbable mesh poses its own complications which include mesh infection, migration, shrinkage and erosion into esophagus or stomach thereby making revisional surgery extremely challenging and hazardous [10].

The current chapter will address an area of controversy i.e., the use of prosthetic material (mesh) at the esophageal hiatus and whenever possible will compare it to suture cruroplasty based on up-to-date clinical literature. The objective of the following discussion is to discuss the clinical outcomes, safety and effectiveness and complications of the two commonly used methods for elective surgical repair of large hiatal hernias.

9.2 Epidemiology

PHH is not an uncommon entity. Surgeons in the twenty-first century encounter PHH in almost 50% of the cases during laparoscopic hiatal hernia repair [1]. PHH predisposes to gastroesophageal reflux disease (GERD) [11] and therefore the incidence of symptomatic cases of PHH is closely related to the diagnosis of GERD. Risk factors for developing PHH include body mass index (BMI) of >25, age > 50 and male sex. Increasing age is not only an independent risk factor for the development of GERD [12], but also increases the incidence of PHH. This is evident in a number of population based studies in various continents [13–16]. There is also a familial preponderance for developing PHH as it confers a 20-fold increased risk of developing PHH in younger siblings of children with this condition [17].

9.3 Patient Selection and Indications for PHH Repair

Patient selection and preoperative evaluation are crucial for successful PHH repair especially in elderly patients with multiple comorbidities. Larusson and his team [18] concluded that age, American Society of Anesthesiologists (ASA) score, and type of operation are significant predictive factors in patients undergoing laparoscopic PHH repair. The investigators advised caution in balancing surgical indications with each patient's comorbidities, age, symptoms, and potentially life-threatening complications. Asymptomatic large PHH or those with minimal symptoms although uncommon, may be observed over a period of time, a strategy called 'watchful waiting' and only after these patients have been counselled regarding the risks of incarceration or strangulation which may require surgery in about 1.2% of the cases and carries mortality of 5.4% [19]. These patients, therefore, should be educated about the appropriate work-up in an elective situation in case emergency surgery is required in the future [20]. However, symptomatic PHH in reasonably fit patients should be offered an elective surgical option [21]. The most common symptoms include gastroesophageal reflux disease (GERD), non-cardiac chest pain, anemia, cardiac arrhythmias, aspiration and shortness of breath. Obstructive symptoms include early satiety, dysphagia and postprandial chest pain.

9.4 Diagnostic Evaluation

Preoperative evaluation for PHH repair requires four main studies which include (1) video esophagogram, a dynamic study which provides information about the overall size and position of the stomach within the hernia; (2) esophagogastroduodenoscopy which can provide information about the mucosa of the stomach and its associated conditions such as Cameron's erosions, erosive esophagitis, and Barrett's esophagus (Fig. 9.2). Additionally, it provides valuable information about Hill's endoscopic classification of hernia (Fig. 9.3), level of esophagogastric junction, length of the esophagus and importantly to rule out malignancy; (3) high resolution impedance manometry (HRIM) proves valuable in planning the antireflux procedure which is part and parcel of hernia repair, whilst knowledge of motility patterns help plan the type of wrap created in these patients; and (4) lastly if GERD is a dominant symptom, 24 h ambulatory pH study will provide an objective score of

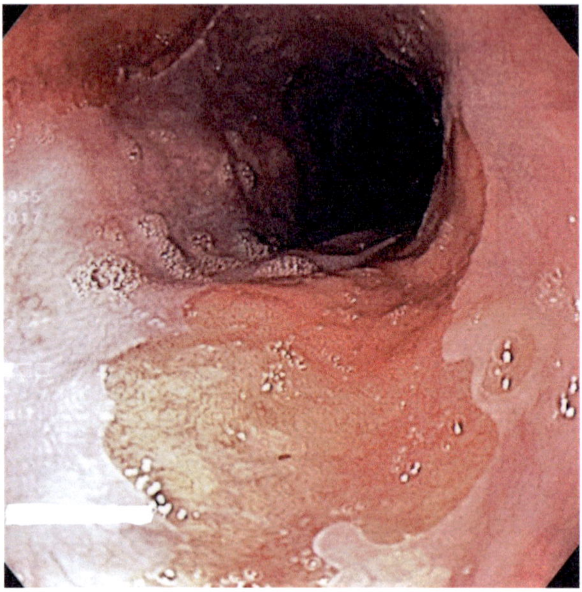

Fig. 9.2 Endoscopic view of Barrett's esophagitis

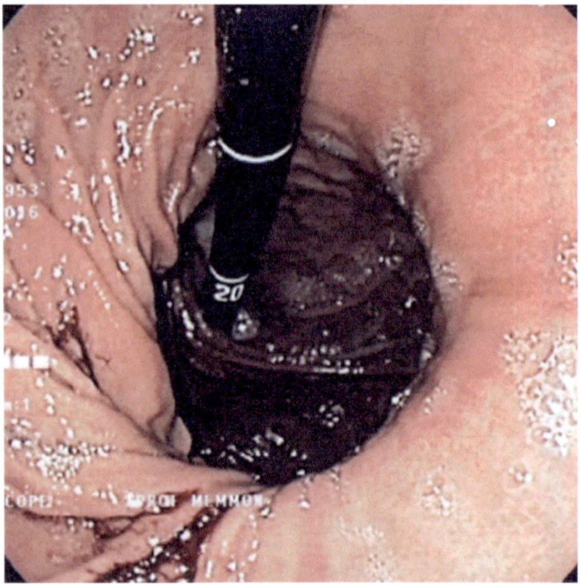

Fig. 9.3 Endoscopic view Hill's grade IV PHH

GERD symptoms (Fig. 9.4). This baseline investigation can be quite useful should symptoms or problems develop in the future postoperatively. In addition to the above baseline foregut studies, depending on patients symptoms and co-morbidities, other investigations which may be of value in the preoperative period include nuclear medicine gastric emptying studies; chest and abdomen computerized

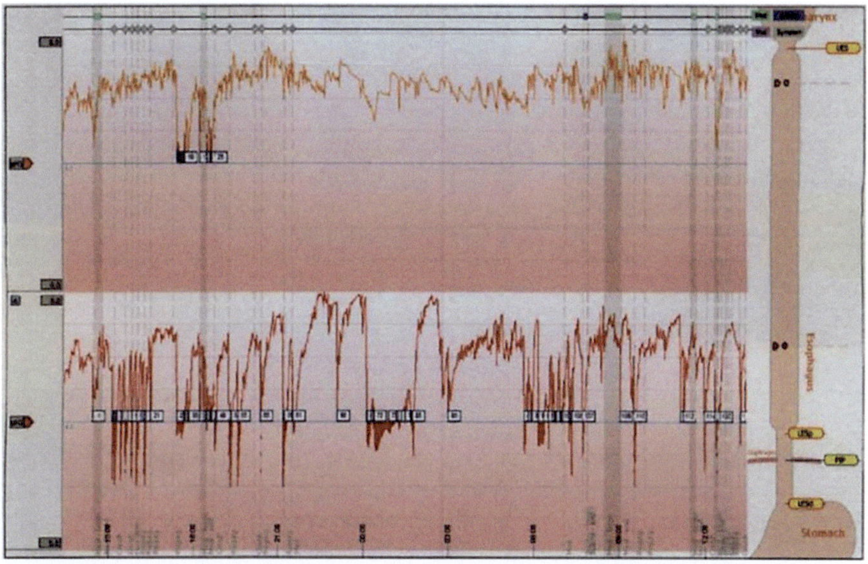

Fig. 9.4 24-h ambulatory pH study showing objective evidence of reflux

tomography, pulmonary function tests, cardiac stress testing and echocardiogram in elderly patients with chest pain.

9.5 Basic Principles for Laparoscopic Repair PHH

Many of the principles of standard fundoplication apply to PHH repair, the most important of which is the tension free repair of the crura [22]. The standard approach in the twenty-first century is laparoscopically via the abdomen although some great results achieved through a transthoracic approach in the twentieth century have to be acknowledged. In a study by Maziak et al. [23], 93% of the patients reported excellent results with a 10 year follow up with only 2 recurrences needing reoperation. However, this technique has fallen into disrepute because of the painful thoracotomy incision, insertion of chest tube, prolonged length of hospital stay and difficult reoperations in cases of complications or recurrence.

The four critical steps of the laparoscopic PHH operation include: (1) excision of the hernia sac in its entirety; (2) adequate mediastinal esophageal mobilization; (3) crural repair and (4) addition of fundoplication [24]. Incomplete dissection of the sac increases the risk of intrathoracic migration of the wrap and recurrence. Some studies have made use of this sac to provide cover to the mesh applied over the crura [7]. Similarly, incomplete mobilization of the esophagus to achieve adequate abdominal length of the esophagus (2–5 cm) or even the addition of Colles gastroplasty to achieve this maneuver in the case of a short esophagus is a vital step in preventing wrap migration and recurrence postoperatively [9]. The crural repair can be achieved either with sutures or a mesh. Cruroplasty is achieved with non-absorbable sutures, either in an interrupted or a continuous fashion (Fig. 9.5). Most of the sutures are placed posterior to the esophagus, although some may need to be placed anteriorly if the crura remains splayed after posterior cruroplasty [8, 25]. It is also common to reduce the intra-abdominal insufflation pressure while approximating the crura, especially for the large PHH. Some surgeons use mesh to reinforce the crural repair and the choice of mesh depends on personal preference of the surgeon and the size of the hiatal defect e.g., some choose to use mesh only when the hiatal defect is large or >5 cm [26, 27]. Mesh cruroplasty may significantly increase operating time (15–50 cm) as reported in a recent meta-analysis [28], but does not necessarily increase the rate of conversion to open [29]. It is standard to perform a fundoplication following crural closure. The type of fundoplication varies from complete to partial anterior or posterior fundoplication. Most common types are Nissen [30–32] (Fig. 9.6) and Toupet [33, 34]. Some surgeons in addition to fundoplication, suture the wrap to the crura or the stomach to the anterior abdominal wall or use tube gastrostomy to further prevent recurrence [7, 35]. The use of a bougie at the time of crural repair or while performing the wrap seems to be practiced by some surgeons [30, 31, 36]. However, it has fallen out of favor and is not considered as standard practice. This is because it possibly contributes to future recurrence by leaving a larger than required gap following cruroplasty [24].

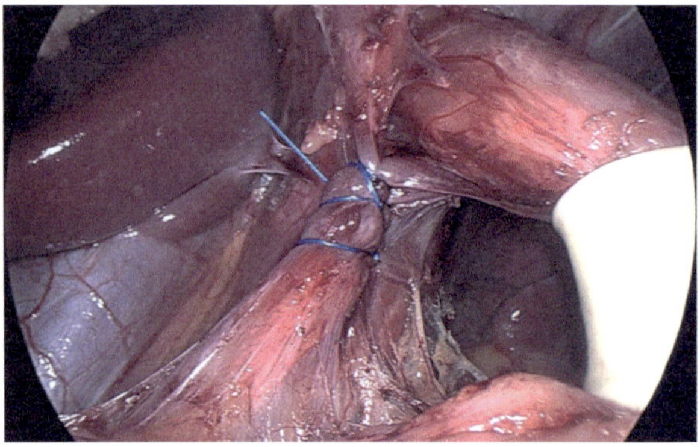

Fig. 9.5 Laparoscopic view of posterior suture cruroplasty using continuous 0 V-Loc™ suture

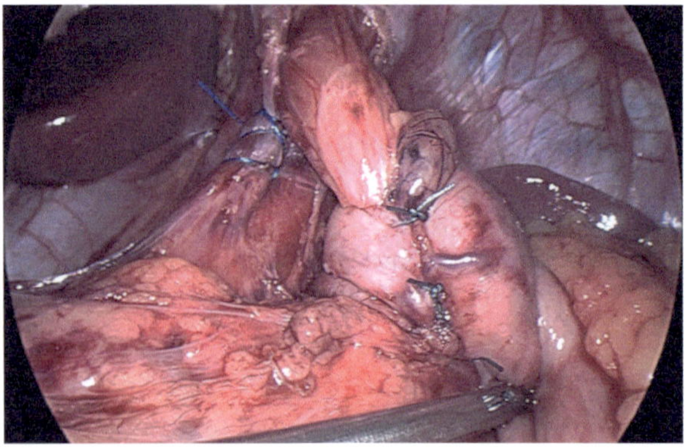

Fig. 9.6 Laparoscopic view of posterior suture cruroplasty and Nissen fundoplication

9.6 Prosthetic Material Versus Sutures for Repair of PHH

An area of controversy is the use of prosthetic material (mesh) at the esophageal hiatus to provide additional support (Figs. 9.7 and 9.8). The majority of surgical mesh are constructed from synthetic materials or animal tissue. Synthetic mesh can be knitted or non-knitted sheet forms and can be absorbable, non-absorbable or a combination of these two. Animal-tissue mesh (bovine or porcine) are either made up of intestine or skin, and are absorbable. Non-absorbable mesh will remain in the body indefinitely and is considered a permanent implant. Absorbable mesh will degrade and lose strength over time. It is not intended to provide long-term

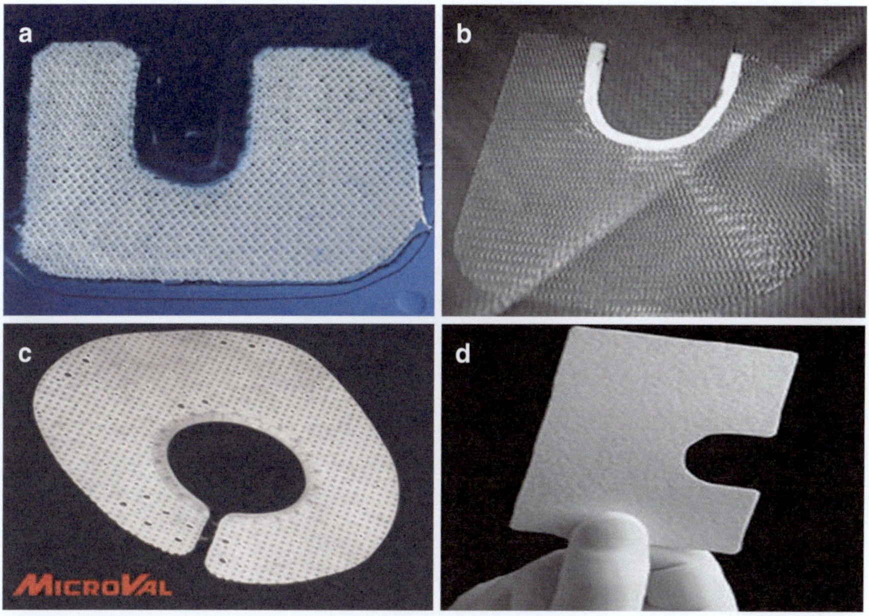

Fig. 9.7 Different types of meshes used to reinforce hiatal defect: (**a**) Covidien Paritex; (**b**) Polypropylene mesh with silicone catheter; (**c**) MicroVal; (**d**) Gore Bio-A tissue reinforcement

Fig. 9.8 Large hiatus hernia reinforced with Gore Bio-A mesh

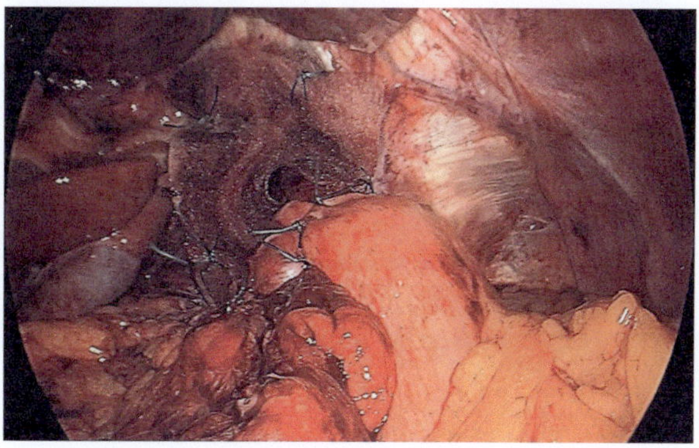

reinforcement to the repair site. As the material degrades, new tissue growth is intended to provide strength to the repair. According to DeMeester [24] the characteristics of an ideal mesh for use at the hiatus include: (1) it should be absorbable with no tendency to erode; (2) easy to use in terms of introducing, positioning, and fixating; (3) provide long-term, effective strengthening of the crural closure and reduce the risk of a recurrent hernia, and (4) it should not preclude a safe reoperation if necessary.

In order to improve upon the high recurrence rate of suture cruroplasty, Carlson and his team, in 1999 [30], reported the very first randomized controlled trial (RCT) of laparoscopic prosthetic reinforcement of large hiatal hernia. Since then, many comparative trials [7–9, 25–27, 31–33, 36–41] and meta-analyses and systematic reviews [28, 42, 43] comparing suture cruroplasty versus mesh repair of large PHH have been published, analyzing various aspects of these two approaches (Table 9.1). Amongst the RCTs, two studies have made use of non-absorbable PTFE meshes [30, 31] and one of prolene mesh [32], while two others have used absorbable (Surgisis® Cook Ireland) meshes with varying results [9, 41]. Similarly, a diverse range of meshes have been used in various other prospective and retrospective studies (Table 9.1). These include vicryl [26], ultrapro [26] and acellular dermal matrix [40]. These meshes have been applied for crural closure in various configurations which include a keyhole or circular configuration [31, 34] where the mesh surrounds the abdominal part of the esophagus, while others have used the mesh in "U" [33, 36], square or rectangular arrangements [7, 39] over the crura posterior to the esophagus. Some have even used the mesh as a bridge when the crural pillars could not be opposed [36, 38]. Although the majority of the surgeons have used staples [27, 30, 36], and tacks [25] to secure the mesh, some have utilized sutures which includes Ethibond® [26, 27, 34, 36, 39], polyster [30], prolene [7], silk [40] or polybutester (V-Loc™) for either cruroplasty or/and to secure the mesh. Lastly fibrin glue has also been increasingly used for mesh fixation to the crura in recent days [44].

9.7 Mesh Complications

The significant complications related to the use of mesh in hiatal hernia surgery, include mesh infection, mesh erosion [45, 46], adhesions and fibrosis, migration of the wrap into the thoracic cavity (recurrence) and fistulae making revisional surgery very challenging even in the hands of the most experienced surgeons. Mesh related complications have been reported to range from 1.3 to 20% [47]. However, a recent systematic review has contradicted such a high rate [43]. Furthermore, a recent meta-analysis confirms comparable low complication rates between suture and mesh cruroplasty in PHH repair [28]. Yet another systematic review has shown a very low complication rate of only 1.9% for the mesh group [42] dispelling the long held belief that mesh repair has a higher complication rate especially over a long period of time. Non-absorbable mesh related

Table 9.1 Salient features of various comparative studies

Author/year	Single/ multicenter	Patients		Follow-up	Age			Type of material	
		Suture	Mesh	Total group	Suture	Mesh	Hiatal defect		
		n	*n*	Months (mean or median with range or SD)	Years (mean with range or SD)	Years (mean with range or SD)	(cm)	Suture	Mesh group (material/fixation/ orientation)
Randomized controlled studies									
Carlson et al. (1999) [30]	Single	15	16	12–36 (only range)	NA	NA	>8	Non absorbable	PTFE/staples/keyhole
Frantzides et al. (2002) [31]	Multi	36	36	39.6 ± 20.4 (mean with SD)	63 (42–81)	58 (36–92)	>8	Non absorbable	PTFE/staples/keyhole
Granderath et al. (2005) [32]	Multi	50	50	12 (mean)	48.7 (24–73)	48.3 (22–71)	Any	Non absorbable	Prolene/sutured/posterior
Oelschlager et al. (2005/2011) [9]	Multi	57	51	58 ± 9.6 for suture group and 60 ± 9.6 for mesh group (median with SD)	64 ± 13	67 ± 11	Any	Non absorbable	Surgisis/NA/NA
Watson et al. (2015) [41]	Multi	43	83	12 (mean)	67.8 (no range)	68 (no range)	Any (>50% stomach in the chest)	Non absorbable	Surgisis/Timesh/Staples/ posterior

(continued)

Table 9.1 (continued)

		Patients		Follow-up	Age			Type of material	
		Suture	Mesh	Total group	Suture	Mesh	Hiatal defect		
Author/year	Single/ multicenter	*n*	*n*	Months (mean or median with range or SD)	Years (mean with range or SD)	Years (mean with range or SD)	(cm)	Suture	Mesh group (material/fixation/ orientation)
Prospective studies									
Leeder et al. (2003) [36]	Single	37	14	46 (18–89) (mean with range)	71 (45–92)	72 (61–85)	Large	Ethibond	Prolene/stapled/posterior "U" shaped
Ringley et al. (2006) [40]	Single	22	22	6.7 (mean with no range)	52.3 (33–75)	57.8 (34–75)	3–10	Silk	Acellular dermal matrix/ sutured/ posterior "U" shaped
Braghetto et al. (2010) [26]	Single	58	23	36 (mean with no range)	NA	NA	>5 for mesh group	Ethibond	Vicryl/ultrapro/surgisis/NA/NA
Retrospective studies									
Hui et al. (2001) [37]	Single	12	12	37 (24–48) (mean with range)	65 (no range)	61 (no range)	Large	Non absorbable	Gortex/prolene/marlex/NA/NA
Morino et al. (2006) [38]	Single	14	61	43 (28–68) (mean with range)	NA	NA	>5	Non absorbable	PTFE/prolene/NA/posterior "U" shaped

Muller-Stich et al. (2006) [27]	Single	40	16	52 (9–117) (mean with range)	NA	NA	Large	Ethibond	Surgipro/vypro/ staples/ posterior butterfly shaped
Zaninotto et al. (2007) [34]	Single	19	35	71 (39–97) (mean)	65 (59–67)	64 (59–69)	Large	Non absorbable	Goretex/prolene/sutured/ keyhole
Soricelli et al. (2009) [7]	Single	93	204	94 (51–135) (mean)	47.6 (no range)	47.5 (no range)	> 3 cm	Prolene	Prolene/staples/ posterior
Gouvas et al. (2011) [25]	Single	48	20	60 (no range) (mean)	NA	NA	Any	Non absorbable	Prolene/PTFE/tacks/keyhole/ posterior "U"
Goers et al. (2011) [39]	Single	33	56	11 (4–15) (mean)	61.8 (52–72)	64.5 (52–76)	Any	Ethibond	Biomesh/sutured/posterior
Dallemagne et al. (2011) [8]	Single	60	25	155 (98–177) (median)	NA	NA	Any	Non absorbable	PTFE/surgisis/NA/ posterior
Asti et al. (2016) [33]	Single	43	41	24 (no range) (median)	65.8 (52–79)	65.9 (55–75)	>5	Non absorbable	Biosynthetic/suture/ posterior "U" shaped

complications occur at an average of 17.3 months (range 1–120) postoperatively and includes dysphagia, heartburn, chest pain, weight loss, epigastric pain and fever from sepsis. Once again it is important to emphasize that these complications are rare [47] (Table 9.2).

9.7.1 Mesh Erosion

Mesh erosion leading to peritonitis, mediastinitis and death may have been observed in non-absorbable mesh [48, 49], but has not been seen in the biological absorbable mesh. These types of complications, although rare, will have significant impact on the patient's quality of life and may require major intervention such as esophageal resection [25]. Mesh erosion is rare and a recent systematic review reported this to be 0.2% [29]. Furthermore, two large studies which used non-absorbable mesh to close the hiatal defect have not shown any mesh complications [31, 50]. The first comparative study to report on biological mesh has not seen any mesh related complications with a follow up of just over 6 months [40]. Since then a few more studies including two RCTs have reported on the long term follow-up of biologic meshes [9, 41]. The longest follow up of biologic mesh was reported by Oelschlager et al. [9] with a mean follow up of 59 (range 40–78) months with no mesh complications. The biggest disadvantage of using biologic mesh seems to be a high recurrence rate of up to 54% over prolonged follow up as reported in the Seattle study [9].

9.7.2 Mesh Related Fibrosis

Extensive fibrosis from use of mesh is probably related to the type of mesh (non-absorbable), its configuration and the position with respect to the esophagus. A recent systematic review estimates it to be around 0.5% [29]. Non-absorbable mesh tends to contract far more than biological mesh leading to fibrosis and possibly esophageal stenosis at the site of insertion. Another reason why biologic mesh causes less complication is because they are less adhesive compared to non-absorbable mesh [29]. Moreover, it is also ill advised to encircle the abdominal esophagus in a circular or keyhole fashion using non-absorable mesh which may lead to esophageal stenosis and erosion of the mesh through the esophagus from mesh contraction. To alleviate this issue some surgeons suggest performing relaxation incisions on the diaphragm which are then reinforced with mesh which would be secured away from the esophagus and stomach. This will prevent possible mesh erosion into these visceras as the ensuing fibrosis will occur away from these hollow organs eliminating the risk of dysphagia [51, 52]. The repair of recurrent hiatus hernia in the presence of previous non-absorbable mesh repair, possess yet another challenge due to the extensive adhesions and fibrosis in the hiatal area. This makes the crura rigid and bringing them

Table 9.2 Salient features of intra- and postoperative variables

Authors/year	Complications		Postoperative Dysphagia		Conversion to Open		Reoperation		Recurrence	
	Suture group	Mesh group	Suture group	Mesh group	Suture group	Mesh group	Suture group	Mesh group	Suture group	Mesh group
	n (%)	*n* (%)	*n*	*n*	*n*	*n*	*n*	*n*	*n* (%)	*n* (%)
Randomized controlled studies										
Carlson et al. (1999) [30]	1	2	NA	NA	NA	NA	3	0	3 (19)	0
Frantzides et al. (2001) [31]	1	0	NA	NA	0	0	5	0	8 (22)	0
Granderath et al. (2005) [32]	0	0	2	2	0	0	NA	4	13 (26)	2 (4)
Oelschlager et al. (2005/2011) [9]	NA	NA	0	0	NA	NA	2	0	20 (59)	14 (54)
Watson et al. (2011) [41]	7	7	2	3	2	0	5	4	10 (23.1)	18 (21): 13 (30.1) for absorbable and 5 (12.8) for non-absorbable
Prospective studies										
Leeder et al. (2003) [36]	3 (8)	3 (21)	1	0	4	0	1	1	1 (3)	2 (14)
Ringley et al. (2006) [40]	4 (18)	4 (18)	1	1	0	0	0	0	2 (9)	0
Braghetto et al. (2010) [26]	NA	NA	NA	NA	NA	NA	0	0	10 (17)	0
Retrospective studies										
Hui et al. (2001) [37]	3 (25)	2 (17)	1	0	0	0	2	1	0	0

(continued)

Table 9.2 (continued)

	Complications		Postoperative Dysphagia		Conversion to Open		Reoperation		Recurrence	
	Suture group	Mesh group	Suture group	Mesh group	Suture group	Mesh group	Suture group	Mesh group	Suture group	Mesh group
Authors/year	*n* (%)	*n* (%)	*n*	*n*	*n*	*n*	*n*	*n*	*n* (%)	*n* (%)
Morino et al. (2006) [38]	NA	NA	3	4	0	0	5	5	10 (77)	13 (35)
Muller-Stich et al. (2006) [27]	8 (20)	5 (19)	6	3	0	0	2	0	7 (19)	0
Zaninotto et al. (2007) [34]	NA	NA	0	1	NA	NA	4	1	8 (42)	3 (8.6)
Soricelli et al. (2009) [7]	NA	NA	NA	NA	2	0	7	3	9 (19)	3 (2.1)
Gouvas et al. (2011) [25]	NA	NA	NA	NA	0	0	0	2	8 (12.7)	4 (4.4)
Goers et al. (2011) [39]	NA	NA	9	23	NA	NA	NA	NA	0	0
Dallemagne et al. (2011) [8]	NA	NA	3	0	0	0	3	0	14 (67)	9 (64)
Asti et al. (2016) [33]	2 (5)	2 (5)	1	1	0	0	0	0	8 (18.6)	4 (9.7)

together in a tension free manner may be impossible. Once again to facilitate a tension free repair in redo surgery, a partial thickness relaxing incision in the right crura followed by application of bioabsorable mesh to cover not only the relaxing incision but to reinforce the crural closure may be the most practical option [21].

9.7.3 Recurrence

In the published literature, there is no common or agreed definition of recurrence. While some described it as any amount of herniation (range 30–50%) of the wrap above the diaphragm [8, 38, 39], others feel that the migration of the wrap needs to be at least 2 cm above the diaphragm [9]. Some have suggested recurrence as the amount of separation between the crural pillars [30, 31]. However, a number of authors have not defined what they mean by recurrence in their studies, further muddying the water [7, 27, 32]. It is unclear whether migration of wrap or crural separation is a sound definition for recurrence or whether symptom recurrence such as heartburn, acid brash, water brash, etc. make up an integral part of the definition of recurrence. In these cases, objective evidence with 24-h ambulatory esophageal pH study should be considered for corroboration of symptoms as relying on subjective definitions for recurrence may result in overestimation of the rate of recurrence.

There are a number of ways to evaluate recurrence objectively. The most commonly adopted method is an esophagogram, which was utilized by almost all the studies evaluating recurrence [8, 9, 25–27, 30–33, 36, 37, 39–41] except for Soricelli et al. [7]. The second most common method was esophagogastroscopy (OGD) [7, 34, 38]. However, ambulatory esophageal pH study, which is considered to be the gold standard for objective evaluation of recurrence of GERD symptoms was utilized the least in the literature [25, 32, 38, 39].

It has been suggested that mesh cruroplasty may have a lower recurrence than suture cruroplasty in repair of PHH. To investigate this, there have been five RCTs and a number of prospective and retrospective studies performed since 1999. Patients with recurrence, present most commonly with chest pain and early satiety [43]. They may also complain of heartburn and regurgitation. While some of the studies [31, 34] report an absolute difference in recurrence favoring mesh repair ranging from 7 to 33%, others show no statistical difference at all between the two groups [8, 9, 26]. Overall, the recurrence rate with the mesh repair was significantly lower compared to suture repair (13% vs 24%) according to a recent systematic review analyzing 13 comparative trials comparing suture cruroplasty versus mesh repair for large PHH. Unfortunately, the authors have tried to pool the data from a varied level of evidence (I to III) producing a lot of heterogeneity making their results unreliable [43]. Furthermore, this disparity in recurrence rate was complicated by the fact that time to evaluation was skewed towards longer follow up after suture cruroplasty. Also only half of the patients in the mesh group were available for follow-up compared to 73% in the suture cohort, further distorting the results. This is in contrast to a recent meta-analysis which has purely looked at type

I evidence i.e., RCTs comparing suture versus mesh cruroplasty [28]. The results of this meta-analysis has shown no significant difference between the two cohorts of patients in terms of recurrence.

As far as the RCTs are concerned, Carlson et al. [30] reported the first RCT analyzing 31 patients with large PHH of 8 cm or greater undergoing suture vs mesh cruroplasty. Their follow-up ranged from 12 to 36 months. The author of this study demonstrated zero recurrence with mesh (PTFE) repair compared to 19% with suture only repair. Frantzides and colleagues [31] who used the same type of mesh in a larger group of patients (n = 72) similarly reported a significantly higher recurrence rate for suture cruroplasty compared to prosthetic repair (22% vs 0% respectively) at a median follow-up of 2.5 years [31]. Five of those eight recurrences needed reoperation with mesh repair, while the rest declined surgery. The hiatal defect in this study was also ≥8 cm. Granderath et al. [32] published their RCT data on 100 patients who were subjected to suture vs mesh cruroplasty. They utilized gastroscopy, 24-h ambulatory pH study and esophagogram at 3 and 12 months to evaluate their recurrence rate. Although a higher rate of recurrence (26%) was noted in the suture group compared to the mesh group (8%), the data regarding their outcome was not available and the follow up was short (12 months). Two further RCTs [9, 41] showed comparable recurrence rates, 59% vs 54% [9] and 23% vs 21% [41] between the suture and mesh groups respectively, at 60 and 12 months' follow-up respectively. The last two RCTs investigated the role of biologic mesh vs suture crural repair [9, 41]. Oelschlagers et al.'s study demonstrated an increasing incidence of recurrence and diminishing durability of the repair with time, irrespective of the material used, although mesh related complications with biologic mesh were nil [9]. This trial reported a 9% rate of recurrent hiatal hernia in the biologic prosthetic group compared to 24% in the suture cruroplasty group at 6 months' follow-up. However, at a median follow-up of 58 months analyzing the same cohort of 72 patients, the recurrence rate in both groups was similar; 59% in the suture cruroplasty group and 54% in the biologic prosthetic group. No statistical significant difference was noted in terms of relevant symptoms or QOL issues between the two groups. No mesh related complications were seen with biologic mesh. The authors of this study concluded that the benefit of biologic prosthesis in reducing hiatal hernia recurrence diminishes at long-term follow-up. These authors emphasized the validity of their results based on the following facts; (1) the objective manner of detecting postoperative recurrence by a blinded third party i.e., radiologists and (2) the participation of experienced laparoscopic surgeons from high volume esophageal surgical centers. However, they conceded that strict criteria used to diagnose the recurrence may have overestimated the recurrence rate. Nonetheless, the authors of this study feel that although the biologic mesh, may not protect against recurrent hiatal hernias, it may reduce the risk of severe hernias resulting in fewer reoperations as evident in their study. They also felt that compared to non-absorbable mesh with its known complications such as erosion into adjacent structures e.g., esophagus or stomach which leads to severe dysphagia, the biologic mesh has no long-term negative consequences. Other comparative studies investigating the role of these meshes in the last decade have shown no difference in the recurrence rate between suture and biological mesh groups [9, 33, 39–41].

Most of the retrospective comparative trials have shown significant lower recurrences in the mesh group (range 2.1–9.7%) compared to the suture group (range 12.7–42%) irrespective of the type of mesh used, its fixation technique, its orientation or the type of wrap performed [7, 25, 26, 34, 38–40], with the exception of studies by Morino et al. [38] and Dallemagne et al. [8]. Dallemagne's group [8] showed a high recurrence rate of 67% vs 64% in both suture and mesh groups respectively after a median follow up of 155 months, whereas Morino's group [38] also showed a higher recurrence rate for both groups although it was significantly higher for the suture group (77%) compared to the mesh cohort (35%) after a mean follow up of 43 months. Despite this high recurrence rate for both groups, the overall number of reoperations in each group were very low. A similar pattern was observed for various other prospective comparative trials with significantly lower recurrence rates in the mesh groups and almost no one needing any reoperation due to recurrence [26, 36, 40].

Recurrence may be concerning as the majority of them may have symptoms, but do they all require reoperation? This remains a moot point. Two studies showed no difference in QOL scores between the groups with and without recurrence after long term follow up [8, 9]. Patients were followed up for a mean period of 58 months in Oelschlager et al.'s study [9], while with Dallemagne et al's study [8], they were followed up for a median of 155 months. While Oelschlager and colleagues [9] used a combination of visual analog scores and a 36-item health survey questionnaire pre- and postoperatively, Dallemagne and colleagues [8] used a 36-item Gastrointestinal Quality of Life Index (GIQLI) developed by Eypasch [53] which was only done postoperatively. Seventy five percent of patients in Dallemagne et al.'s study reported significant improvement in their QOL and symptom improvement, scoring high on GIQLI [8]. Furthermore, although radiological recurrence was detected in two thirds of their patients, it had no impact on patients' QOL. Oelschlagers et al.'s study [9] on a long term follow-up of their patients undergoing suture and mesh cruroplasty, found no difference in the QOL score between the two cohorts. One can therefore conclude that subjective or even objective symptom recurrence may not be the indication for revisional surgery.

9.7.4 Reoperation

Obeid and Velanovich [54] defines reoperation as an operation required to address anatomical or symptomatic recurrence or other problems related to the index paraesophageal hiatal hernia repair. Reoperation rate after cruroplasty has been reported at 6% in the suture group and 3.7% in the mesh group in a systematic review by Tam et al. [43] It also estimates that the patients are 60% less likely to have reoperations following mesh cruroplasty compared to suture cruroplasty. A meta-analysis by Memon et al. [28], which analyzed only the RCTs, showed a significantly higher rate of reoperation for suture repair compared to the mesh group. A similar result was obtained by Muller-Stich et al. [42] in another systematic review where the reoperation rate for mesh repair was 2.4% compared to the suture group which was 8%. They also estimated that the chance of a patient needing reoperation in the first

3 years following mesh repair of PHH is half that of those repaired with sutures only. The main reasons for reoperation appear to be recurrence, mesh related complications, migration of wrap and dysphagia in the long term. Reoperation cannot be taken lightly as it has many disadvantages and difficulties. It carries higher mortality and morbidity, longer operative time, longer post-operative hospital stay, higher costs to patients and insurers and possibly a higher incidence of complications as a result of prolonged hospital stay [28].

Almost all of the reoperations were reported within the first postoperative year. The true incidence of reoperation over a longer period of time is not available for most studies simply because few authors have published their longitudinal data. Oelschlager et al. [9] published a median follow-up of 58 months analyzing the cohort of 72 patients undergoing suture and mesh repair for large PHH. They reported only 2 patients requiring reoperation, both in the suture group, despite the fact that over 50% of the patients had recurrence in both cohorts of patients. It is unclear if PPIs were used as treatment for some of these recurrences or not. The probable explanation for the persistence of improvement despite the anatomic recurrence may be that the average recurrence is relatively small when compared with the initial anatomic defect. Most of the studies reported on recurrences which were not operated upon or were managed conservatively with proton pump inhibitors. In Frantzides et al.'s [31] study 5 out of 8 patients in the suture cruroplasty group underwent further surgery and placement of PTFE mesh to close the hiatal defect. In Granderath et al.'s RCT [32] although there was statistically significant intrathoracic wrap migration in the suture cruroplasty group (13 patients) versus the prosthetic mesh repair group (4 patients), the authors have provided reoperation details of 4 patients in the latter group, two of whom had further circular hiatal mesh placement. No such information is available regarding the fate of 13 patients in the suture cruroplasty group. Adelaide's RCT [41] revealed 4 revisional surgeries in the suture cruroplasty group within 30 days for (a) tight hiatal repair (n = 1), (b) acute hiatal hernia (n = 3) and one at 7 months for recurrent hiatal hernia (n = 1). In the prosthetic mesh group, no surgery was required in the absorbable mesh group whereas 3 revisional surgeries occurred within 30 days for (a) tight hiatal repair (n = 2) and acute hiatal hernia and gastric perforation (n = 1). One reoperation was carried out at 8 months for persistent dysphagia.

9.7.5 *Dysphagia*

Persistent dysphagia is one of the important indications for reoperation. Not many studies provide details of this complication, and therefore the true incidence of dysphagia both in the short and long term remains speculative for both suture and mesh repair. Granderath and colleagues [32] reports dysphagia in 3 patients in the mesh group and 1 in the suture group, but only the outcome of 2 patients in the mesh group is reported. While Carlson et al. [30] and Frantzides et al. [31], both, have failed to provide any data on dysphagia rate in either groups. Oelschlager et al. [9]

reported no dysphagia in either of the groups. Watson et al. [41] on the other hand reports dysphagia in 2 patients in the suture and 3 in the mesh group (all with non-absorbable mesh), but no outcomes have been detailed.

While most of the studies reported dysphagia based solely on subjective clinical symptoms reported by the patients, other studies undertook further evaluation in the form of QOL score [8], GIQLI score [9] or dysphagia score [41]. When clinically dysphagia was suspected, it was confirmed with barium studies. Watson et al's study is the only one to detail the pre- and post-operative dysphagia score which was a combination of zero to ten analogue score, Visick score and SF-36 QOL score [41]. Furnee et al. [29] in his systematic review concluded that more patients with mesh repair experienced dysphagia in the first 3 months compared to their suture counterparts. This seemed to be transient and the difference between the mesh and suture group disappeared at 1 year except in cases of esophageal stenosis or mesh erosion.

9.8 Conclusions

Based on the current literature in particular some of the recent meta-analyses and systematic reviews, it seems that prosthetic hiatal herniorrhaphy and suture cruroplasty produce comparable results for repair of large PHH. In the future, a number of issues need to be addressed to determine the clinical outcomes, safety and effectiveness of these two methods for elective surgical treatment of large PHHs. These include (1) standardized definition of large PHH; (2) standardized techniques for suture and prosthetic repair; (3) type of prosthesis used—biologic versus non-absorbable; (4) standardized method of securing the mesh such as use of sutures, tacks or biologic glues; (5) standardized classification of recurrent hiatal hernia post repair; (6) standardized method of detecting recurrence e.g., gastroscopy, barium swallow or CT; (7) objective assessment of recurrent hiatal hernia via 24 h ambulatory impedance pH monitoring and lastly (8) long term postoperative longitudinal data collection of at least 5 years to detect the true incidence of hiatal hernia recurrence between suture cruroplasty and prosthetic hiatal herniorrhaphy. We believe the use of prosthetic hiatal herniorrhaphy for large PHH needs to be individualized based on the operative findings and the surgeon's recommendation.

What Is the Current Knowledge and What Future Direction Is Required

- Large PHH account for almost 50% of the cases encountered during contemporary laparoscopic hiatal hernia repair.
- Patient selection and preoperative evaluation are crucial for successful PHH repair especially in elderly patients with multiple comorbidities.
- An area of controversy is the use of prosthetic material (mesh) at the esophageal hiatus to provide additional support.

- Mesh related complications have been exaggerated. A number of recent meta-analysis and systematic reviews have shown comparable low complication rates between suture and mesh cruroplasty in PHH repair.
- In the published literature, there is no common or agreed definition of recurrence.
- The results of several meta-analysis and systematic reviews have shown comparable recurrence rate for patients undergoing either suture or prosthetic cruroplasty and most of these recurrences can easily be managed by conservative management.
- The use of prosthetic hiatal herniorrhaphy for large PHH needs to be individualized based on the operative findings and the surgeon's recommendation.

References

1. Engstrom C, Cai W, Irvine T, Devitt PG, Thompson SK, Game PA, Bessell JR, Jamieson GG, Watson DI. Twenty years of experience with laparoscopic antireflux surgery. Br J Surg. 2012;99:1415–21.
2. Akerland A, Onnell H, Key E. Hernia diaphragmatica hiatus oesophagei vom anastomischen und rontgenologischen gesichtspunct. Acta Radiol. 1926;6:3–22.
3. Cuschieri A, Shimi S, Nathanson LK. Laparoscopic reduction, crural repair, and fundoplication of large hiatal hernia. Am J Surg. 1992;163:425–30.
4. Schieman C, Grondin SC. Paraesophageal hernia: clinical presentation, evaluation, and management controversies. Thorac Surg Clin. 2009;19:473–84.
5. Hashemi M, Peters JH, DeMeester TR, Huprich JE, Quek M, Hagen JA, Crookes PF, Theisen J, DeMeester SR, Sillin LF, Bremner CG. Laparoscopic repair of large type III hiatal hernia: objective follow-up reveals high recurrence rate. J Am Coll Surg. 2000;190:554–61.
6. Mattar SG, Bowers SP, Galloway KD, Hunter J, Smith C. Long-term outcome of laparoscopic repair of paraoesopahgeal hernia. Surg Endosc. 2002;16:745–9.
7. Soricelli E, Basso N, Genco A, Cipriano M. Long-term results of hiatal hernia mesh repair and antireflux laparoscopic surgery. Surg Endosc. 2009;23:2499–504.
8. Dallemagne B, Kohnen L, Perretta S, Weerts J, Markiewicz S, Jehaes C. Laparoscopic repair of paraesophageal hernia: long-term follow-up reveals good clinical outcome despite high radiological recurrence rate. Ann Surg. 2011;253:291–6.
9. Oelschlager BK, Pellegrini CA, Hunter JG, Brunt ML, Soper NJ, Sheppard BC, Polissar NL, Neradilek MB, Mitsumori LM, Rohrmann CA, Swanstrom LL. Biologic prosthesis to prevent recurrence after laparoscopic paraesophageal hernia repair: long-term follow-up from a multicenter, prospective, randomized trial. J Am Coll Surg. 2011;213:461–8.
10. Tatum RP, Shalhub S, Oelschlager BK, Pellegrini CA. Complications of PTFE mesh at the diaphragmatic hiatus. J Gastrointest Surg. 2008;12:953–7.
11. Oor JE, Koetje JH, Roks DJ, Nieuwenhuijs V, Hazebroek E. Laparoscopic hiatal hernia repair in the elderly patient. World J Surg. 2016;40:1404–11.
12. Bashashati M, Sarosiek I, McCallum RW. Epidemiology and mechanisms of gastroesophageal reflux disease in the elderly: a perspective. Ann N Y Acad Sci. 2016;1380:230–4.
13. Hallan A, Bomme M, Hveem K, Møller-Hansen J, Ness-Jensen E. Risk factors on the development of new-onset gastroesophageal reflux symptoms. A population-based prospective cohort study: the HUNT study. Am J Gastroenterol. 2015;110:393–400.
14. Okimoto E, Ishimura N, Morito Y, Mikami H, Shimura S, Uno G, Tamagawa Y, Aimi M, Oshima N, Kawashima K, Kazumori H, Sato S, Ishihara S, Kinoshita Y. Prevalence of

gastroesophageal reflux disease in children, adults, and elderly in the same community. J Gastroenterol Hepatol. 2015;30:1140–6.
15. Ahmadi B, Alimohammadian M, Yaseri M, Majidi A, Boreiri M, Islami F, Poustchi H, Derakhshan MH, Feizesani A, Pourshams A, Abnet CC, Brennan P, Dawsey SM, Kamangar F, Boffetta P, Sadjadi A, Malekzadeh R. Multimorbidity: epidemiology and risk factors in the Golestan cohort study, Iran: a crosssectional analysis. Medicine. 2016;95:e2756.
16. Petrick JL, Nguyen T, Cook MB. Temporal trends of esophageal disorders by age in the Cerner health facts database. Ann Epidemiol. 2016;26:151–4.
17. Carré IJ, Johnston BT, Thomas PS, Morrison PJ. Familial hiatal hernia in a large five generation family confirming true autosomal dominant inheritance. Gut. 1999;45:649–52.
18. Larusson HJ, Zingg U, Hahnloser D, Delport K, Seifert B, Oertli D. Predictive factors for morbidity and mortality in patients undergoing laparoscopic paraesophageal hernia repair: age, ASA score and operation type influence morbidity. World J Surg. 2009;33:980–5.
19. Stylopoulos N, Gazelle GS, Rattner DW. Paraesophageal hernias: operation or observation? Ann Surg. 2002;236:492–500.
20. Sheff SR, Kothari SN. Repair of the giant hiatal hernia. J Long-Term Eff Med Implants. 2010;20:139–48.
21. Jutric Z, Louie BE. Laparoscopic paraesophageal hernia repair. Surg Laparosc Endosc Percutan Tech. 2013;23:436–41.
22. Fisichella PM. A synopsis of techniques for paraesophageal hernia repair: different approaches to current controversies. Surg Laparosc Endosc Percutan Tech. 2013;23:423–4.
23. Maziak DE, Todd TR, Pearson FG. Massive hiatus hernia: evaluation and surgical management. J Thorac Cardiovasc Surg. 1998;115:53–60.
24. DeMeester SR. Laparoscopic paraesophageal hernia repair: critical steps and adjunct techniques to minimize recurrence. Surg Laparosc Endosc Percutan Tech. 2013;23:429–35.
25. Gouvas N, Tsiaoussis J, Athanasakis E, Zervakis N, Pechlivanides G, Xynos E. Simple suture or prosthesis hiatal closure in laparoscopic repair of paraesophageal hernia: a retrospective cohort study. Dis Esophagus. 2011;24:69–78.
26. Braghetto I, Korn O, Csendes A, Burdiles P, Valladares H, Brunet L. Postoperative results after laparoscopic approach for treatment of large hiatal hernias: is mesh always needed? Is the addition of an antireflux procedure necessary? Int Surg. 2010;95:80–7.
27. Muller-Stich BP, Holzinger F, Kapp T, Klaiber C. Laparoscopic hiatal hernia repair: long-term outcome with the focus on the influence of mesh reinforcement. Surg Endosc. 2006;20:380–4.
28. Memon MA, Memon B, Yunus RM, Khan S. Suture Cruroplasty versus prosthetic hiatal Herniorrhaphy for large hiatal hernia: a meta-analysis and systematic review of randomized controlled trials. Ann Surg. 2016;263:258–66.
29. Furnee E, Hazebroek E. Mesh in laparoscopic large hiatal hernia repair: a systematic review of the literature. Surg Endosc. 2013;27:3998–4008.
30. Carlson MA, Richards CG, Frantzides CT. Laparoscopic prosthetic reinforcement of hiatal herniorrhaphy. Dig Surg. 1999;16:407–10.
31. Frantzides CT, Madan AK, Carlson MA, Stavropoulos GP. A prospective, randomized trial of laparoscopic polytetrafluoroethylene (PTFE) patch repair vs simple cruroplasty for large hiatal hernia. Arch Surg. 2002;137:649–52.
32. Granderath FA, Schweiger UM, Kamolz T, Asche KU, Pointner R. Laparoscopic Nissen fundoplication with prosthetic hiatal closure reduces postoperative intrathoracic wrap herniation: preliminary results of a prospective randomized functional and clinical study. Arch Surg. 2005;140:40–8.
33. Asti E, Lovece A, Bonavina L, Milito P, Sironi A, Bonitta G, Siboni S. Laparoscopic management of large hiatus hernia: five-year cohort study and comparison of mesh-augmented versus standard crura repair. Surg Endosc. 2016;30:5404–9.
34. Zaninotto G, Portale G, Costantini M, Fiamingo P, Rampado S, Guirroli E, Nicoletti L, Ancona E. Objective follow-up after laparoscopic repair of large type III hiatal hernia. Assessment of safety and durability. World J Surg. 2007;31:2177–83.
35. Mimatsu K, Oida T, Kida K, Fukino N, Kawasaki A, Kano H, Kuboi Y, Amano S. Simultaneous laparoscopic Nissen fundoplication and percutaneous endoscopic gastrostomy to treat an elderly patient with a large paraesophageal hernia: a case report. Asian J Endosc Surg. 2014;7:165–8.

36. Leeder PC, Smith G, Dehn TC. Laparoscopic management of large paraesophageal hiatal hernia. Surg Endosc. 2003;17:1372–5.
37. Hui TT, Thoman DS, Spyrou M, Phillips EH. Mesh crural repair of large paraesophageal hiatal hernias. Am Surg. 2001;67:1170–4.
38. Morino M, Giaccone C, Pellegrino L, Rebecchi F. Laparoscopic management of giant hiatal hernia: factors influencing long-term outcome. Surg Endosc. 2006;20:1011–6.
39. Goers TA, Cassera MA, Dunst CM, Swanström LL. Paraesophageal hernia repair with biomesh does not increase postoperative dysphagia. J Gastrointest Surg. 2011;15:1743–9.
40. Ringley CD, Bochkarev V, Ahmed SI, Vitamvas ML, Oleynikov D. Laparoscopic hiatal hernia repair with human acellular dermal matrix patch: our initial experience. Am J Surg. 2006;192:767–72.
41. Watson DI, Thompson SK, Devitt PG, Smith L, Woods SD, Aly A, Gan S, Game PA, Jamieson GG. Laparoscopic repair of very large hiatal hernia with sutures versus absorbable mesh versus nonabsorbable mesh: a randomized controlled trial. Ann Surg. 2015;261:282–9.
42. Müller-Stich BP, Kenngott HG, Gondan M, Gondan M, Stock C, Linke GR, Fritz F, Nickel F, Diener MK, Gutt CN, Wente M, Büchler MW, Fischer L. Use of mesh in laparoscopic Paraesophageal hernia repair: a meta-analysis and risk-benefit analysis. PLoS One. 2015;10:1–17.
43. Tam V, Winger DG, Nason KS. A systematic review and meta-analysis of mesh vs suture cruroplasty in laparoscopic large hiatal hernia repair. Am J Surg. 2016;211:226–38.
44. Tanrikulu Y, Kar F, Yalcin B, Yilmaz G, Temi V, Cagsar M. The importance of the mesh shape in preventing recurrence after Nissen fundoplication. Int J Clin Exp Med. 2015;8:9684–91.
45. Carlson MA, Condon RE, Ludwig KA, Schulte WJ. Management of intrathoracic stomach with polypropylene mesh prosthesis reinforced transabdominal hiatus hernia repair. J Am Coll Surg. 1998;187:227–30.
46. Schneider R, Herrington JL Jr, Granda AM. Marlex mesh in repair of a diaphragmatic defect later eroding into the distal esophagus and stomach. Am Surg. 1979;45:337–9.
47. Stadlhuber RJ, Sherif AE, Mittal SK, Fitzgibbons RJ Jr, Michael Brunt L, Hunter JG, Demeester TR, Swanstrom LL, Daniel Smith C, Filipi CJ. Mesh complications after prosthetic reinforcement of hiatal closure: a 28-case series. Surg Endosc. 2009;23:1219–26.
48. Antoniou SA, Koch OO, Antoniou GA, Pointner R, Granderath FA. Mesh-reinforced hiatal hernia repair: a review on the effect on postoperative dysphagia and recurrence. Langenbeck's Arch Surg. 2012;397:19–27.
49. Frantzides CT, Carlson MA, Loizides S, Papafili A, Luu M, Roberts J, Zeni T, Frantzides A. Hiatal hernia repair with mesh: a survey of SAGES members. Surg Endosc. 2010;24:1017–24.
50. Grubnik VV, Malynovskyy AV. Laparoscopic repair of hiatal hernias: new classification supported by long-term results. Surg Endosc. 2013;27:4337–46.
51. Huntington TR. Laparoscopic mesh repair of the esophageal hiatus. J Am Coll Surg. 1997;184:399–400.
52. Kehdy F. Current management of paraesophageal hernia. Am Surg. 2011;77:1565–73.
53. Eypasch E, Williams JI, Wood-Dauphinee S, Ure BM, Schmülling C, Neugebauer E, Troidl H. Gastrointestinal quality of life index: development, validation and application of a new instrument. Br J Surg. 1995;82:216–22.
54. Obeid NM, Velanovich V. The choice of primary repair or mesh repair for paraesophageal hernia: a decision analysis based on utility scores. Ann Surg. 2013;257:655–64.

Chapter 10
Lower Esophageal Sphincter Efficacy Following Laparoscopic Antireflux Surgery with Hiatal Repair: Role of Fluoroscopy, High-Resolution Impedance Manometry and FLIP in Detecting Recurrence of GERD and Hiatal Hernia

Vivien Wong, Barry McMahon, and Hans Gregersen

10.1 Introduction

Gastroesophageal reflux disease (GERD) is a global public health problem affecting more than 20% of the population. Hiatus hernia, a quite frequent condition in elderly, is known to be an important risk factor for the development of GERD. In subjects who are symptomatic hiatal hernia promotes gastric acid access to the esophagus and impairs its clearance. The overall consequence of increased esophageal acid exposure is reflux esophagitis. Medical therapy with PPI is the first choice of treatment but does not help all patients. The first surgical repair for hiatus hernia was reported by Soresi in 1926 [1]. Since then there have been many diagnostic and therapeutic advancements but there is still a need for development of current techniques due to the physiological and anatomical complexity of the region. The esophago-gastric junction (EGJ) has a complex anatomical and mechanical function in normal subjects as well as in patients with hiatus hernia, and in those with surgically repaired EGJ and hernia (see later).

Efficacy is the ability to produce a desired result or effect. Speaking about the lower esophageal sphincter (LES), efficacy under physiological conditions as well as pathophysiological conditions such as in herniation and after hiatus repair relates to its ability to avoid any pathological consequences of reflux of gastric contents. These complex issues will be discussed later in the chapter. Firstly, LES is part of a

V. Wong • H. Gregersen (✉)
Department of Surgery, Prince of Wales Hospital,
4/F, Clinical Science Building, Shatin, NT, Hong Kong
e-mail: hag@giome.org

B. McMahon
Trinity Academic Gastroenterology Group, Trinity College, Dublin, Ireland

M.A. Memon (ed.), *Hiatal Hernia Surgery*,
https://doi.org/10.1007/978-3-319-64003-7_10

wider barrier mechanism to prevent reflux of gastric contents into the esophagus. Other structures such as the crura of the diaphragm and the FLAP valve contribute to the barrier mechanism as well. The anatomy gets even more complicated when normal tissues structures are remodeled such as in herniation and when surgical or endoscopic fundoplication procedures are carried out. Secondly, efficacy can be evaluated in terms of several variables and parameters including symptoms, pH in esophagus, EGJ pressure profiles, clearance, and flow through the EGJ. Therefore, diagnostic technologies such as hypersensitivity testing, high-resolution manometry (HRM), intraluminal impedance, pH-metry, fluoroscopy, functional luminal imaging (FLIP) and endoscopy are relevant and of value. However, we may not fully comprehend how these tests complement each other.

This chapter provides an insight into the complex anatomy and physiology of the EGJ including the LES under normal conditions and under remodeled conditions as observed in herniation and during operational procedures. The chapter deals in particular with efficacy evaluation of the surgical repair and recurrence based on fluoroscopy, impedance manometry, and FLIP.

10.2 Anatomy of the EGJ

The EGJ consists of several structures that regulate transport of swallowed substances to the stomach and serves as a barrier against reflux of gastric contents [2, 3] (Fig. 10.1). The reflux barrier is predominantly maintained by the LES and the crural fibers of the diaphragm [4, 5].

LES is a tonically contracted segment of the EGJ that together with the clasp and sling fibers of the gastric cardia form an integrated sphincter mechanism [2, 3]. LES anatomy is fascinating since a distinct anatomical sphincter with muscle thickening has not been clearly identified [2, 3, 6, 7]. Rather, manometric studies have shown

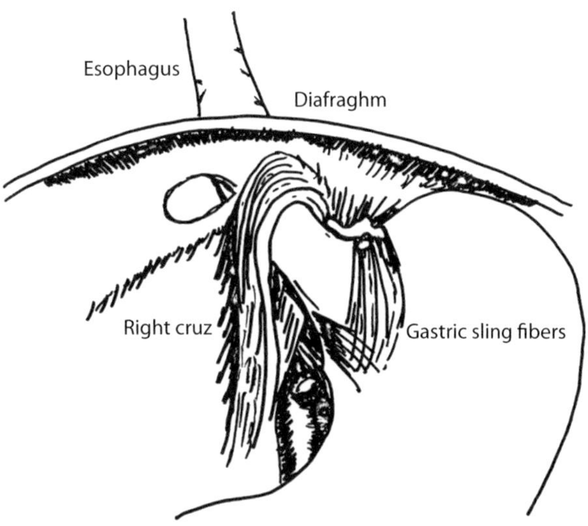

Fig. 10.1 The anatomy of the normal esophago-gastric junction showing the esophagus, stomach, diaphragm and the clasp and sling fibers (modified and reproduced with permission from ref. [2])

the high-pressure zone in the lower esophagus [8, 9]. LES is not an annular sphincter but rather formed by two crossing muscle bundles, i.e. the semicircular "clasp" and the oblique "sling" muscular fibers derived from the oblique fibers of the stomach [2, 3, 6, 7, 10]. Closure of the EGJ appears to be due to contraction of these muscle bundles in conjunction with crural fibers of the diaphragm [7, 9, 11–16].

Another important anti-reflux structure is the gastroesophageal flap valve formed by a musculo-mucosal fold that maintains a pressure gradient between the stomach and lower esophagus to keep gastric contents away from the EGJ [3, 14, 17–21]. The sling fibers of the stomach located below the LES are associated with a valve mechanism whereby pressure in the gastric fundus creates a flap that presses against the lower end of the esophagus [20].

The gastroesophageal flap valve is located at the gastric cardia where it maintains the acute angle of His [7, 20].

Brasseur and co-workers described three distinct components of the barrier mechanism in the gastro-esophageal segment and how they can be differentiated. The components are the extrinsic crural sphincter and the intrinsic LES and sling/clasp muscle unit. Efficacy is maintained by a delicate interplay between the components [22].

Hiatus hernia is characterized by proximal displacement of the EGJ causing the intrinsic sphincter to lie proximal to the hiatus formed by the crural diaphragm [23] (Fig. 10.2). This is likely caused by rupture or weakening of the phreno-esophageal ligament [25]. Patients with hiatus hernia have more reflux episodes and greater esophageal acid exposure than patients without hiatus hernia and they have more severe esophagitis [26]. Furthermore, larger hiatal hernia is associated with a greater esophageal acid exposure and prolonged acid clearance times [27]. This is likely a reflection of the remodeled mechanical properties of the barrier mechanism [28]. Referring again to the work by Brasseur, hiatus hernia with its distinct mechano-morphometric changes disrupts the integrity of the physiological barrier mechanism [22].

Surgical or endoscopic fundoplication aims to restore the lost efficacy observed in herniation. The geometry of the EGJ and mechanically defect LES can be somewhat restored by antireflux surgery. The LES length and the FLAP valve are to some degree regenerated which increases the baseline LES pressure [29]. In addition to the contribution to the pressure increase, the lengthened LES better resist the effect

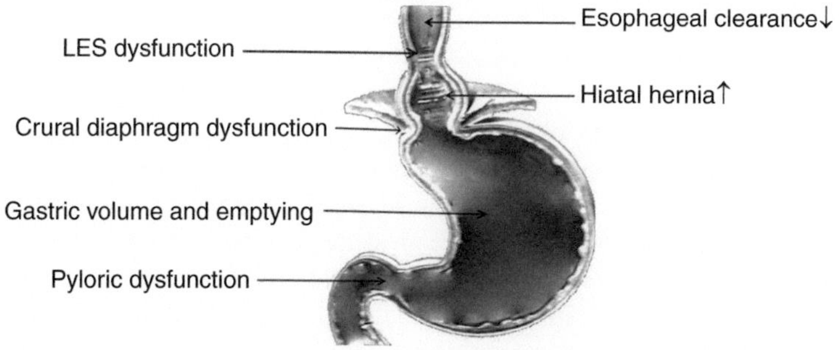

Fig. 10.2 Mechanisms contributing to reflux disease including the hiatal hernia (reproduced with permission from ref. [24])

of gastric wall tension in opening the LES. This is complemented by the recreation of the FLAP valve which tends to occlude the lumen and increase pressure [30]. If the wrap is defect or recurrence occur, then the full geometric-mechanical effect is not obtained and efficacy will be impaired.

10.3 Physiology of Esophago-Gastric Junction with Focus on LES Efficacy

From studies performed up to 20 years ago and summarized elegantly by reviews from Mittal & Balaban [3] and Kahrilas [31], it is evident that the core tenants of the barrier function at the EGJ are now well established. The thickened muscle area at the distal end of the esophagus represent the LES intrinsic barrier whereas the diaphragmatic hiatus, which is located as a narrow opening in the diaphragm where the distal esophagus exits the thoracic cavity and enters the abdominal cavity, represents an extrinsic barrier. Studies indicate that the proximal 2 cm of the 4 cm-long LES is where the so-called extrinsic "pinch cock" effect of the diaphragm overlaps the intrinsic circular valve effect of the LES [32]. The physiology described in these reviews still forms the basis for surgical treatment options as mentioned in the recent review by Patti and coworkers [33].

The role of the LES at the EGJ has been quite well understood for a considerable time. In normal subjects the LES exerts a circular muscle force at the distal end of the esophagus just as it enters the stomach. This is part of the barrier that ensures stomach contents do not travel back into the esophagus. When swallowing is initiated the LES relaxes allowing ingested material to travel from the esophagus into the stomach [34]. Much of our understanding of this comes from manometric studies. These type of studies were further enhanced in the 1970's by Dent and coworkers, who using a variant of manometry known as the Dent sleeve, demonstrated that the LES relaxes at other times as well [35]. These events are known as transient lower esophageal sphincter relaxations (TLESRs). It has been shown that the number of transient relaxations is higher in patients suffering from GERD [32].

The more recent work of Miller and Brasseur used a very precise manometric pull-through technique concurrent with high frequency ultrasound and studied the high-pressure zone at the EGJ [22]. Their aim was to separate and manometrically quantify in vivo the skeletal and smooth muscle components at the EGJ in an attempt to gather more physiological detail in the LES region. This was achieved using atropine in one group of healthy volunteers to suppress the cholinergic smooth muscle sphincter effect and cistracurium in another group to neuromuscularly block the crural sphincter. Hence, the muscle contributions could be studied separately. The main and significant finding from this study is that the pressure profiles generated by manometric pull-through of the region, if carried out with great precision and with the interventions above, can obtain more information on the physiology and function of the LES.

From this work new information that suggests the LES has two subcomponents is evident. The authors conclude that one component is a proximal smooth muscle component. They describe this as the lower esophageal circular muscle, which tends to move with the movement of the crural diaphragm component probably due to its attachment to the phreno-esophageal ligament. The other component is described as the smooth muscle component distal to the diaphragm and from ultrasound appeared to be located approximately at the position of the sling-clasp muscle fibers [36].

10.4 Laparoscopic Antireflux Surgery with Hiatal Repair Surgical Aspects

The anti-reflux effect of fundoplication was discovered after a 16-year follow-up of a patient with partial esophagectomy done using a fundoplication wrap around the anastomosis with the purpose of preventing leakage [37]. It became the most commonly practiced effective surgical treatment for GERD. However, how the procedure has augmented the effect of the lower esophageal complex to act as a valve against reflux is still under discussion.

Fundoplication is shown to increase the nadir lower esophageal pressure [38, 39] and thereby better resists the intra-gastric pressure that produces reflux, while preserving its ability to relax (though less completely) upon wet swallows [38]. While this increase in pressure is shown to be exerted by the gastric wrap in animal studies excluding the LES by myotomy [40], the fact that this new high pressure zone behaves similarly to the physiological LES is interpreted as improvement of the LES smooth muscles by some authors [41].

The relaxation pattern of the LES is also altered after fundoplication. Increased TLESR is found in many patients with GERD [42–45]. The relaxation is initiated by gastric cardiac distension, the most sensitive zone as shown in animal studies [46]. The fundoplication wrap alters the distensibility at the region. Ireland and coworkers have demonstrated a significant decrease in TLESR frequency detected after fundoplication and gastroesophageal reflux associated with the episodes [39].

10.5 Recurrence of GERD and Hiatal Hernia Clinical Features

10.5.1 Clinical Features and Fundoplication Failures

The rate of long-term resumption of acid-reducing medication after fundoplication is shown to vary widely from 5.8 to 62%, with most reports showing a rate of $<20\%$ [47]. Level I evidence showed a symptom resolution rate of 67% at 7-year follow up [47]. Recurrence with new reflux symptoms usually indicates a breakdown of the fundoplication [48]. A systematic review on surgical re-intervention after anti-reflux surgery showed that over 80% of failed procedure is due to disruption of the post-operative anatomy [49].

Upon symptom recurrence after fundoplication, the approach to investigate for indication of re-operation is similar to that for the primary procedure. Investigations aim to show objective evidence of acid reflux recurrence and to show the integrity of the previous repair. Most patients who received re-operations were worked up with endoscopy, fluoroscopy and/or pH monitoring studies [49]. In particular, endoscopy and fluoroscopy help visualize the status of the wrap and hiatal repair.

A successful anti-reflux surgery comprises of a proper fundoplication and an intact hiatal hernia repair. Various types of fundoplication wrap disruptions have been described [50], according to the status of the wrap itself and the presence of any recurrence of the hiatus hernia. The wrap can be incompetent due to loosening or breakdown, or intact but slipped so part of the stomach is herniated through the wrap. Hiatus hernia may recur in any of the scenarios, and the wrap itself may also herniate through the diaphragm (Fig. 10.3).

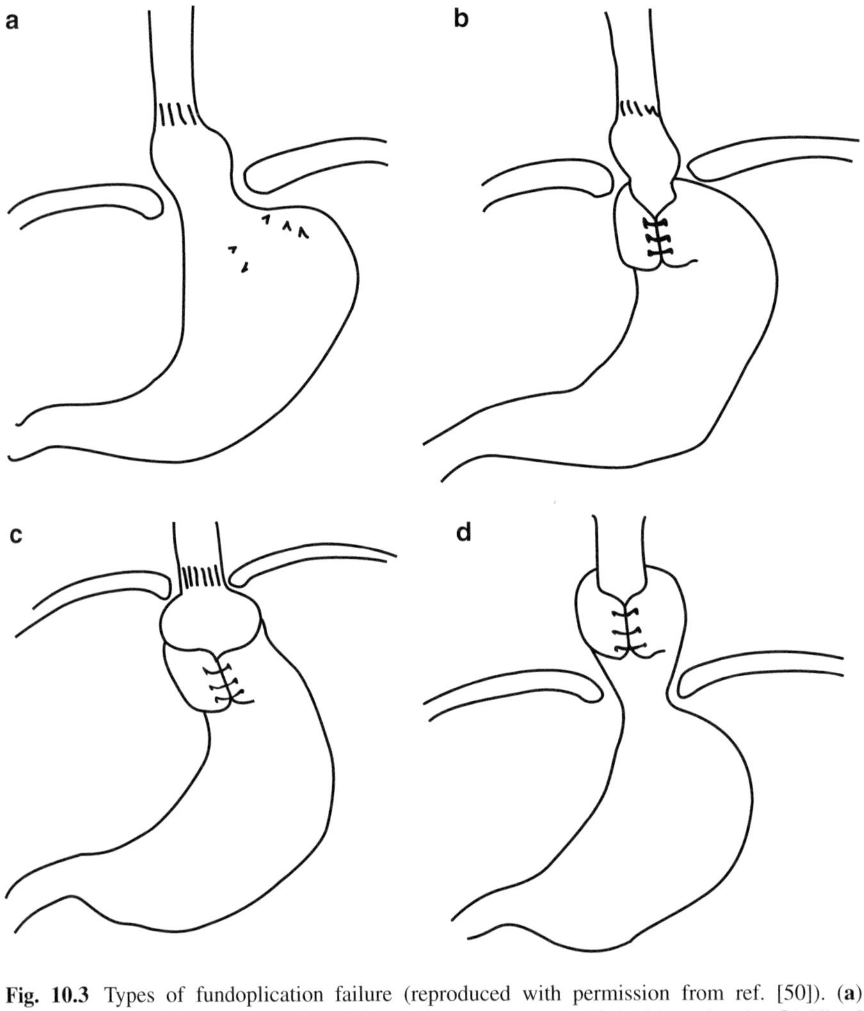

Fig. 10.3 Types of fundoplication failure (reproduced with permission from ref. [50]). (**a**) Complete or partial wrap disruption with or without recurrence of the hiatus hernia. (**b**) Hiatal herniation of the stomach via the intact fundoplication wrap. (**c**) Slippage of the wrap causing gastric herniation through the wrap only but not the diaphragm. (**d**) Hiatal herniation of the intact fundoplication wrap

10.5.2 Role of Fluoroscopy

Barium esophagography is a simple investigation that allows surgeons to assess the morphology of the wrap, albeit interpretation can be challenging even for radiologists unless full understanding of the surgical procedure itself is acquired [51]. Double-contrast study is preferred. Three components can be observed: (1) the wrap, (2) hiatus hernia, and (3) presence of reflux. Barium esophagogram after fundoplication would show a smooth well-circumscribed filling defect at the gastric fundus surrounding the narrowed distal esophagus, located below the diaphragm. The wrap can occasionally be filled with barium contrast (Fig. 10.4). Normally, above the wrap would be the esophagus and below the stomach. A slipped wrap would show the presence of the gastric fundus above the wrap (Fig. 10.5). Noting the level of diaphragm, recurrence of hiatus hernia can be identified, even in the case of herniation of the whole wrap (Fig. 10.6). Occasionally, contrast reflux is observed during fluoroscopy, confirming the presence of an incompetent LES.

In the situation of reflux recurrence after fundoplication, endoscopy (esophagogastroduodenoscopy) is another important investigation. It plays the role of identifying failed procedure and ruling out any other organic causes of the new symptoms. Endoscopic features to identify a failed fundoplication was described by Jailwala and coworkers, including presence of esophagitis, ease of endoscope passage through the EGJ, location of wrap relative to diaphragmatic hiatus, location of the squamocolumnar junction and the appearance of the wrap [53].

A competent fundoplication should give an endoscopic appearance, upon retroflexion, a good seal around the endoscope by the wrap, and its resultant lengthened intra-abdominal portion of the LES.

Compared with barium esophagography, endoscopy is able to pick up 10–15% more structural abnormalities upon investigation for recurrence [53] whereas it is less informative upon workup for dysphagia. However, fluoroscopy is still recommended in the planning of revision surgery as an image guide to the relative anatomy of different structures.

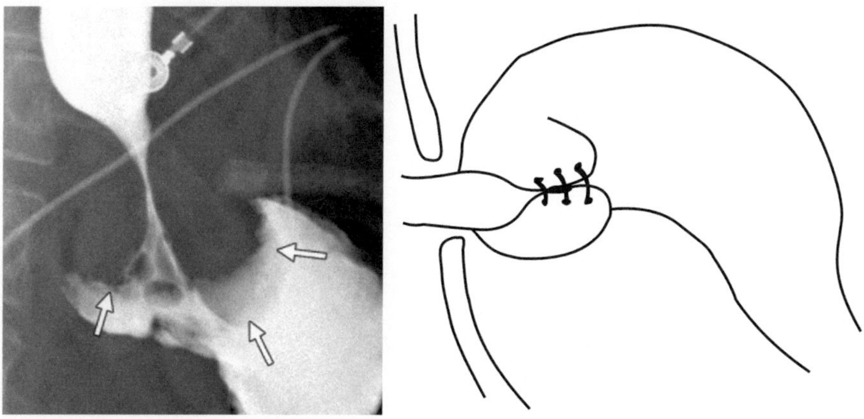

Fig. 10.4 Barium esophagogram after fundoplication (reproduced with permission from ref. [52]) with the well-circumscribed filling defects seen around the narrowed distal esophagus, and a schematic diagram of the corresponding anatomy

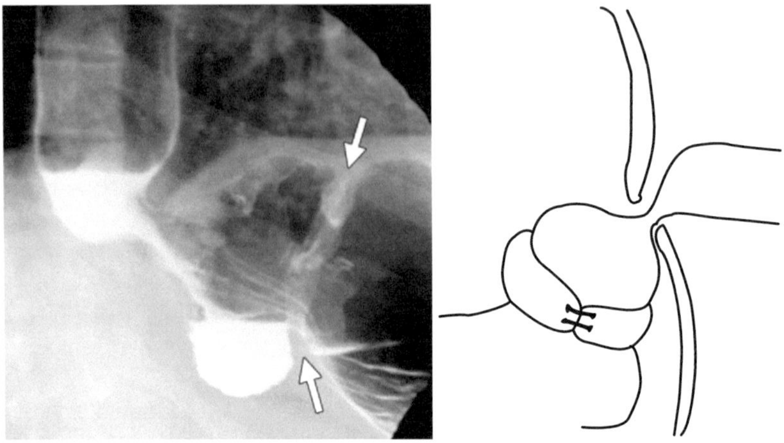

Fig. 10.5 Barium esophagogram showing a slipped wrap, indicated by the *arrows*, and part of the stomach is now above the wrap (reproduced with permission from ref. [52]). Schematic diagram of corresponding anatomy

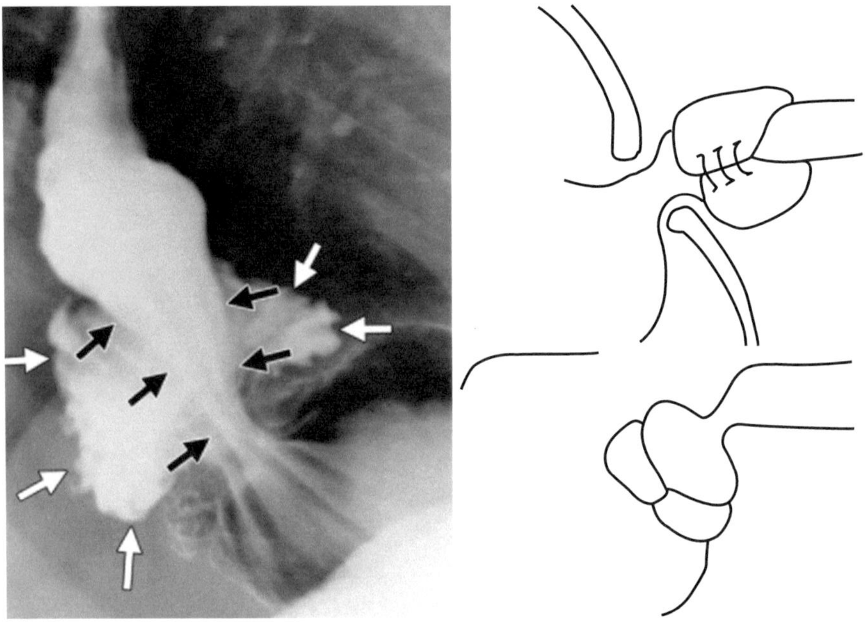

Fig. 10.6 Barium esophagogram showing herniation of the whole fundoplication wrap above the diaphragm (reproduced with permission from ref. [52]). The wrap is filled with contrast. Schematic diagram of corresponding anatomy

10.5.3 Role of High-Resolution Impedance-Manometry

Invariably for type I sliding hernia, the LES has moved through the diaphragmatic hiatus and has herniated in the thoracic cavity [54]. High-resolution manometry can identify what is sometimes referred to as the double hump or double high-pressure zone [55]. This can be seen clearly in Fig. 10.7. Evaluating hernia size indirectly based on the distance between the double high-pressure zone on high-resolution manometry tracings is fast coming the accepted practice in clinics globally [56]. This is very useful for general diagnosis and orientation of a hiatal hernia but it does not give precise information on structure and function. It is recommended as part of patient work up before surgery [57].

As high-resolution manometry has evolved over the last 20 years so too has the concept of intraluminal impedance and the combined concept of high-resolution impedance manometry (HRIM). Studies have shown that intraluminal impedance provides a much better understanding of the solid, liquid or gaseous state of the refluxate [58]. However, although the technique has proven to be a useful tool in this regard, and despite predictions on its development into clinical practice, this has not

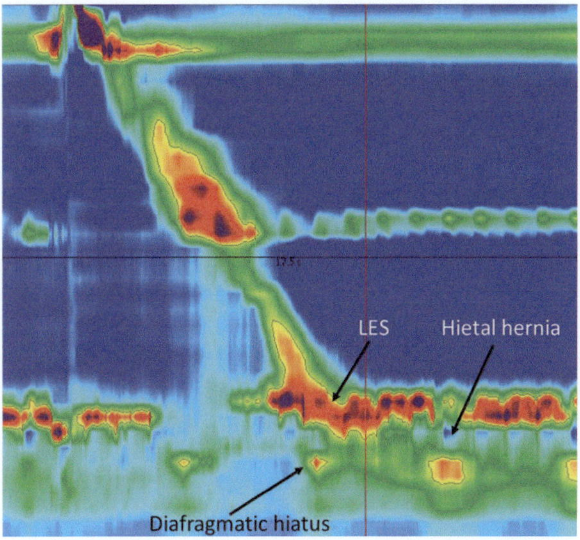

Fig. 10.7 High resolution manometry tracing of a single swallow by a patient with a small size hiatal hernia. The hernia is indicated by the spacing between the green color suggesting a higher pressure where there is a squeeze present from the tone of the LES and the pinchcock effect of the diaphragmatic hiatus. The *X*-axis represents time, *Y*-axis is position in the esophagus and color represents pressure going from *blue* for low pressure through *green* toward *red* for high pressure. Precise values are not shown as this figure is for illustrative purposes only

materialized. Arguably it will not be useful to help diagnose patients with hiatal hernia or the recurrence of GERD and hiatal hernia after antireflux surgery [59]. This is mostly because repair of hiatal hernia by antireflux surgery alters biomechanical activity in the region of the EGJ. As intraluminal impedance does not provide objective measures of function, it cannot directly evaluate improvements in the junction barrier after surgery. Early information indicates that intraluminal impedance may have a role in assessing the acid pocket and this relates to the hypothesis that in patients with hiatal hernia the acid pocket may appear in the hiatus [60]. Further studies need to be carried out to evaluate if using intraluminal impedance to assess the makeup of the refluxate in the hiatus and to assess if this is altered, improved, or eradicated after anti-reflux surgery or to determine recurrence.

Since the physiological concept of TLESR is widely accepted and can currently be more easily assessed using high-resolution manometry, its assessment role with respect to hiatal hernia patients is worth a mention [61]. However, studies back in the year 2000 are conflicting. Van Herwaarden and coworkers claimed that TLESRs in patients with HH were comparible to those without HH and in the same year and journal Kahrilas and coworkers claimed TLESRs were increases in patients with GERD and hiatal hernia [62, 63]. However, there is no evidence from the literature of TLESR evaluation being important before or after antireflux surgery to evaluation efficacy. This of course makes some sense since very often it is not a lack of tone or pressure in the LES that is observed with hiatal hernia but a separation on the two main mechanism of the barrier, i.e. the LES and the crural diaphragm.

10.5.4 Role of the Functional Luminal Imaging Probe

New work using the functional luminal imaging probe (FLIP) to measure function in the region of the LES and the wider EGJ segment suggests it may have a role in antireflux surgery in general and in the evaluation of hiatal hernia in particular. In brief FLIP provides serial measures of cross-sectional areas inside a long bag and the lumen geometry and distensibility can be derived from the measurements.

De Haan and coworkers provided some insights into the role of FLIP in the evaluation of reflux surgery, Nissen and Toupet in a series of 75 patients (48 of which were redos). The authors suggested that there is ongoing variability in the outcomes of antireflux procedures despite their existence for more than 50 years. This has hampered the ability to assess adequately predictors of clinical and symptomatic outcomes. In their study they showed that the esophagogastric segment is less distensible after anti-reflux surgery and that Nissen procedures are less distensible than Toupet procedures. Based on this they suggested FLIP provides a method to tailor fundoplication distensibility by observing geometry and pressure intraoperatively. Although further studies are needed, this could help create more uniformity in technique, improve the long-term symptomatic outcomes and further minimize side effects [64].

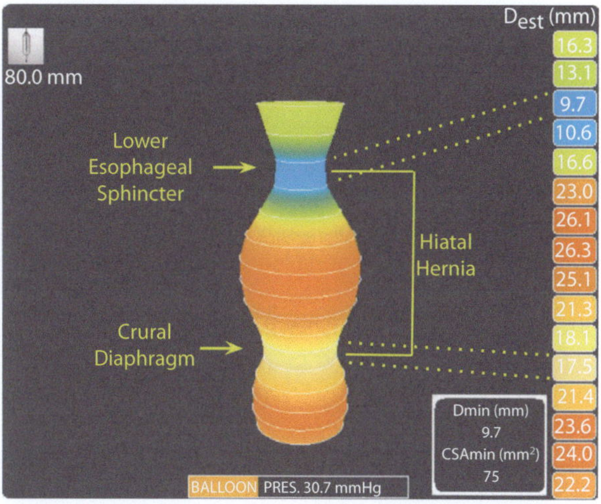

Fig. 10.8 EndoFLIP® image demonstrating how the probe can straddle two narrow regions created by a small hiatal hernia. In this case the distance between the two narrow regions, the upper one being the effect of the LES and the lower one being the crural diaphragm (CD) is approximately 4 cm. This image has been kindly provided by Dr. Christian Lottrup

It follows that enquiry into the role of FLIP as a distensibility technique may teach us something about the separation of the intrinsic effect of the LES and the extrinsic effect of the diaphragmatic hiatus when they are no longer co-located to form the EGJ.

Recent work by Lottrup and coworkers indicated that more subtle information on hernia may help develop a better understanding of its role in reflux disease. Therefore, it may assist with tailoring and improving antireflux surgery for hiatal hernia as recommended by Tatarian and coworkers in their review [65, 66]. Work has been initiated to evaluate FLIP as a tool to provide better functional measurement of the different parts of the EGJ when a hiatal hernia is present, to compare the distensibility of the EGJ components in HH patients and controls, and to attempt to diagnose HH. It is evident from Fig. 10.8 that FLIP is capable of distinguishing two narrow regions in patients with smaller hernias. The study concluded that FLIP allows for a separate assessment of LES and crural diaphragm components, where distensibility and compliance can be evaluated along with visualization of the region. The work further confirms the importance of the superimposition of these two components to achieve competence of the gastroesophageal segment in many patients. This is clearly missing in hiatal hernia patients.

Concepts and thinking on the physiology of the EGJ region have been available for more than 10 years and are eloquently described in Gordon's review paper in 2004 [67]. New techniques need to be developed and evolved or adapted to highlight and understand the physiological changes that occur with hiatal hernia. In this way, we can understand the causes better and ultimately provide better preventions or treatments. The paper also touches on early studies by Pandolfino and coworkers evaluating changes in cross-sectional area in the LES segment with hiatal hernia [68]. These studies underpin more recent concepts using FLIP as a distensibility technique. FLIP in its present or a future form may provide one of these new techniques.

10.6 Conclusions and Perspectives

It is indisputable that surgical repair of the EGJ with hiatal hernia is an effective treatment but recurrence may occur. Continued improvement of surgical technology and evaluation of efficacy are important. Some technologies for evaluating efficacy have been around for many years and still play an important role in clinical decision-making. HRM and fluoroscopy will likely continue to have an important role in clinical evaluation of hernia, surgical repair and recurrence. New technologies like FLIP are evolving and show potential since it provides data on the geometry and distensibility of the EGJ. Kwiatek and coworkers indicated that the FLIP method will be a valuable method to assess the outcome of antireflux surgery as a supplement to other measured outcomes [69] but more work is needed before the clinical value is clear.

The physiology of the EGJ is complex and has been studied for many years. Advanced physiological studies have contributed significantly [22] which also may impact on the understanding of hiatal hernia pathophysiology and the remodeling created during surgical repairs. We are starting to be introduced to bioengineering studies using geometric and mechanical 2D and 3D models of the EGJ based on detailed anatomical data using high-resolution microscopic imaging [70, 71]. Similar to other organs, such models will increase our understanding of the interplay between anatomy, geometry, mechanics and function. In vivo advanced models may be based on diffusion tensor magnetic resonance imaging (DT-MRI) technology that provides a non-destructive and high-resolution method for reconstructing the fiber orientation throughout the LES region. This technique is used to measure the anisotropic diffusion properties of biological tissues as a function of the spatial position within the sample. Better understanding of the precise myoarchitecture of the LES and its relationship to EGJ function will be beneficial for our understanding of physiology, reflux pathophysiology, and clinical outcomes of anti-reflux surgery.

What Is the Current Knowledge and What Future Direction Is Required

- Efficacy of the esophagogastric junction (EGJ) under physiological and pathophysiological conditions such as in herniation and after hiatus repair relates to its ability to avoid any pathological consequences of reflux of gastric contents.
- Efficacy of the EGJ barrier can be evaluated with endoscopy, pH-metry, fluoroscopy, impedance manometry, and the functional luminal imaging probe.
- Surgical or endoscopic fundoplication aims to restore the lost efficacy observed in herniation by restoring the geometry of the EGJ and mechanically defect lower esophageal sphincter. It is indisputable that surgical

repair of the EGJ with hiatal hernia is an effective treatment but recurrence may occur.

- Upon symptom recurrence after fundoplication, the approach to investigate for indication of re-operation is similar to that for the primary procedure. Investigations aim to show objective evidence of acid reflux recurrence and to show the integrity of the previous repair.
- Continued improvement of surgical technology and evaluation of efficacy are important due to the anatomical and physiological complexity of the esophago-gastric junction in health and disease.
- HRM and fluoroscopy will likely continue to have an important role in clinical evaluation of hernia, surgical repair and recurrence. New technologies like FLIP are evolving and show potential since it provides data on the geometry and distensibility of the EGJ.

References

1. Stylopoulos N, Rattner DW. The history of hiatal hernia surgery: from Bowditch to laparoscopy. Ann Surg. 2005;241:185–93.
2. Miller LS, Vegesna AK, Brasseur JG, et al. The esophagogastric junction. Ann N Y Acad Sci. 2011;1232:323–30.
3. Mittal RK, Balaban DH. The esophagogastric junction. N Engl J Med. 1997;336:924–32.
4. Zaninotto G, DeMeester TR, Schwizer W, Johansson KE, Cheng SC. The lower esophageal sphincter in health and disease. Am J Surg. 1988;155:104–11.
5. Banki F, Mason RJ, Hagen JA, Bremner CG, Streets CG, Peters JH, DeMeester TR. The crura and crura-sphincter pressure dynamics in patients with isolated upright and isolated supine reflux. Am Surg. 2001;67:1150–6.
6. Bombeck CT, Dillard DH, Nyhus LM. Muscular anatomy of the gastroesophageal junction and role of phrenoesophageal ligament; autopsy study of sphincter mechanism. Ann Surg. 1966;164:643–54.
7. Liebermann-Meffert D, Allgower M, Schmid P, et al. Muscular equivalent of the lower esophageal sphincter. Gastroenterology. 1979;76:31–8.
8. Stelzner F, Stelzner M. Manometry data support a novel concept of the lower esophageal sphincter system. Langenbecks Arch Surg. 2010;395:1083–91.
9. Pettersson GB, Bombeck CT, Nyhus LM. The lower esophageal sphincter: mechanisms of opening and closure. Surgery. 1980;88:307–14.
10. Korn O, Csendes A, Burdiles P, et al. Anatomic dilatation of the cardia and competence of the lower esophageal sphincter: a clinical and experimental study. J Gastrointest Surg. 2000;4:398–406.
11. Curcic J, Roy S, Schwizer A, et al. Abnormal structure and function of the esophagogastric junction and proximal stomach in gastroesophageal reflux disease. Am J Gastroenterol. 2014;109:658–67.
12. DeMeester TR, Wernly JA, Bryant GH, et al. Clinical and in vitro analysis of determinants of gastroesophageal competence. A study of the principles of antireflux surgery. Am J Surg. 1979;137:39–46.
13. Friedland GW. Progress in radiology: historical review of the changing concepts of lower esophageal anatomy: 430 B.C.--1977. AJR Am J Roentgenol. 1978;131:373–8.

14. Vantrappen G, Texter EC Jr, Barborka CJ, et al. The closing mechanism at the gastroesophageal junction. Am J Med. 1960;28:564–77.
15. Odze RD. Unraveling the mystery of the gastroesophageal junction: a pathologist's perspective. Am J Gastroenterol. 2005;100:1853–67.
16. Mittal RK, Fisher M, McCallum RW, et al. Human lower esophageal sphincter pressure response to increased intra-abdominal pressure. Am J Phys. 1990;258:G624–30.
17. Hill LD, Kozarek RA, Kraemer SJ, et al. The gastroesophageal flap valve: in vitro and in vivo observations. Gastrointest Endosc. 1996;44:541–7.
18. Hill LD, Kozarek RA. The gastroesophageal flap valve. J Clin Gastroenterol. 1999;28:194–7.
19. Takeuchi R, Kato K, Mizuno S, et al. Abnormal gastroesophageal flap valve is highly associated with endoscopic reflux esophagitis after helicobacter pylori eradication. Helicobacter. 2004;9:1–8.
20. Thor KB, Hill LD, Mercer DD, et al. Reappraisal of the flap valve mechanism in the gastroesophageal junction. A study of a new valvuloplasty procedure in cadavers. Acta Chir Scand. 1987;153:25–8.
21. Paterson WG. The normal antireflux mechanism. Chest Surg Clin N Am. 2001;11:473–83.
22. Brasseur JG, Ulerich R, Dai Q, Patel DK, Soliman AMS, Miller LS. Pharmacological dissection of the human gastrooesophageal segment into three sphincteric components. J Physiol. 2007;580:961–75.
23. van Herwaarden MA, Samsom M, Smout AJ. The role of hiatus hernia in gastro-oesophageal reflux disease. Eur J Gastroenterol Hepatol. 2004;16:831–5.
24. Bashashati M, Sarosiek I, McCallum RW. Epidemiology and mechanisms of gastroesophageal reflux disease in the elderly: a perspective. Ann N Y Acad Sci. 2016;1380:230–4.
25. Curci JA, Melman LM, Thompson RW, Soper NJ, Matthews BD. Elastic fiber depletion in the supporting ligaments of the gastroesophageal junction: a structural basis for the development of hiatal hernia. J Am Coll Surg. 2008;207:191–6.
26. Patti MG, Goldberg HI, Arcerito M, Bortolasi L, Tong J, Way LW. Hiatal hernia size affects lower esophageal sphincter function, esophageal acid exposure, and the degree of mucosal injury. Am J Surg. 1996;171:182–6.
27. Jones MP, Sloan SS, Jovanovic B, Kahrilas PJ. Impaired egress rather than increased access: an important independent predictor of erosive oesophagitis. Neurogastroenterol Motil. 2002;14:625–31.
28. Gregersen H, Christensen J. Clinical biomechanics. An Introduction. Sharjah: Bentham Science Publishers; 2016.
29. Mason RJ, DeMeester TR, Lund RJ, Peters JH, Crookes P, Ritter M, Gadenstatter M, Hagen JA. Nissen fundoplication prevents shortening of the sphincter during gastric distention. Arch Surg. 1997;132:719–24.
30. Bonavina L, Siboni S, Saino GI, Cavadas D, Braghetto I, Csendes A, Korn O, Figueredo EJ, Swanstrom LL, Wassenaar E. Outcomes of esophageal surgery, especially of the lower esophageal sphincter. Ann N Y Acad Sci. 2013;1300:29–42.
31. Kahrilas PJ. Anatomy and physiology of the gastroesophageal junction. Gastroenterol Clin N Am. 1997;26(3):467–86.
32. Dent J, Holloway RH, Toouli J, Dodds WJ. Mechanisms of lower oesophageal sphincter incompetence in patients with symptomatic gastrooesophageal reflux. Gut. 1998;29(8):1020–8.
33. Patti MG. An evidence-based approach to the treatment of gastroesophageal reflux disease. JAMA Surg. 2016;151(1):73–8.
34. Liu J, Parashar VK, Mittal RK. Asymmetry of lower esophageal sphincter pressure: is it related to the muscle thickness or its shape? Am J Phys. 1997;272:G1509–17.
35. Dent J. A new technique for continuous sphincter pressure measurement. Gastroenterology. 1976;71(2):263–7.
36. Miller L, Dai Q, Vegesna A, Korimilli A, Ulerich R, Schiffner B, et al. A missing sphincteric component of the gastro-oesophageal junction in patients with GORD. Neurogastroenterol Motil. 2009;21(8):813–e52.
37. Nissen R, Eine E, Einfat HE. Operation zur Beeinflussung der R defluxochitis Schweiz. Schweiz Med Wochenschr. 1956;86:590–2.

38. Lundell L, Myers JC, Jamieson GG. The effect of antireflux operations on lower oesophageal sphincter tone and postprandial symptoms. Scand J Gastroenterol. 1993;28(8):725–31.
39. Ireland AC, Holloway RH, Toouli J, Dent J. Mechanisms underlying the antireflux action of fundoplication. Gut. 1993;34(3):303–8.
40. Condon RE, Kraus MA, Wollheim D. Cause of increase in "lower esophageal sphincter" pressure after fundoplication. J Surg Res. 1976;20(5):445–50.
41. Higgs RH, Castell DO, Farrell RL. Evaluation of the effect of fundoplication on the incompetent lower esophageal sphincter. Surg Gynecol Obstet. 1975;141(4):571–5.
42. Dodds WJ, Dent J, Hogan WJ, Helm JF, Hauser R, Patel GK, et al. Mechanisms of gastroesophageal reflux in patients with reflux esophagitis. N Engl J Med. 2010;307(25):1547–52.
43. Dent J, Dodds WJ, Friedman RH, Sekiguchi T, Hogan WJ, Arndorfer RC, et al. Mechanism of gastroesophageal reflux in recumbent asymptomatic human subjects. J Clin Invest. 1980;65(2):256–67.
44. Mittal RK, Holloway RH, Penagini R, Blackshaw LA. Transient lower esophageal sphincter relaxation. Gastroenterology. 1995;109(2):601–10.
45. Penagini R, Schoeman MN, Dent J, Tippett MD, Holloway RH. Motor events underlying gastro-oesophageal reflux in ambulant patients with reflux oesophagitis. Neurogastroenterol Motil. 1996;8(2):131–41.
46. Franzi SJ, Martin CJ, Cox MR, Dent J. Response of canine lower esophageal sphincter to gastric distension. Am J Phys. 1990;259:G380–5.
47. The SAGES Guidelines Committee, Stefanidis D, Hope WW, Kohn GP, Reardon PR, Richardson WS, et al. Guidelines for surgical treatment of gastroesophageal reflux disease. Surg Endosc. 2010;24(11):2647–69.
48. O'Hanrahan T, Marples M, Bancewicz J. Recurrent reflux and wrap disruption after Nissen fundoplication: detection, incidence and timing. Br J Surg. 1990;77(5):545–7.
49. Furnée EJB, Draaisma WA, Broeders IAMJ, Gooszen HG. Surgical reintervention after failed antireflux surgery: a systematic review of the literature. J Gastrointest Surg. 2009;13(8):1539–49.
50. Hill LD, Ilves R, Stevenson JK, Pearson JM. Reoperation for disruption and recurrence after Nissen fundoplication. Arch Surg. 1979;114(4):542–8.
51. Raeside MC, Madigan D, Myers JC, Devitt PG, Jamieson GG, Thompson SK. Post-fundoplication contrast studies: is there room for improvement? Br J Radiol. 2012;85(1014):792–9.
52. Carbo AI, Kim RH, Gates T, D'Agostino HR. Imaging findings of successful and failed fundoplication. Radiographics. 2014;34(7):1873–84.
53. Jailwala J, Massey B, Staff D, Shaker R, Hogan W. Post-fundoplication symptoms: the role for endoscopic assessment of fundoplication integrity. Gastrointest Endosc. 2001;54(3):351–6.
54. Kahrilas PJ, Kim HC, Pandolfino JE. Approaches to the diagnosis and grading of hiatal hernia. Best Pract Res Clin Gastroenterol. 2008;22(4):601–16.
55. Klaus A, Raiser F, Swain JM, Hinder RA. Manometric components of the lower esophageal double hump. Dig Dis. 2000;18(3):172–7.
56. Savarino E, de Bortoli N, Bellini M, Galeazzi F, Ribolsi M, Salvador R, et al. Practice guidelines on the use of esophageal manometry - A GISMAD-SIGE-AIGO medical position statement. Dig Liver Dis. 2016;48(10):1124–35.
57. Jobe BA, Richter JE, Hoppo T, Peters JH, Bell R, Dengler WC, et al. Preoperative diagnostic workup before antireflux surgery: an evidence and experience-based consensus of the esophageal diagnostic advisory panel. J Am Coll Surg. 2013;217(4):586–97.
58. Herbella FA. Critical analysis of esophageal multichannel intraluminal impedance monitoring 20 years later. ISRN Gastroenterol. 2012;2012:903240.
59. Hyun JJ, Bak YT. Clinical significance of hiatal hernia. Gut Liver. 2011;5(3):267–77.
60. Boeckxstaens GE. Alterations confined to the gastro-oesophageal junction: the relationship between low LOSP, TLOSRs, hiatus hernia and acid pocket. Best Pract Res Clin Gastroenterol. 2010;24(6):821–9.
61. Kessing BF, Conchillo JM, Bredenoord AJ, Smout AJ, Masclee AA. The clinical relevance of transient lower oesophageal sphincter relaxations in gastro-oesophageal reflux disease. Aliment Pharmacol Ther. 2011;33(6):650–61.

62. Kahrilas PJ, Shi G, Manka M, Joehl RJ. Increased frequency of transient lower esophageal sphincter relaxation induced by gastric distention in reflux patients with hiatal hernia. Gastroenterology. 2000;118(4):688–95.
63. van Herwaarden MA, Samsom M, Smout AJ. Excess gastroesophageal reflux in patients with hiatus hernia is caused by mechanisms other than transient LES relaxations. Gastroenterology. 2000;119(6):1439–46.
64. DeHaan RK, Davila D, Frelich MJ, Gould JC. Esophagogastric junction distensibility is greater following Toupet compared to Nissen fundoplication. Surg Endosc. 2017;31(1):193–8.
65. Lottrup C, McMahon BP, Ejstrud P, Ostapiuk MA, Funch-Jensen P, Drewes AM. Esophagogastric junction distensibility in hiatus hernia. Dis Esophagus. 2016;29(5):463–71.
66. Tatarian T, Pucci MJ, Palazzo F. A modern approach to the surgical treatment of Gastroesophageal reflux disease. J Laparoendosc Adv Surg Tech A. 2016;26(3):174–9.
67. Gordon C, Kang JY, Neild PJ, Maxwell JD. The role of the hiatus hernia in gastro-oesophageal reflux disease. Aliment Pharmacol Ther. 2004;20(7):719–32.
68. Pandolfino JE, Shi G, Trueworthy B, Kahrilas PJ. Esophagogastric junction opening during relaxation distinguishes nonhernia reflux patients, hernia patients, and normal subjects. Gastroenterology. 2003;125(4):1018–24.
69. Kwiatek MA, Kahrilas PJ, Soper NJ, et al. Esophagogastric junction distensibility after fundoplication assessed with a novel functional luminal imaging probe. J Gastrointest Surg. 2010;14(2):268–76.
70. Yassi R, Cheng LK, Al-Ali S, et al. Three-dimensional high-resolution reconstruction of the human gastro-oesophageal junction. Clin Anat. 2010;23:287–96.
71. Gregersen H, Liao D, Brasseur JG. The Esophagiome: concept, status, and future perspectives. Ann N Y Acad Sci. 2016;1380(1):6–18.

Chapter 11
Adverse Outcome and Failure Following Laparoscopic Anti-reflux Surgery for Hiatal Hernia: Is One Fundoplication Better than Other?

Ciro Andolfi and Marco P. Fisichella

11.1 Introduction

The management of hiatal hernia (HH) is one of the most debated in surgery. Trends regarding indications, approach (open, laparoscopic, thoracoscopic), sac excision, mesh placement, and routine performance of fundoplication have changed over time. Today, most surgeons lean to perform a laparoscopic HH repair that entails the excision of the sac, liberal use of a mesh to buttress the hiatus, and the addition of an anti-reflux procedure. The rationale of including an anti-reflux procedure is to treat coexistent reflux or to prevent the onset of "de novo" postoperative reflux [1, 2]. In fact, many studies have shown that in the majority of patients a HH is associated with symptoms—even subtle—of dysphagia, bloating, or gastroesophageal reflux disease (GERD), and that an extensive hiatal dissection could exacerbate GERD postoperatively by impairing the anatomical anti-reflux barrier [3]. Already in 1996, a work by Wo et al. [4] showed that 68% of patients with type III PEH had a history of heartburn. Interestingly, many of these patients (41%) no longer had GERD symptoms at the time the operation, and the authors attributed this finding to the flap valve created by the stomach above the gastro-esophageal junction, suggesting that, in most patients, a type III paraesophageal hernia may be an enlarging sliding hernia. A recent double-blinded randomized controlled trial by Muller-Stich et al. [5] has validated the addition of an anti-reflux procedure by showing that a fundoplication during a PEH repair results in a net improvement in patients'

C. Andolfi, M.D.
Department of Surgery, The University of Chicago Pritzker School of Medicine, Chicago, IL, USA

M.P. Fisichella, M.D. (✉)
Department of Surgery, Brigham and Women's Hospital and Boston VA Healthcare System, Harvard Medical School, 1400 VFW Parkway, West Roxbury, Boston 02132, MA, USA
e-mail: piero.fisichella@va.gov

M.A. Memon (ed.), *Hiatal Hernia Surgery*,
https://doi.org/10.1007/978-3-319-64003-7_11

symptoms with reduced acid exposure and esophagitis. However, very little has been written on which type of fundoplication should be performed in these patients based on the outcome. In general, a total fundoplication is the preferred approach in patients with GERD, as it provides a better control of reflux than a partial fundoplication [6, 7]. Conversely, recent trends have highlighted how in patients with PEH a partial fundoplication could provide—especially in the absence of preoperative manometric data—a satisfactory balance between prevention/control of GERD and prevention of postoperative dysphagia. We have set as the goal of our chapter that to provide an evidence based overview of how the type of fundoplication can affect the outcome of a hiatal hernia repair.

11.2 Laparoscopic Anti-reflux Surgery Failure

Most experts would agree that failure of a fundoplication is generally owing to 1 of the following causes: (1) wrong indications for the operation; (2) wrong preoperative workup; and (3) wrong type of fundoplication.

11.2.1 Indications

Indications for surgery result from an accurate clinical and diagnostic evaluation of the patient hiatal hernia. Whether the patient has GER symptoms or not, when choosing to add a fundoplication, it is important to perform a complete work-up and also consider patient's comorbidities into account. For instance, it has been extensively shown that in the setting of morbid obesity a hiatal hernia repair with fundoplication has the highest chance of recurrence. In these patients, the surgical treatment, independent from the primary achievement of weight loss, may result in the failure of the procedure, a more difficult conversion to a bariatric operation at a later time, and would not resolve other comorbidities.

11.2.2 Preoperative Workup

Hiatal hernia repair and antireflux surgery have excellent long-term outcome but has been reported with large variations in hiatal hernia recurrence, post-operative reflux symptoms and dysphagia. The appreciation of the excellent outcomes of primary antireflux surgery and the introduction of minimal invasive approaches have led to increased number of primary antireflux procedures with subsequent increased numbers of failure and demand for revision. Recent data show that 10–20% of patients will eventually experience recurrence of their symptoms or new onset of dysphagia.

There seems to be little agreement on the best preoperative evaluation of patients with HH. Generally, an esophagram (or a CT scan) and an upper endoscopy (EGD) are requested to evaluate the type of hernia and to exclude concomitant foregut pathologies (Figs. 11.1 and 11.2). Regarding preoperative esophageal testing, the presence of esophagitis Los Angeles classification C or D, or Barrett's esophagus, can be considered an objective evidence of gastroesophageal reflux and might avoid further pH testing, which is usually performed to detect reflux prior to performing a fundoplication. Some authors limit the performance of a fundoplication to patients with gastroesophageal reflux (GER) symptoms [8–12]. However, other authors prefer to implement their patient's selection by adding objective measures of reflux (pH monitoring or EGD findings) [8, 9, 11]. Leeder et al. [12] elected to perform a fundoplication in all patients since 1998, due to the excessive amount of reflux symptoms in the follow-up of patients who underwent a HH repair without a fundoplication. However, the debate whether to add or not a fundoplication still persists. Proponents of the addition of a fundoplication cite that GER symptoms have poor sensitivity and specificity [13–17] and are unreliable when deciding whether to perform a fundoplication or not. A preoperative pH monitoring would be

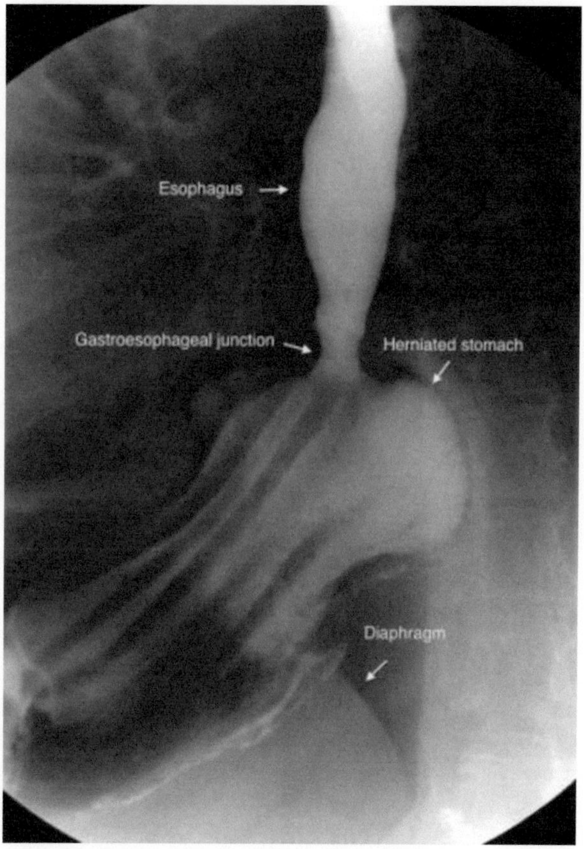

Fig. 11.1 Barium swallow

Fig. 11.2 Upper endoscopy

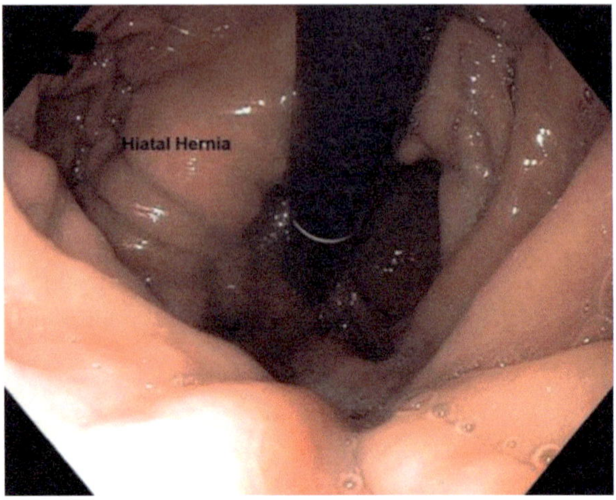

the most appropriate tool in this decision-making, as it provides a more sensitive and specific assessment of the presence and severity of GERD. In addition, proponents of these addition of a fundoplication cite that an extensive hiatal dissection, even in patients without preoperative reflux, impairs the gastroesophageal barrier with resulting "de novo" GERD [5, 18]. Many authors believe that pH monitoring had little value, as a fundoplication should have been routinely performed [1, 19–34]. Esophageal manometry plays a more important role than pH testing in planning a fundoplication [14, 16, 35, 36]. The primary purpose of performing an esophageal manometry before an anti-reflux procedure is to exclude achalasia or other primary esophageal motility disorders, which would contraindicate total fundoplication and favor a cardiomyotomy. Esophageal manometry also helps detecting those patients with severe degree of hypomotility of the esophageal body that would contraindicate a total fundoplication in favor of a partial. In fact, several authors have convened that when the esophageal contraction amplitude (or, in another words, the pressure needed to pass a food bolus past a total fundoplication) is 30–40 mmHg, then a partial fundoplication should be considered to prevent postoperative dysphagia [37, 38].

11.2.3 Is One Fundoplication Better than Another?

Carrott et al. [39] suggested that symptoms associated with paraesophageal hernia are varied, and that truly asymptomatic patients are rare. In this single-center review of 270 consecutive patients undergoing surgical repair of paraesophageal hernia, Carrott et al. found that symptoms included heartburn (65%), early satiety (50%), chest pain (48%), dyspnea (48%), dysphagia (48%), and regurgitation (47%). Due to the difficulty in evaluating the esophageal motor function in some of these patients and the common preoperative complaint of dysphagia [2, 38, 39],

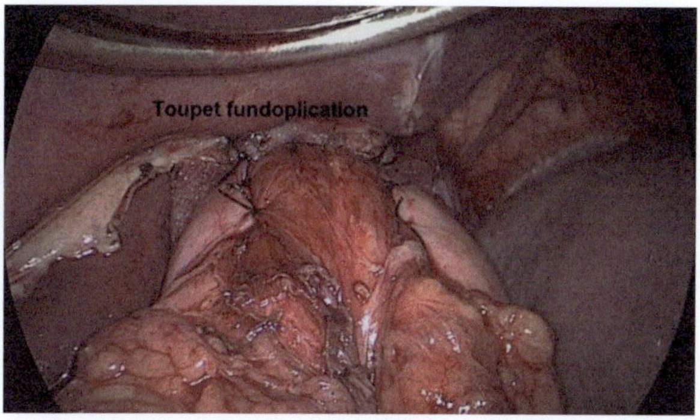

Fig. 11.3 Partial posterior fundoplication

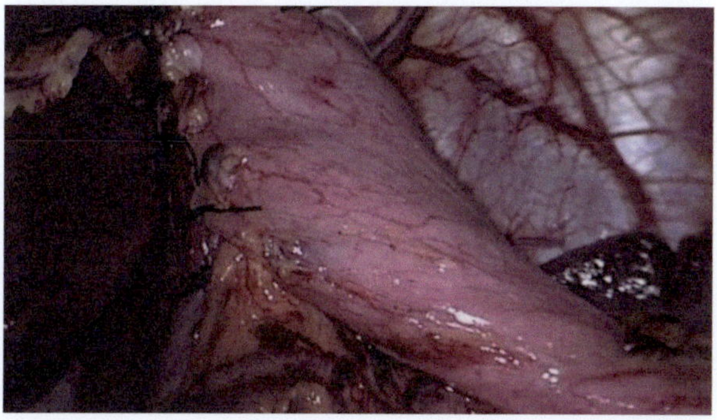

Fig. 11.4 Partial anterior fundoplication

some surgeons prefer to perform a partial fundoplication (Figs. 11.3 and 11.4), rather than a total fundoplication [23, 24]. In fact, a partial fundoplication might be associated with fewer functional problems—leading to persistent dysphagia postoperatively—than a total fundoplication in those patients who might have undiagnosed impaired esophageal motility [38]. However, there has been little objective evidence to support this trend, and one might argue that the overall durability of a partial fundoplication in the control of reflux might be less reliable than that of a total fundoplication [40–43]. Currently, there is a large agreement to perform a partial fundoplication (either posterior or anterior) in patients with impaired esophageal motility. Allaix et al. [44] suggested performing a total fundoplication as the procedure of choice, while reserving a partial fundoplication in cases of severe esophageal dismotility or during emergencies, when the patient presents with signs and symptoms of incarceration or strangulation. The rationale of this approach was that patients are frequently elderly, often they do not have preoperative esophageal manometry, and a partial fundoplication might also be an effective form of gastropexy. Conversely, Arafat et al. [30] routinely performed manometry in all patients, and in those with a challenging insertion, they placed the manometry catheter with the help of an endoscope. Arafat et al. suggested performing a partial fundoplication when manometry showed aperistalsis or severe dismotility, yet not objectively defined. Auyang et al. [45] suggested performing a partial fundoplication in patients with 90% or more failed peristaltic contractions. Cohn et al. shunned from a total fundoplication in all patients with aperistalsis and those with severe dysphagia with inability to pass the manometry catheter. DeMeester and other authors reported that a fundoplication should always be added to all HH repairs and the type of fundoplication should be selected on the basis of the patient's esophageal motility [32–34].

In the studies by Ponsky and Stiven, of 142 patients undergoing HH repair with a partial fundoplication–141 partial posterior (270 Toupet) and 1 partial anterior (180 Dor, due to the anatomical difficulties in performing a posterior wrap)—at a mean follow-up of 17 months, no patient reported reflux symptoms, while 4 (3%) patients (1 in the Ponsky and 3 in the Stiven study) presented with postoperative dysphagia requiring endoscopic dilation [23, 24]. In two studies, by Mittal et al. [10] and Van Der Westhuizen et al. [10, 11] no fundoplication was performed in patients with impaired esophageal peristalsis, and in patients with normal motility, the type of fundoplication was chosen according to gastric anatomy and fundus compliance. Overall, on a combined number of 225 patients, 150 (66.5%) underwent total fundoplication, 18 (8%) partial posterior fundoplication, 1 (0.5%) partial anterior fundoplication, 4 (2%) a gastric bypass for obesity (BMI[40 kg/m^2), and 52 (23%) had no fundoplication. Postoperatively, at a mean follow-up of 29 months, 18 patients (12%) who underwent a total fundoplication presented with dysphagia, with 10 requiring endoscopic dilation. Eleven patients presented postoperatively with symptoms of reflux, seven after a total fundoplication (4.6%), and four after PEH repair alone (7.7%), yet no postoperative pH monitoring was performed [10, 11]. Interestingly, Dallemagne et al. and Leeder et al. routinely performed a preoperative manometry and stated that they considered a total fundoplication as the procedure choice in all patients, while they reserved a partial fundoplication only to those with little compliance of the gastric fundus [12, 26]. Overall, on a combined number of 118 patients (96 total fundoplication, 11 partial anterior, and 11 partial posterior), among patients with total fundoplication, three had postoperative dysphagia (3%); two required a conversion to a Toupet fundoplication and 1 improved after endoscopic dilation. Among these 118 patients, 21 (18%) had postoperative reflux symptoms. Gouvas et al. [21] divided the 16 patients with abnormal esophageal motility in two subgroups: one group of nine patients who received a total fundoplication, and another group of seven patients who received a partial posterior fundoplication. At 12 months of follow-up, they showed that four patients (44%) after a total fundoplication and two patients (29%) after a partial fundoplication presented with postoperative dysphagia. Conversely, four patients (57%) presented with reflux symptoms after a partial fundoplication, while one patient (11%) presented with GER symptoms after a total fundoplication. In addition, all 16 patients underwent postoperative esophageal pH monitoring and all of those with a partial fundoplication had an abnormal amount of reflux (mean DeMeester score of 33), while 4 out of 9 patients (44%) after a total fundoplication had an abnormal amount of reflux (mean DeMeester score of 39).

11.3 Conclusions

These data have shown that in the majority of surgeons prefer to add a fundoplication to all HH repairs, preferably a total fundoplication in patients with normal esophageal motility. Despite this widespread tailored approach, as of today there is no evidence in literature that a fundoplication is better than another in preventing reflux and avoiding dysphagia in patients undergoing hiatal hernia repair, and the small prospective/retrospective and non-comparative studies in the literature do not help in drawing definitive conclusions. Based on our experience, we strongly suggest performing esophageal testing, when possible, and adopt a tailored approach performing a total fundoplication only in patients with effective esophageal motility.

What Is the Current Knowledge and What Future Direction Is Required

- Most of the authors agree that a fundoplication should be added to a hiatal hernia repair.
- When possible, a complete workup including pH monitoring and high-resolution manometry should be performed before planning an operation.
- The majority of surgeons embrace a tailored approach when choosing the antireflux procedure, performing a total fundoplication only in patients with effective esophageal peristalsis.
- A partial anterior or posterior fundoplication should be considered for patients with esophageal motility disorders.
- Further study is required to validate this tailored approach.

References

1. Swanstrom LL, Jobe BA, Kinzie LR, Horvath KD. Esophageal motility and outcomes following laparoscopic paraesophageal hernia repair and fundoplication. Am J Surg. 1999;177:359–63.
2. Andolfi C, Jalilvand A, Plana A, Fisichella PM. Surgical treatment of paraesophageal hernias: a review. J Laparoendosc Adv Surg Tech A. 2016;26(10):778–83.
3. Maziak D, Todd T, Pearson F. Massive hiatus hernia: evaluation and surgical management. J Thorac Cardiovasc Surg. 1998;115:53–60.
4. Wo JM, Branum GD, Hunter JG, Trus TN, Mauren SJ, Waring JP. Clinical features of type III (mixed) paraesophageal hernia. Am J Gastroenterol. 1996;91(5):914–6.
5. Muller-Stich BP, Achtstatter V, Diener MK, Gondan M, Warschkow R, Marra F, et al. Repair of paraesophageal hiatal hernias—is a fundoplication needed? A randomized controlled pilot trial. J Am Coll Surg. 2015;221(2):602–10.
6. Patti MG, Robinson T, Galvani C, Gorodner MV, Fisichella PM, Way LW. Total fundoplication is superior to partial fundoplication even when esophageal peristalsis is weak. J Am Coll Surg. 2004;198(6):863–9. discussion 869–70

7. Ottignon Y, Pelissier EP, Mantion G, et al. Gastroesophageal reflux. Comparison of clinical, pH-metric and manometric results of Nissen's and of Toupet's procedures. Gastroenterol Clin Biol. 1994;18:920–6.
8. Medina L, Peetz M, Ratzer E, Fenoglio M. Laparoscopic paraesophageal hernia repair. JSLS. 1998;2(3):269–72.
9. Furnee EJ, Draaisma WA, Gooszen HG, Hazebroek EJ, Smout AJ, Broeders IA. Tailored or routine addition of an antireflux fundoplication in laparoscopic large hiatal hernia repair: a comparative cohort study. World J Surg. 2011;35(1):78–84. https://doi.org/10.1007/s00268-010-0814-8.
10. Mittal SK, Bikhchandani J, Gurney O, Yano F, Lee T. Outcomes after repair of the intrathoracic stomach: objective follow-up of up to 5 years. Surg Endosc. 2011;25(2):556–66.
11. Van der Westhuizen L, Dunphy KM, Knott B, Carbonell AM, Smith DE, Cobb WS. The need for fundoplication at the time of laparoscopic paraesophageal hernia repair. Am Surg. 2013;79(6):572–7.
12. Leeder PC, Smith G, Dehn TC. Laparoscopic management of large paraesophageal hiatal hernia. Surg Endosc. 2003;17(9):1372–5.
13. Patti MG, Diener U, Tamburini A, Molena D, Way LW. Role of esophageal function tests in diagnosis of gastroesophageal reflux disease. Dig Dis Sci. 2001;46(3):597–602.
14. Andolfi C, Vigneswaran Y, Kavitt RT, Herbella FA, Patti MG. Laparoscopic antireflux surgery: importance of patient's selection and preoperative workup. J Laparoendosc Adv Surg Tech A. 2017;27(2):101–5.
15. Herbella FA, Andolfi C, Vigneswaran Y, Patti MG, Pinna BR. Importance of esophageal manometry and pH monitoring for the evaluation of otorhinolaryngologic (ENT) manifestations of GERD. A multicenter study. J Gastrointest Surg. 2016;20(10):1673–8.
16. Jobe BA, Richter JE, Hoppo T, Peters JH, Bell R, Dengler WC, DeVault K, Fass R, Gyawali CP, Kahrilas PJ, Lacy BE, Pandolfino JE, Patti MG, Swanstrom LL, Kurian AA, Vela MF, Vaezi M, DeMeester TR. Preoperative diagnostic workup before antireflux surgery: an evidence and experience-based consensus of the esophageal diagnostic advisory panel. J Am Coll Surg. 2013;217(4):586–97. https://doi.org/10.1016/j.jamcollsurg.2013.05.023.
17. Andolfi C, Bonavina L, Kavitt RT, Konda VJ, Asti E, Patti MG. Importance of esophageal manometry and pH monitoring in the evaluation of patients with refractory gastroesophageal reflux disease: a multicenter study. J Laparoendosc Adv Surg Tech A. 2016;26(7):548–50.
18. Casabella F, Sinanan M, Horgan S, Pellegrini CA. Systematic use of gastric fundoplication in laparoscopic repair of paraesophageal hernias. Am J Surg. 1996;17(5):485–9.
19. Perdikis G, Hinder RA, Filipi CJ, Walenz T, McBride PJ, Smith SL, et al. Laparoscopic paraesophageal hernia repair. Arch Surg. 1997;132(6):586–9. discussion 90–1
20. El Khoury R, Ramirez M, Hungness ES, Soper NJ, Patti MG. Symptom relief after laparoscopic paraesophageal hernia repair without mesh. J Gastrointest Surg. 2015;19(11):1938–42.
21. Gouvas N, Tsiaoussis J, Athanasakis E, Zervakis N, Pechlivanides G, Xynos E. Simple suture or prosthesis hiatal closure in laparoscopic repair of paraesophageal hernia: a retrospective cohort study. Dis Esophagus. 2011;24(2):69–78.
22. Wiechmann RJ, Ferguson MK, Naunheim KS, McKesey P, Hazelrigg SJ, Santucci TS, et al. Laparoscopic management of giant paraesophageal herniation. Ann Thorac Surg. 2001;71(4):1080–6. discussion 6–7
23. Ponsky J, Rosen M, Fanning A, Malm J. Anterior gastropexy may reduce the recurrence rate after laparoscopic paraesophageal hernia repair. Surg Endosc. 2003;17(7):1036–41.
24. Stiven PN, Hansen R, Richardson A, Leibman S, Smith GS. Postoperative dysphagia in laparoscopic paraesophageal hernia repair: the effect of distal esophageal angulation. Surg Laparosc Endosc Percutan Tech. 2013;23(5):449–52.
25. Alicuben ET, Worrell SG, DeMeester SR. Impact of crural relaxing incisions, collis gastroplasty, and non-cross-linked human dermal mesh crural reinforcement on early hiatal hernia recurrence rates. J Am Coll Surg. 2014;219(5):988–92.
26. Dallemagne B, Kohnen L, Perretta S, Weerts J, Markiewicz S, Jehaes C. Laparoscopic repair of paraesophageal hernia. Long-term follow-up reveals good clinical outcome despite high radiological recurrence rate. Ann Surg. 2011;253(2):291–6.

27. Terry M, Smith CD, Branum GD, Galloway K, Waring JP, Hunter JG. Outcomes of laparoscopic fundoplication for gastroesophageal reflux disease and paraesophageal hernia. Surg Endosc. 2001;15(7):691–9.
28. Gantert WA, Patti MG, Arcerito M, Feo C, Stewart L, DePinto M, Bhoyrul S, Rangel S, Tyrrell D, Fujino Y, Mulvihill SJ, Way LW. Laparoscopic repair of paraesophageal hiatal hernias. J Am Coll Surg. 1998;186(4):428–32. (discussion 432–3)
29. Edye MB, Canin-Endres J, Gattorno F, Salky BA. Durability of laparoscopic repair of paraesophageal hernia. Ann Surg. 1998;228(4):528–35.
30. Arafat FO, Teitelbaum EN, Hungness ES. Modern treatment of paraesophageal hernia: preoperative evaluation and technique for laparoscopic repair. Surg Laparosc Endosc Percutan Tech. 2012;22(4):297–303.
31. Cohn TD, Soper NJ. Paraesophageal hernia repair: techniques for success. J Laparoendosc Adv Surg Tech A. 2017;27(1):19–23.
32. DeMeester SR. Laparoscopic paraesophageal hernia repair: critical steps and adjunct techniques to minimize recurrence. Surg Laparosc Endosc Percutan Tech. 2013;23(5):429–35.
33. Oleynikov D, Jolley JM. Paraesophageal hernia. Surg Clin North Am. 2015;95(3):555–65.
34. Soper NJ, Teitelbaum EN. Laparoscopic paraesophageal hernia repair: current controversies. Surg Laparosc Endosc Percutan Tech. 2013;23(5):442–5.
35. Cai W, Watson DI, Lally CJ, Devitt PG, Game PA, Jamieson GG. Ten-year clinical outcome of a prospective randomized clinical trial of laparoscopic Nissen versus anterior 180 (degrees) partial fundoplication. Br J Surg. 2008;95(12):1501–5. https://doi.org/10.1002/bjs.6318.
36. Broeders JA, Roks DJ, Ahmed Ali U, Watson DI, Baigrie RJ, Cao Z, Hartmann J, Maddern GJ. Laparoscopic anterior 180-degree versus Nissen fundoplication for gastroesophageal reflux disease: systematic review and meta-analysis of randomized clinical trials. Ann Surg. 2013;257(5):850–9. https://doi.org/10.1097/SLA.0b013e31828604dd.
37. Minjarez RC, Jobe BA. Surgical therapy for gastroesophageal reflux disease. GI Motil Online. 2006. https://doi.org/10.1038/gimo56
38. Patti MG, De Bellis M, De Pinto M, Bhoyrul S, Tong J, Arcerito M, Mulvihill SJ, Way L. Partial fundoplication for gastroesophageal reflux. Surg Endosc. 1997;11(5):445–8.
39. Carrott PW, Hong J, Kuppusamy M, Koehler RP, Low DE. Clinical ramifications of giant paraesophageal hernias are underappreciated: making the case for routine surgical repair. Ann Thorac Surg. 2012;94(2):421–6. https://doi.org/10.1016/j.athoracsur.2012.04.058.
40. Thor KB, Silander T. A long-term randomized prospective trial of the Nissen procedure versus a modified Toupet technique. Ann Surg. 1989;210:719–24.
41. Lundell L, Abrahamsson H, Ruth M, et al. Long-term results of a prospective randomized comparison of total fundic wrap (Nissen-Rossetti) or semi-fundoplication (Toupet) for gastro-oesophageal reflux. Br J Surg. 1996;83:830–5.
42. Chrysos E, Tsiaoussis J, Zoras OJ, et al. Laparoscopic surgery for gastroesophageal reflux disease patients with impaired esophageal peristalsis: total or partial fundoplication? J Am Coll Surg. 2003;197:8–15.
43. Erenoglu C, Miller A, Schirmer B. Laparoscopic Toupet versus Nissen fundoplication for the treatment of gastroesophageal reflux diesease. Int Surg. 2003;88:219–25.
44. Allaix ME, Patti MG. Laparoscopic paraesophageal hernia repair. Surg Laparosc Endosc Percutan Tech. 2013;23(5):425–8.
45. Auyang ED, Pellegrini CA. How i do it: laparoscopic paraesophageal hernia repair. J Gastrointest Surg. 2012;16(7):1406–11.

Chapter 12
Post-operative HRIM and FLIP for Dysphagia Following Antireflux Procedures

John Pandolfino and Dustin Carlson

12.1 Introduction

Post-operative dysphagia after an antireflux procedure is a common problem that requires a thorough evaluation of anatomy and physiology to determine whether the complaint is due to obstruction at the esophagogastric junction or a defect in peristalsis that was either missed or underestimated during the pre-operative assessment. Many tools are helpful in this assessment and the first step is to assess the anatomy of the EGJ as antireflux procedures focus primarily on attempting to augment the barrier function of this anatomic zone. This can be accomplished with a careful endoscopy or a barium esophagram to determine whether the antireflux procedure is intact or potentially disrupted with or without herniation. Additionally, these tools are also important in ruling out strictures and other mechanical problems related to the various endoscopic and surgical approaches.

High-resolution impedance-manometry (HRIM) and Functional lumen imaging probe (FLIP) evaluation should be performed when there is no overt cause of post-operative dysphagia found on endoscopy and barium esophagram. High-resolution impedance manometry can assess the ability of the lower esophageal sphincter (LES) to relax and can also provide surrogate information regarding obstruction via an assessment of intrabolus pressure. Additionally, peristaltic function and bolus clearance can also be assessed during HRIM to determine whether there are severe abnormalities in motor function that will lead to severe bolus retention once the antireflux barrier is improved. The FLIP procedure is a complementary approach that can be used endoscopically to assess the opening dynamics of the EGJ. Although the FLIP has been primarily utilized in the evaluation of achalasia, this approach

J. Pandolfino (✉) • D. Carlson
Division of Gastroenterology and Hepatology, Department of Medicine,
Feinberg School of Medicine, Northwestern University,
676 St Clair St, Suite 1400, Chicago, IL 60611-2951, USA
e-mail: j-pandolfino@northwestern.edu

M.A. Memon (ed.), *Hiatal Hernia Surgery*,
https://doi.org/10.1007/978-3-319-64003-7_12

can be applied to the evaluation of post-fundoplication dysphagia as the primary focus is documenting normal EGJ opening.

The current chapter will focus on the work-up of post-operative dysphagia after antireflux procedures with the assumption that there are no overt abnormalities in anatomy noted on endoscopy or barium esophagram. Additionally, the approach to these patients will be generalized across both the endoscopic and surgical approaches as the primary goal of HRIM and FLIP are to rule out a major motor disorder and obstruction at the EGJ.

12.2 Algorithm: Evaluation of Dysphagia After an Antireflux Procedure

It is not uncommon for a patient to note some degree of dysphagia after an antireflux procedure and the difficult part of the early evaluation is determining whether the complaint is transient or will persist. A feeling of food hanging up or that there is a foreign body sensation is expected during the early post-procedure period (first 30 days) because the anatomy has been altered to prevent reflux and thus, inherently this area will be more obstructive to passage of liquid and food. As long as patients are maintaining their weight, not requiring narcotics for pain or regurgitating (especially at night), I will monitor the patient closely during this early post-procedure time-frame. After 30 days, if the patient continues to have symptoms or the symptoms are progressive or associated with weight loss and nocturnal regurgitation, evaluation with endoscopy and/or barium esophagram should be performed to assess the anatomy (Fig. 12.1). If there is no overt herniation or disruption, or there is a suggestion that an obstruction is occurring due to these abnormalities, the next step should focus on assessing EGJ opening. This can be accomplished by performing an EndoFLIP™ evaluation during the endoscopic evaluation. Alternatively, this can be accomplished with a barium esophagram using a 12.5 mm barium tablet if FLIP is not available. If there is an obstruction noted and the anatomy is conducive to dilation [no frank herniation or disruption], I will typically perform a through-the-scope (TTS) balloon dilation to 20 mmHg with the caveat that this will likely need to be repeated and escalated if no change in symptoms occur to a higher diameter using either the EsoFLIP dilator balloon or the standard pneumatic balloon dilators from 30 to 35 mm. Patients without evidence of obstruction should undergo HRIM evaluation and in most instances I will typically place this during endoscopy to expedite the work-up and improve patient adherence. The typical swallow protocol will be used to determine whether peristaltic function has changed and whether an underlying primary motor disorder was undiagnosed before the operation. It is important to realize that the operation can alter motor function and pseudoachalasia may be difficult to discern from primary achalasia that was missed. The pre-operative manometry is usually very helpful as it is unlikely that achalasia has

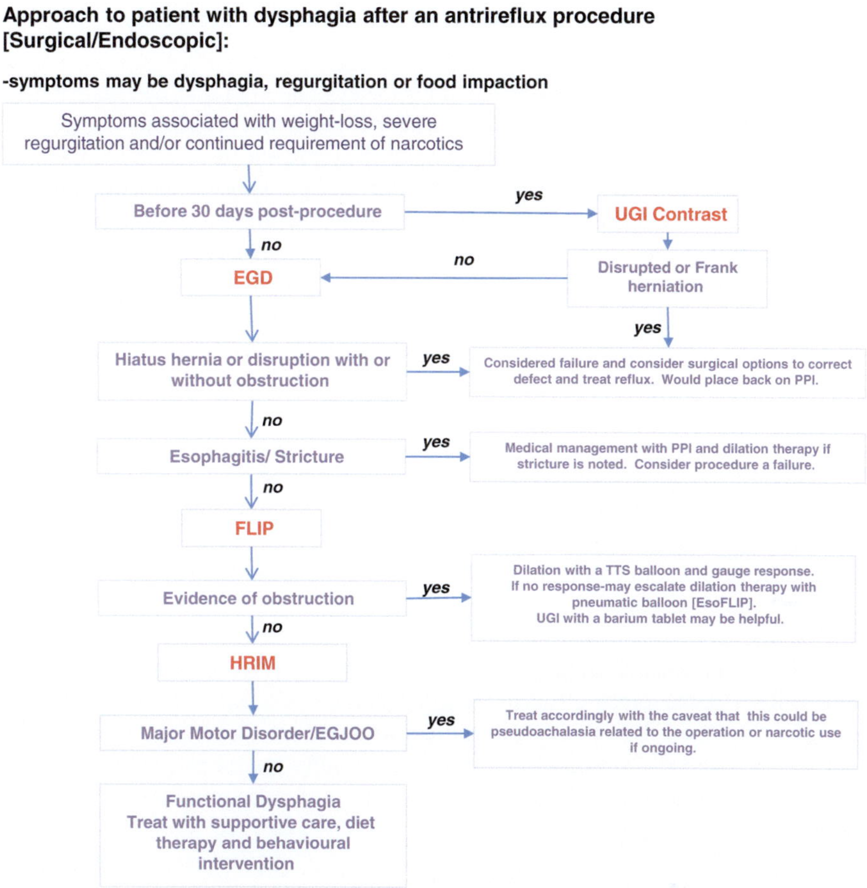

Fig. 12.1 Management algorithm for patients presenting with dysphagia after an antireflux procedure. Patients presenting with symptoms that are severe requiring pain medication and/or associated with regurgitation and weight loss require some evaluation to primarily rule out an anatomic or mechanical problem related to herniation or disruption. A step-wise approach is used that ultimately will lead to a diagnosis consistent with functional dysphagia if both FLIP analysis and HRIM are negative

evolved over a short time period and occasionally, interventions with amyl nitrite can be helpful to differentiate a mechanical obstruction (no relaxation to amyl nitrite) from achalasia (relaxation in response to amyl nitrite). Additionally, narcotics can be associated with a type III achalasia pattern or an EGJOO and repeat manometry off these medications should be attempted if possible. Patients without evidence of obstruction or a major motor disorder will typically be treated as if they meet criteria for functional dysphagia and will be referred for cognitive behavioral therapy, hypnosis and dietary consultation.

12.3 High-Resolution Impedance Manometry (HRIM)

Esophageal manometry is recommended for the evaluation of non-obstructive dysphagia and prior to anti-reflux surgery [1]. Although not a primary indication, manometry has been used to assess persistent dysphagia in post-fundoplication patients and extrapolating from protocols for dysphagia appears to be reasonable. High-resolution manometry (HRM) utilizes catheters with pressure sensors spaced 1–2 cm apart that are positioned spanning from the hypopharynx to the stomach to simultaneously measure pressures generated along the entire length of the esophagus. Sophisticated software processes the HRM pressure output to generate esophageal pressure topography (EPT) plots that represent esophageal motility and sphincter function on color-coded, pressure-space-time plots [2]. Analysis of EPT plots is facilitated by objective metrics of esophageal function that can be applied to classify individual swallows and generate esophageal motility diagnosis according to a consensus-generated scheme: the Chicago Classification [3, 4]. Once again, the Chicago Classification was not meant to assess post-fundoplication dysphagia, however, it is reasonable to utilize the current metrics given the fact that asymptomatic post-fundoplication patients appear to have similar normal values when compared to controls [5, 6].

Over the last 5 years, there has been an increased interest in combining HRM technology with impedance and to leverage the information on bolus transit from impedance with the improved accuracy and detail of HRM. Basically, this approach gives you the "best of both worlds" and allows for more sophisticated analysis of esophageal function. Impedance electrodes are usually spaced at 2 cm intervals to straddle pressure sensors and provide an assessment of bolus transit/retention and a more robust assessment of IBP.

12.3.1 HRIM Study Protocol

After catheter calibration and application of topical anesthetic to the patient's nare and/or throat, the HRM catheter is placed transnasally and positioned with the pressure sensors spanning form the hypopharynx, through the esophagus, and 3–5 cm into the stomach. After a brief period for patient acclimation, a baseline of resting pressures can be obtained over approximately 30 s of easy breathing and without swallows. Confirmation of correct placement of the catheter traversing the esophagogastric junction (EGJ) can be confirmed during this period by recognition of the presence of the pressure inversion point (PIP), i.e., the point at which the inspiration-associated negative intrathoracic pressure inverts to the positive intra-abdominal pressure. Having the patient take deep breaths facilitates identification of the PIP by augmenting the EGJ pressure and exaggerating the intra-thoracic and intra-abdominal pressures. This can be helpful in patients after hernia repair to determine whether there is recurrence, however, this should usually be noted during endoscopy.

The Chicago classification is based on the analysis of ten supine, liquid (5-mL water) swallows and is validated for use in the non-surgical patient. Since one of the primary objectives in assessing patients after antireflux procedures focuses on defining subtle obstruction, additional components can be added to the manometric protocol to supplement clinical interpretation. Inclusion of upright swallows can be useful to help distinguish if abnormal pressure signals, particularly at the EGJ, are related to anatomic abnormalities, such as vascular artifact or hiatal hernia [7]. Incorporating swallows of different bolus textures (thick liquids or solid) or a test meal may also be beneficial to uncover symptoms and/or abnormal findings of esophageal function [8]. Multiple, rapid swallows (generally 5 swallows of 2-mL water spaced 2–3 s) can also be included to elucidate defects in deglutitive inhibition (if esophageal contractions occur during the course of the multiple swallows) and to assess for *peristaltic reserve* [9, 10]. Peristaltic reserve can be identified by augmentation of the esophageal contractile vigor following the multiple swallows and may help predict risk of developing post-fundoplication dysphagia or detect an etiology for symptoms in an otherwise normal manometry study [9, 10].

Our institutions standard protocol includes (1) Ten supine, liquid swallows, (2) five upright liquid (5-mL water) swallows, (3) one multiple, rapid swallows (five swallows of 2-mL water spaced 2–3 s), and (4) provocative swallows with a thick liquid (applesauce) and solid (crackers) food bolus based on suspicion for obstruction and a final 200 mL mixed saline swallow to mimic a timed barium esophagram.

12.3.2 HRIM Interpretation

Interpretation of EPT studies in the patient presenting with dysphagia after an antireflux procedure can be performed in a stepwise, hierarchical fashion directed by the Chicago Classification (Figs. 12.2 and 12.3) [4]. There are, however, several caveats to note when applying the Chicago Classification to EPT analysis for patients who have undergone an antireflux procedure. First, the absolute values reported in the Chicago Classification (and in the remainder of this review) are based on normative values generated from supine swallows of 5-mL water using the Sierra HRM assembly (Medtronic Inc., Shoreview, MN). Thus, interpretation using different catheter assemblies, patient positions, and/or boluses, needs to account for expected differences in normative values of EPT metrics, which are summarized in a review by Herregods and colleagues [11]. Additionally, there are studies that have presented data on HRM metric values in patients who are asymptomatic after fundoplication. These values are very similar to what is seen in the published normative ranges for non-surgical controls, however, small elevations in IRP are probably within what would be expected and a careful assessment of bolus transit may help determine whether a slightly elevated IRP is contributing to the current symptoms.

More recently, a new analysis paradigm has been introduced that combines the analysis of HRM and impedance. Automated impedance manometry (AIM) utilizes

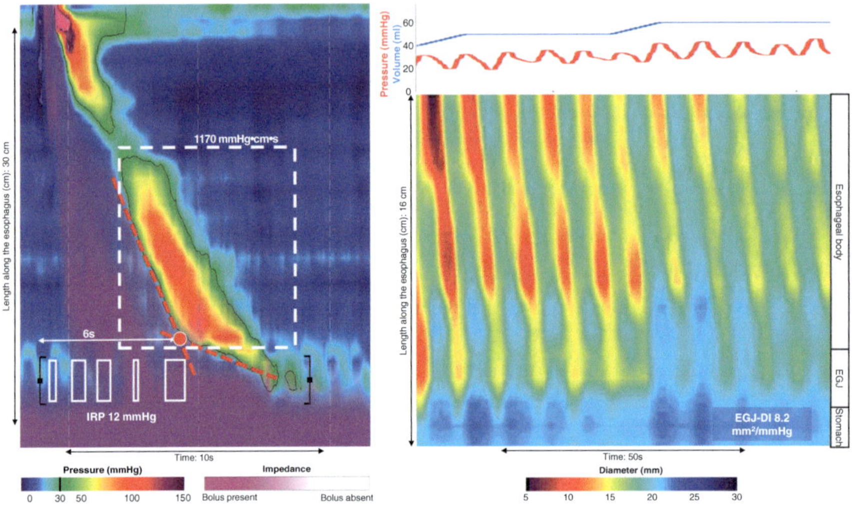

Fig. 12.2 Analysis of esophageal pressure topography and impedance using color isocontours**,** (*Left*) An example of a normal swallow with intact peristaltic integrity is provided. The color scales for pressure and impedance are noted on the bottom below the topography plot. Deglutitive lower esophageal sphincter (LES) relaxation is measured by the integrated relaxation pressure (**IRP**), the mean pressure of the EGJ during the four contiguous or non-contiguous seconds of maximal relaxation (i.e., lowest pressure) during the deglutitive window (10 s after the swallow). The value is 12 mmHg and this is within the normal range, The contractile deceleration point (CDP; *red circle*) is localized by identifying the point along the 30-mmHg isobaric contour at the intersect of lines (*dashed-red*) tangent to (1) the trailing edge of the propagating contractile wave distal to the transition zone and (2) the terminal portion of the wave front proximal to the esophagogastric junction (EGJ). The **distal latency** is then measured as the time from the onset of swallow to the CDP and is normal at 6 s. Peristaltic vigor is measured by the distal contractile integral (**DCI**), a composite metric of pressure amplitude × duration × axial length (mmHg•s•cm) of the distal esophageal contraction (i.e., between the transition zone and the proximal border of the EGJ). The value for this swallow is approximately 1100, which is normal. (*Right*) An example of a FLIP topography plot with the diameter color scale on the bottom and the pressure and volume tracings on the top. This is a normal study with evidence of repetitive antegrade contractions which represent peristaltic contractions in response to volumetric distention. The distensibility index measured through the EGJ is 8.2 mm^2/mmHg and suggests minimal resistance to flow through the EGJ. Values less than 2.8 are consistent with obstruction

the temporal association of peak pressure, nadir impedance and detailed measures of IBP to determine bolus transit dynamics and this approach does appear to have some value in the post-fundoplication patients with dysphagia. This approach led to the development of other metrics focused on utilization of impedance data with and without pressure information, such as the bolus flow time (BFT) and the esophageal impedance integral (EII).

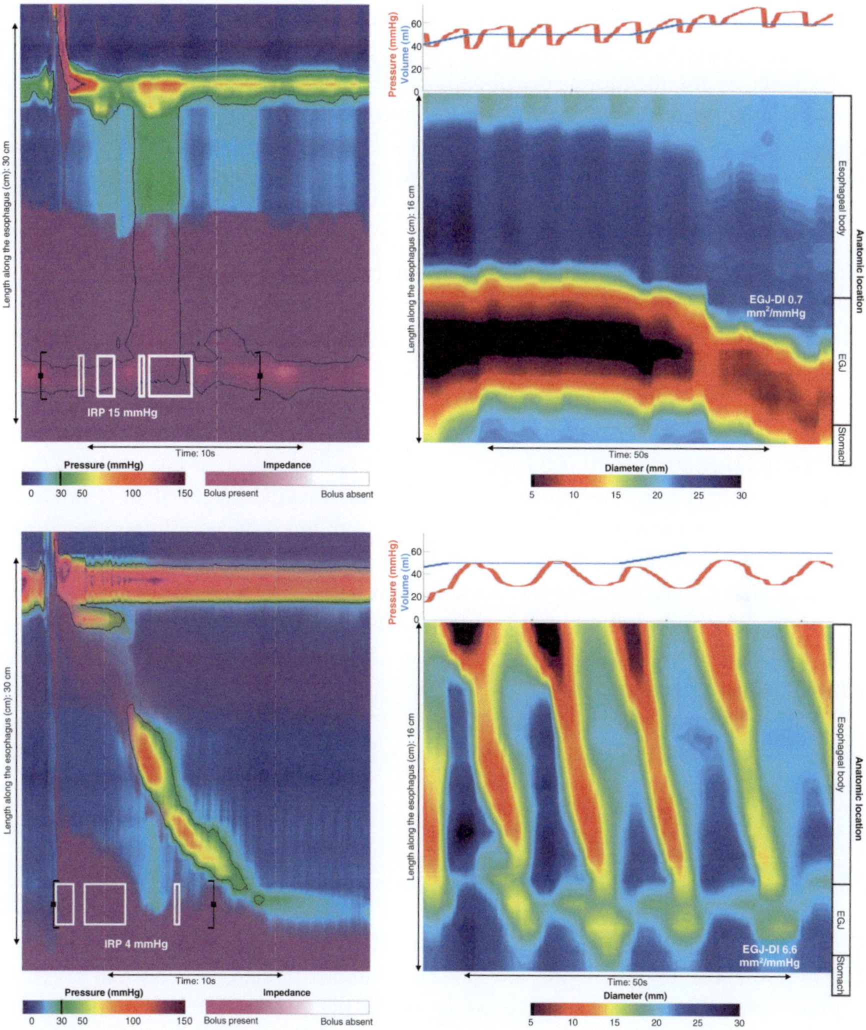

Fig. 12.3 HRIM and FLIP topography in two patients after fundoplication. Figure 12.3a represents data from a patient with an obstruction related to a tight wrap. The patient has no evidence of peristalsis on both the HRIM study and the FLIP topography. Additionally, both the HRIM and FLIP study support an obstruction. The HRIM supports a severe obstruction at the EGJ with a borderline IRP and abnormal pressurization on the esophageal topography plot with severe bolus retention. The FLIP study supports obstruction with a very low distensibility index and the inability to reach a diameter above 12.5 mm at pressures greater than 30 mmHg. This patient would benefit from dilation or reoperation. Figure 12.3b represents data acquired in a patient with normal function on both HRIM and FLIP topography and the dysphagia symptoms in this patient are likely functional

12.3.2.1 Individual High-Resolution Manometry Metrics

The Chicago Classification is based on the assessment of patients without previous foregut surgery, and thus technically should not be applied to these patients. However, with acknowledgement of these factors, the *concepts* of EPT interpretation based on the Chicago Classification can be broadly applied.

12.3.2.2 Basal EGJ and Upper Esophageal Sphincter Assessment

Though not incorporated in the Chicago Classification of esophageal motility diagnoses, EGJ morphology and basal pressure are important parameters in the assessment of dysphagia after an anti-reflux procedure. The basal EGJ should be assessed during a period of quiet breathing and absent of swallows. Because the crural diaphragm (CD) contributes to EGJ pressure, both the separation of the LES-CD (i.e., EGJ morphology) and the effect of the respiratory cycle on basal EGJ pressure should be appreciated; greater LES-CD separation and reduced CD augmentation pressures are associated with increased reflux [12, 13]. Elevated basal EGJ pressures are also be observed, but the clinical relevance of this finding remains unclear. Reporting EGJ morphology and basal pressures is more important in the patient with dysphagia after antireflux procedures as the procedure specifically targets the antireflux barrier and the components of the EGJ. Large separation of the LES and CD will be seen in disruption and signifies reherniation. Additionally, abnormal basal EGJ pressure values or high EGJCI values can be associated with obstruction.

12.3.2.3 Deglutitive LES Relaxation

Deglutitive LES relaxation is measured with HRM/EPT using the IRP. Because the IRP is referenced to gastric pressure, the IRP can be affected by abnormal pressurization within the stomach. Thus, we typically place the gastric reference 2 cm below the EGJ, though may adjust the placement of the gastric reference to reflect the esophageal outflow resistance pressure in patients. This measurement is the most important parameter in patients with dysphagia as patients with post-fundoplication as this is where the primary alteration occurred and studies support that patients with post-procedure dysphagia have significantly elevated IRP values compared to controls and asymptomatic post-fundoplication patients [6].

12.3.2.4 Distal Latency

The contractile deceleration point (CDP) has been recognized as an important landmark that represents the physiologic transition from esophageal peristalsis to ampullary formation and emptying [14]. Clinically, identification of this landmark draws its primary importance in defining the *distal latency* (Fig. 12.1), the essential metric defining spastic contractions [15]. The CDP should represent the transition to the *terminal* propagating velocity and should be within 3 cm of the EGJ [4, 14]. This metric should not be altered after an antireflux procedure and evidence of abnormal latency intervals may be related to a missed diagnosis of a spastic disorder or narcotic induced.

12.3.2.5 Peristaltic Vigor

Peristaltic vigor is measured in HRM/EPT by the distal contractile integral (DCI; Fig. 12.1). As one of the goals of the most recent update of the Chicago Classification was to simplify the esophageal motility assessment using EPT, the DCI claimed greater importance in the schema for individual swallow assessment [4]. Hypercontractile swallows are defined by a DCI > 8000 mmHg•s•cm, a value previously exceeding any observed DCI in studies of normal controls. Swallows with a DCI < 450 mmHg•s•cm showed strong agreement with ineffective swallows identified on conventional manometry and thus a lower DCI threshold has been incorporated into the classification scheme to define ineffective swallows [4, 16]. One interesting phenomenon of antireflux procedures is the finding of increased peristaltic vigor after the procedure. This augmentation is likely due to the esophagus responding to an increase in outflow resistance [Mittal- animal model paper]. In fact, overt jackhammer esophagus can be related to a tight or disrupted fundoplication and this will improve if the obstruction is removed. Thus, all patients who present with jackhammer esophagus after antireflux procedures should be presumed to have an obstruction until proven otherwise.

12.3.2.6 Peristaltic Integrity

In swallows with a normal DCI, the integrity of the peristaltic wave is assessed by measuring the length of axial breaks in the 20 mmHg isobaric contour. Previous versions of the Chicago Classification differentiated breaks into small (3–5 cm) and large (>5 cm), though the most recent update only classifies swallows with large peristaltic breaks (i.e., >5 cm) as fragmented swallows. Once again, these weak contractions will lead to altered bolus transport that may be accentuated in the context of an antireflux procedure.

12.3.2.7 Pressurization Pattern

The final step in assessing individual swallows in determination of the pressurization pattern. With the IBC set at 30 mmHg, swallows are assessed for panesophageal pressurization, i.e. simultaneous esophageal pressurization extending from the upper esophageal sphincter (UES) to the EGJ, and/or compartmentalized pressurization, i.e., when distal esophageal pressurization extends from the contractile front to the EGJ. An assessment of the degree of compartmentalized pressurization is an important component of the HRIM evaluation of patients with dysphagia after antireflux procedures as this is a more accurate methodology to define obstruction at the EGJ. Although there is no validated approach, using the isobaric contour tool, one is able to scroll up and down to determine the minimal pressurization within the compartmentalized area between the LES and propagating wave. If this value is above 30 mmHg, the patient likely has a significant obstruction. These patients are usually referred for an UGI with a 12.5 mm barium tablet of an endoscopy with FLIP if this was not done previously.

12.3.2.8 Individual Impedance Based Metrics

Bolus Flow Time

A study using concurrent HRIM and esophageal intraluminal ultrasound demonstrated that impedance measurement can assess EGJ opening and esophageal emptying [17]. Based on this concept, our group developed and validated a novel HRIM metric to specifically assess flow across the EGJ: the bolus flow time (BFT) [18]. Utilizing simultaneous videofluoroscopy with HRIM, bolus flow across the EGJ was observed on fluoroscopy when two criteria were met: (1) bolus was present, which was associated with a decrease in impedance and (2) A preferential trans-EGJ pressure gradient existed such that pressure in the distal esophagus was greater than at the crural diaphragm. Both of these criteria were incorporated into a computer-based algorithm for automated calculation of the BFT. To measure the BFT, three impedance and three manometry signals are placed through the EGJ at 1-cm intervals (thus, impedance and pressure signals were interpolated by the analysis software). The distal impedance and manometry signal is positioned within the hiatus as identified by crural contractions [18, 19]. Using the impedance signals, the duration of bolus presence is determined: The onset of bolus presence is defined as the point at which the impedance dropped to 90% of the nadir; the offset of bolus presence is defined as the return to 50% of the impedance baseline. Using the three manometry signals, periods of a trans-EGJ flow-permissive pressure gradient (i.e., when the esophageal pressure was greater than both the crural and intra-gastric pressure signals) are determined. The BFT is then derived as the sum of all periods meeting the criteria of both bolus presence and a flow-permissive pressure gradient time. If the impedance drop is not greater than 50% at each axial location and/or a flow-permissive pressure gradient is not achieved, the BFT is considered to be zero. The median BFT value of the five upright swallows is utilized for each patient. Previous study of asymptomatic volunteers demonstrated a median (interquartile range, IQR) BFT of 3.2 s (2.3–3.9 s) for upright swallows; lower BFT values indicate reduced esophageal emptying [19]. We recently reported that the BFT was a useful measure in patients with suspected achalasia and borderline IRP measures and that BFT had a better symptom-association than basal EGJ pressure (EGJP) or IRP in patients with achalasia prior to intervention [19].

Measures of Bolus Residual/Retention

Two measures of esophageal bolus residual can be calculated: the *esophageal impedance integral (EII) ratio* and the nadir impedance to peak pressure *impedance ratio* (IR).

The EII ratio is measured by creating a measurement region-of-interest (ROI) ranging from the distal border of the upper esophageal sphincter to the proximal border of the EGJ and starting at the upper esophageal sphincter relaxation and lasting to the completion of peristalsis or 12 s [20]. A best-fit diagonal straight line that demarcated the present or expected peristaltic wave front is defined to divide the swallow ROI into swallow (Z1) and post-swallow (Z2) impedance domains. The amount of bolus present within each domain (Z1 and Z2) is then quantified by measuring the esophageal impedance integral (EII), which represented the volume of intra-esophageal liquid present within each domain (Z1 and Z2). The EII is measured by first determining the times of bolus presence by assessing the mean baseline impedance and the nadir impedance at all times within the ROI; domains of bolus presence are defined when the impedance value decreased to 50% from baseline. The amount of bolus (i.e., EII) is then quantified by measuring the impedance-pixel density (impedance value × time × axial length). Finally, the EII ratio is calculated as the EII-Z2 divided by EII-Z1; i.e., the ratio of residual bolus volume (Z2) relative to the intra-esophageal bolus volume following the swallow, but before the peristaltic wave. A greater EII ratio indicates a greater degree of bolus retention [20].

The IR is measured by creating an analysis region-of-interest ranging from the distal border of the upper esophageal sphincter to the proximal border of the EGJ and starting at the upper esophageal sphincter relaxation and lasting to the completion of peristalsis [21]. The contractile peaks of the peristaltic wave and corresponding nadir impedance time points preceding the peaks (corresponding to maximum distension) are identified along the ROI. To determine the IR the nadir impedance value is divided by the impedance value mapped to the timing of peak contraction (peak pressure impedance). IR is calculated at each position along the ROI and the average IR was then calculated for the whole esophagus. A greater IR indicates a greater degree of bolus retention [21].

12.3.2.9 Pressure-Flow Measures of Distension Pressure, Flow Timing and Bolus Pressurization

Pressure-flow parameters are measured for the distal esophagus proximal of the EGJ. A measurement ROI is defined from the mid-point of the transition zone to the proximal border of the EGJ (Fig. 12.2b) [21]. Note, the transition zone midpoint is defined by the lowest pressure between proximal and distal esophageal pressure segments or the distal margin of the proximal esophageal segment in the case of large 20 mmHg iso-contour pressure defects (>5 cm). The peaks of the peristaltic contraction and corresponding nadir impedance time points preceding the peaks (indicative of maximal luminal cross-sectional area) are identified along the ROI. Guided by the timing of nadir impedance and peak pressure, four pressure-flow variables can be determined as described below:

1. The *pressure at nadir Impedance* (PNadImp) is used to define the discrete intrabolus distension pressure occurring at the point of maximal luminal distention.
2. The *intrabolus pressure slope* (IBP slope) is defined by calculating the average gradient of pressure change from the nadir impedance point to the midpoint in time between nadir impedance and peak pressure. This quantifies the rate of pressure change (or pressure "ramp") during the isotonic/auxotonic phase of esophageal contraction preceding luminal occlusion.
3. The *time from nadir impedance to peak pressure* (TNIPP) is used to define the flow latency from maximum distension to maximum contraction.
4. Finally, the *pressure-flow index* (PFI) is calculated using the formula PFI = (intrabolus distension pressure × IBP slope)/(TNIPP—peak pressure). The *intrabolus distension pressure* is defined by calculating the median distension pressure from the nadir impedance point to the midpoint in time between nadir impedance and peak pressure. The peak pressure was the pressure recorded at the maximum wave amplitude.

12.3.3 *The Utilization of Pressure Flow Metrics in the Analysis of Post-fundoplication Dysphagia*

In a study from Myers et al., liquid and viscous swallows were evaluated using the Pressure-Flow analysis paradigm in 19 patients with reflux disease before and after surgery. Automated impedance manometry (AIM) analysis calculated a range of pressure and bolus movement variables and compared these to standard measures of esophago-gastric junction pressure and total bolus transit time were also evaluated. At 5 months postop, 15 patients reported some dysphagia, including 7 with new-onset dysphagia. Three AIM-derived pressure-flow variables: time from nadir esophageal impedance to peak esophageal pressure (TNadImp-PeakP), median intra-bolus pressure (IBP, mmHg), and the rate of bolus pressure rise (IBP slope, mmHgs(−1)). These variables were combined to form a dysphagia risk index (DRI = IBP × IBP_slope/TNadImp-PeakP). DRI values derived from preoperative measurements were significantly elevated in those with postoperative dysphagia (DRI = 58, IQR = 21–408 vs no dysphagia DRI = 9, IQR = 2–19, $P < 0.02$). A DRI >14 was optimally predictive of dysphagia (sensitivity 75% and specificity 93%). Although this approach is promising, it is currently only utilized by specialized centers with specialized manual extraction protocols and customized software packages.

12.4 Functional Lumen Imaging Probe (Flip)

Assessment of esophageal *distensibility* is somewhat limited with traditional methods of esophageal disease evaluation (i.e., upper endoscopy, manometry, and barium-radiography) [22]. Devices employing impedance planimetry, which measures luminal cross-sectional area (CSA), combined with intra-luminal pressure sensors allow for evaluation of esophageal mechanical properties and distensibility. Initial studies applying impedance planimetry to the esophagus demonstrated the feasibility and utility in evaluating the esophagogastric junction (EGJ) and esophageal hypersensitivity [23, 24]. Multiple impedance planimetry electrodes measuring serial, adjacent CSAs in a tubular lumen (essentially high-resolution impedance planimetry) allowed for anatomic and biomechanical characterization of the esophagus: a functional lumen imaging probe (FLIP) [25].

Recently, a commercially-available device, the EndoFLIP (Crospon, Inc. Galway, Ireland) has increased the availability of FLIP. Subsequently, research and clinical utilization of FLIP to assess esophageal function and disease has increased. The FLIP has demonstrated the potential to become a valuable tool for functional evaluation in esophageal diseases associated with abnormalities of EGJ competence (e.g., achalasia and gastroesophgeal reflux disease, GERD) and mechanical properties of the esophageal body (e.g., eosinophilic esophagitis, EoE) [26]. The FLIP consists of a 240-mm long, 3-mm outer diameter catheter with a balloon mounted on the distal end. The balloon houses 16 paired impedance planimetry electrodes spaced at consistent intervals and a solid-state pressure transducer located at the distal end. Excitation electrodes at either end of the balloon emit a continuous low electric current. As the balloon is filled with a conductive fluid, the voltage (which is proportional to impedance) is measured across the paired impedance planimetry electrodes providing measurement of CSA. The balloon is infinitely compliant (within allotted fill volumes) to allow conformation to the esophageal lumen and subsequent measurement of distensive properties of the tubular lumen. Two primary device sizes are commercially available with FLIP measurement segments of 8 or 16-cm. Some studies report use of earlier models that consisted of a 10–14 cm balloon that housed the 16-paired electrodes spaced at 4-mm intervals for a 6.4-cm measurement length [27–31].

12.4.1 FLIP: Protocol

During a FLIP study, measurements of 16-sequential CSAs and one intra-bag pressure are simultaneously measured at a 10-Hz sampling rate during volume-controlled distension of the bag. Luminal d*iameter* measurements, which simplify use for clinical application, are generated from the CSA measures by assuming a circular lumen: $CSA = \pi(diameter/2)^2$. The FLIP is placed into the esophagus either trans-orally or trans-nasally in a sedated or awake patient. Due to patient tolerance, our institutional practice is to place the catheter orally either during endoscopy with conscious sedation (typically using the 16-cm measurement device) or intra-operatively during general anesthesia (typically using the 8-cm measurement device). The FLIP is positioned within the esophagus by identifying the waist on the real-time, semi-3D display at a low fill volume (typically 20–30 mL). With the 16-cm bag, the distal esophageal body can be evaluated simultaneously with the EGJ; the EGJ then serves as a reference point to control for catheter movement during the study. Marking the catheter with an endoscopically or manometrically measured distance to the EGJ can also assist with placement, though maintenance of stable FLIP positioning by visualizing landmarks on the real-time display during the course of the study remains paramount.

During stable positioning of the catheter, volume-controlled distension of the bag is performed. CSA and pressure (thus distensibility) measurements may vary depending on the degree of volume distension, thus measurements should be obtained at a stable distension volume and over a time sufficient to allow accounting for measurement fluctuation related to respiration and esophageal contractions/peristalsis. Additionally, measurements should be obtained at a volume that can generate sufficient intra-bag pressure to distend the esophageal body to allow an evaluation of the luminal CSA/pressure relationship. Our practice is to perform step-wise volumetric distension with the 16-cm bag during endoscopic evaluation using 10 mL increments; we focus on the EGJ distensibility measures at the 60-ml fill volume. For intra-operative use, we typically make EGJ measures at the 40-mL fill volume with the 8-cm bag.

12.4.2 FLIP Analysis

Though both CSA (diameter) and pressure are simultaneously measured (and often reported independently in studies), assessing the relationship between luminal CSA and distending (intra-bag) pressure arguably reflects the greatest value provided by the FLIP for the esophageal evaluation (Figs. 12.2 and 12.3). The distensibility index (DI) has been the typical measure of sphincter distensibility and is calculated by dividing the median narrowest CSA (within the sphincter of interest) divided by median intra-bag pressure over a set timeframe (or distension volume). The FLIP measurements are dynamic with both CSA and pressure fluctuation occurring during a stable distension volume, thus various methods using the FLIP Analytics software (Crospon) or other external software methods (e.g., MATLAB, The Math Works, Natick, MA) have been reported to generate metrics.

The FLIP is indicated (and FDA approved for use in the United States) for clinical use as a pressure and dimension measurement device, as an adjunctive test in patients with symptoms consistent with esophageal hypersensitivity and to estimate the size of a stoma produced by a gastric band. Thus, clinical applications for FLIP are varied. Studies utilizing FLIP have consistently demonstrated an abnormal reduced EGJ-DI (i.e., more narrowed EGJ lumen at greater distending-pressure) in treatment naïve achalasia patients [28, 32–34]. Further, studies assessing achalasia treatment response (e.g., after pneumatic dilation or LES myotomy) have reported lower EGJ-DI in patients with poor symptomatic outcomes (particularly below a threshold of 2.8–2.9 $mm^2/mmHg$ than in patients with good symptomatic outcomes [28, 32]; they also suggest that EGJ-DI may have a stronger association with symptoms and esophageal retention (per timed-barium esophagram) than manometric measures of LES pressures.

Although there is little data on FLIP in post-fundoplication, it is logical to apply the cut-offs for normal ranges and EGJ outlflow obstruction utilized in achalasia. Patients with DI values less than 3.0 $mm^2/mmHg$ may have obstruction and values less than 1.0 are highly suspicious for a tight wrap or mechanical obstruction in the patient after an antireflux procedure. We utilize the DI to determine whether dilation will be performed and response to therapy.

Additionally, evaluation of esophageal *contractility* (described in more detail below) with achalasia may also provide some complementary clinical information to the standard assessment with esophageal manometry [34]. This has been incorporated into a live display that can substantially help diagnose obstruction and dysmotility in the post-fundoplication patient (Figs. 12.2 and 12.3).

12.5 Conclusions

The approach to the patient with dysphagia after an antireflux procedure requires a multidisciplinary approach using multiple diagnostic tools which provide complementary information. The choice of initial test is typically focused on ruling out severe complications and this requires an assessment of anatomy and bolus retention. In patients presenting during the early post-operative phase (within 30 days), it is best to start with an UGI to determine whether there is evidence of disruption, herniation or frank obstruction. Patients with positive or equivocal results will usually require an upper endoscopy to reconfirm the anatomy and assess whether other complications, such as esophagitis, stricture or a tight wrap are contributing to the symptoms. The FLIP device provides a more accurate methodology to assess EGJ obstruction during endoscopy and we have included this in our endoscopic protocol whenever we are evaluating patients with dysphagia after an antireflux procedure. If the FLIP supports an obstruction, we would proceed with dilation and will escalate the dilation target based on the results of the FLIP. We have relied less on manometry to assess EGJ obstruction and its primary role is focused on assessing motility in patients with normal EGJ distensibility to determine whether dramatic changes in peristalsis have occurred or a primary motor disease was missed in the pre-operative evaluation. The utilization of amyl nitrite to assess mechanical versus underlying achalasia is well described, but used less in the context of FLIP testing. Although this algorithm provides a framework, the clinical presentation and availability of the tools will certainly determine the sequence in which they are utilized.

What Is the Current Knowledge and What Future Direction Is Required

- Dysphagia is a common symptom after antireflux procedures.
- Pre-operative assessment of symptomatic dysphagia and motility are important in the work –up of patients referred for antireflux surgery.
- The causes of dysphagia after antireflux procedures are very heterogeneous and range from surgical complications related to anatomic disruption to functional dysphagia related to visceral hypersensitivity.
- Obstruction related to surgical complications should always be ruled out with a careful endoscopy complemented by radiographic evaluation.
- New technologies, such as HRIM and FLIP may help improve detection of abnormal EGJ opening and obstruction as a potential cause of post-procedure dysphagia.
- Using FLIP based dilation techniques could be helpful in patients with mechanical obstruction related to a tight wrap using a staged graded dilation.

Acknowledgements This work was supported by T32 DK101363 (JEP) and R01 DK079992 (JEP) from the Public Health service.

Disclosures: John E. Pandolfino: Given Imaging/Medtronic (Consultant, Grant, Speaking), Sandhill Scientific (Consulting, Speaking), Takeda (Speaking), Astra Zeneca (Speaking), Torax (Speaking, Consulting), Impleo (Consultant).

Dustin A. Carlson: none.

References

1. Pandolfino JE, Kahrilas PJ, American GA. American Gastroenterological Association medical position statement: clinical use of esophageal manometry. Gastroenterology. 2005;128(1):207–8.
2. Clouse RE, Staiano A. Topography of the esophageal peristaltic pressure wave. Am J Phys. 1991;261(4 Pt 1):G677–84.
3. Pandolfino JE, Ghosh SK, Rice J, et al. Classifying esophageal motility by pressure topography characteristics: a study of 400 patients and 75 controls. Am J Gastroenterol. 2008;103(1):27–37.
4. Kahrilas PJ, Bredenoord AJ, Fox M, et al. The Chicago classification of esophageal motility disorders, v3.0. Neurogastroenterol Motil. 2015;27(2):160–74.
5. Weijenborg PW, Savarino E, Kessing BF, et al. Normal values of esophageal motility after antireflux surgery; a study using high-resolution manometry. Neurogastroenterol Motil. 2015;27(7):929–35.
6. Wilshire CL, Niebisch S, Watson TJ, et al. Dysphagia postfundoplication: more commonly hiatal outflow resistance than poor esophageal body motility. Surgery. 2012;152(4):584–92. discussion 92-4
7. Xiao Y, Read A, Nicodeme F, et al. The effect of a sitting vs supine posture on normative esophageal pressure topography metrics and Chicago classification diagnosis of esophageal motility disorders. Neurogastroenterol Motil. 2012;24(10):e509–16.
8. Sweis R, Anggiansah A, Wong T, et al. Normative values and inter-observer agreement for liquid and solid bolus swallows in upright and supine positions as assessed by esophageal high-resolution manometry. Neurogastroenterol Motil. 2011;23(6):509–e198.

9. Fornari F, Bravi I, Penagini R, et al. Multiple rapid swallowing: a complementary test during standard oesophageal manometry. Neurogastroenterol Motil. 2009;21(7):718–e41.
10. Shaker A, Stoikes N, Drapekin J, et al. Multiple rapid swallow responses during esophageal high-resolution manometry reflect esophageal body peristaltic reserve. Am J Gastroenterol. 2013;108(11):1706–12.
11. Herregods TV, Roman S, Kahrilas PJ, et al. Normative values in esophageal high-resolution manometry. Neurogastroenterol Motil. 2015;27(2):175–87.
12. Pandolfino JE, Bianchi LK, Lee TJ, et al. Esophagogastric junction morphology predicts susceptibility to exercise-induced reflux. Am J Gastroenterol. 2004;99(8):1430–6.
13. Pandolfino JE, Ghosh SK, Zhang Q, et al. Quantifying EGJ morphology and relaxation with high-resolution manometry: a study of 75 asymptomatic volunteers. Am J Physiol Gastrointest Liver Physiol. 2006;290(5):G1033–40.
14. Pandolfino JE, Leslie E, Luger D, et al. The contractile deceleration point: an important physiologic landmark on oesophageal pressure topography. Neurogastroenterol Motil. 2010;22(4):395–400. e90
15. Roman S, Lin Z, Pandolfino JE, et al. Distal contraction latency: a measure of propagation velocity optimized for esophageal pressure topography studies. Am J Gastroenterol. 2011;106(3):443–51.
16. Xiao Y, Kahrilas PJ, Kwasny MJ, et al. High-resolution manometry correlates of ineffective esophageal motility. Am J Gastroenterol. 2012;107(11):1647–54.
17. Hong SJ, Bhargava V, Jiang Y, et al. A unique esophageal motor pattern that involves longitudinal muscles is responsible for emptying in achalasia esophagus. Gastroenterology. 2010;139(1):102–11.
18. Lin Z, Imam H, Nicodeme F, et al. Flow time through esophagogastric junction derived during high-resolution impedance-manometry studies: a novel parameter for assessing esophageal bolus transit. Am J Physiol Gastrointest Liver Physiol. 2014;307(2):G158–63.
19. Lin Z, Carlson DA, Dykstra K, et al. High-resolution impedance manometry measurement of bolus flow time in achalasia and its correlation with dysphagia. Neurogastroenterol Motil. 2015;27(9):1232–8.
20. Lin Z, Nicodeme F, Lin CY, et al. Parameters for quantifying bolus retention with high-resolution impedance manometry. Neurogastroenterol Motil. 2014;26(7):929–36.
21. Omari TI, Wauters L, Rommel N, et al. Oesophageal pressure-flow metrics in relation to bolus volume, bolus consistency, and bolus perception. United European Gastroenterol J. 2013;1(4):249–58.
22. Pandolfino JE, Shi G, Trueworthy B, et al. Esophagogastric junction opening during relaxation distinguishes nonhernia reflux patients, hernia patients, and normal subjects. Gastroenterology. 2003;125(4):1018–24.
23. Rao SS, Hayek B, Summers RW. Impedance planimetry: an integrated approach for assessing sensory, active, and passive biomechanical properties of the human esophagus. Am J Gastroenterol. 1995;90(3):431–8.
24. McMahon BP, Frokjaer JB, Drewes AM, et al. A new measurement of oesophago-gastric junction competence. Neurogastroenterol Motil. 2004;16(5):543–6.
25. McMahon BP, Frokjaer JB, Liao D, et al. A new technique for evaluating sphincter function in visceral organs: application of the functional lumen imaging probe (FLIP) for the evaluation of the oesophago-gastric junction. Physiol Meas. 2005;26(5):823–36.
26. Hirano I, Pandolfino JE, Boeckxstaens GE. Functional lumen imaging probe for the management of esophageal disorders: expert review from the clinical practice updates committee of the AGA Institute. Clin Gastroenterol Hepatol. 2017;15(3):325–34.
27. Kwiatek MA, Pandolfino JE, Hirano I, et al. Esophagogastric junction distensibility assessed with an endoscopic functional luminal imaging probe (EndoFLIP). Gastrointest Endosc. 2010;72(2):272–8.
28. Rohof WO, Hirsch DP, Kessing BF, et al. Efficacy of treatment for patients with achalasia depends on the distensibility of the esophagogastric junction. Gastroenterology. 2012;143(2):328–35.

29. Verlaan T, Rohof WO, Bredenoord AJ, et al. Effect of peroral endoscopic myotomy on esophagogastric junction physiology in patients with achalasia. Gastrointest Endosc. 2013;78(1):39–44.
30. Tucker E, Sweis R, Anggiansah A, et al. Measurement of esophago-gastric junction cross-sectional area and distensibility by an endolumenal functional lumen imaging probe for the diagnosis of gastro-esophageal reflux disease. Neurogastroenterol Motil. 2013;25(11):904–10.
31. Mikami H, Ishimura N, Fukazawa K, et al. Effects of metoclopramide on Esophageal motor activity and Esophagogastric junction compliance in healthy volunteers. J Neurogastroenterol Motil. 2016;22(1):112–7.
32. Pandolfino JE, de Ruigh A, Nicodeme F, et al. Distensibility of the esophagogastric junction assessed with the functional lumen imaging probe (FLIP) in achalasia patients. Neurogastroenterol Motil. 2013;25(6):496–501.
33. Rieder E, Swanstrom LL, Perretta S, et al. Intraoperative assessment of esophagogastric junction distensibility during per oral endoscopic myotomy (POEM) for esophageal motility disorders. Surg Endosc. 2013;27(2):400–5.
34. Carlson DA, Lin Z, Kahrilas PJ, et al. The functional lumen imaging probe detects Esophageal contractility not observed with manometry in patients with achalasia. Gastroenterology. 2015;149(7):1742–51.

Chapter 13
Preoperative Assessment of Failed Fundoplication with Recurrent Hiatal Hernia

Kenan Ulualp, Kathleen Simon, and Jon C. Gould

Hiatal hernia repair and fundoplication provide excellent long-term results. However, even with the application of the time-tested surgical principles, recurrence rates in postoperatively-unscreened and screened patient groups may be as high as 14% and 25% respectively [1–3]. Also, recurrent hiatal hernia is recognized as the most common cause of the failure of an antireflux procedure with an incidence of approximately 50% of all cases [4, 5]. Failed fundoplication and recurrent hiatal hernia may be associated with a myriad of symptoms that may necessitate urgent surgical care and present a challenging clinical problem that requires in depth understanding of the condition.

13.1 Definition and Anatomy

Failed fundoplication is an anatomical deviation from the desired postoperative configuration that should provide optimum result as a gastroesophageal junction enhancement procedure. Failed fundoplication may be classified as *slipped*, *malpositioned* or *loose* and may or may not be together with an hiatal hernia. Similarly, ***failed diaphragmatic hernia repair*** refers to a deviation from the targeted optimum anatomic configuration at the time of the diaphragmatic repair that would prevent herniation of the abdominal organs to the thoracic cavity but at the same time do not interfere with the normal physiology. Anatomically it may be classified as a recurrence with *intact hiatus*, *lateral defect*, *anterior defect*, *posterior defect* or

K. Ulualp, M.D. • K. Simon, M.D. • J.C. Gould, M.D. (✉)
Division of General Surgery, Department of Surgery, Medical College of Wisconsin, Milwaukee, WI 53226, USA
e-mail: jgould@mcw.edu

M.A. Memon (ed.), *Hiatal Hernia Surgery*,
https://doi.org/10.1007/978-3-319-64003-7_13

Table 13.1 Types of failed fundoplication and hiatal hernia repair

Slipped fundoplication and hiatal hernia
Slipped fundoplication
Malpositioned fundoplication
Malpositioned fundoplication and hiatal hernia
Tight fundoplication
Hiatal hernia alone
Loose fundoplication
Tight cruroplasty

anteroposterior defect, listed in increasing order of frequency [6]. Above definitions therefore include intact fundoplications and cruroplasties that are symptomatic but require treatment due to over-tightness (Table 13.1).

13.2 Pathophysiology

Despite having been recognized over two centuries ago particularly by the work of Bochdalek and Morgagni, pathophysiology of the hiatal hernia still remains to be elucidated [7]. Limited data in the literature suggest; (a) unrelenting motion of the diaphragm, (b) increased intraabdominal pressure, (c) esophageal shortening and (d) structural changes in the diaphragm and adjacent ligaments as three main pathophysiologic mechanisms leading to hiatal hernia (Table 13.2) [7–12].

Technical reasons and mesh related complications may be added to this list as other contributing factors in the patients with previous repairs. Pathophysiologic mechanisms leading to recurrence act by interfering with antegrade pumping of the bolus, wound healing and principle of tension-free hernia repair.

13.3 Clinical Presentation

According to traditional understanding a recurrent hiatal hernia may or may not be symptomatic, and asymptomatic cases are usually discovered incidentally during a work-up for another reason. However, recent reports challenge this notion by suggesting that symptoms associated with silent hernias are much broader than previously thought and truly asymptomatic patients are rare [13–15]. Symptoms like insidious alterations in eating habits, early satiety and postprandial dyspnea that gradually increase over time—particularly in the elderly population—may in fact be related with a recurrent hiatal hernia and should not be assumed to arise due to aging [16]. Moreover, pulmonary symptoms in the patients with hiatal hernia may also remain underappreciated likely because in elderly population symptoms such as dyspnea is often attributed to arise from other comorbidities [17]. Therefore a careful history taking is necessary in the patients that are assumed to be

Table 13.2 Pathophysiologic mechanisms and etiology of hiatal hernia

Mechanism	Etiology
Increased intraabdominal pressure	Obesity
	Pregnancy
	Straining
	Chronic constipation
	Weight lifting
Esophageal shortening	Congenital short esophagus
	Esophageal/periesophageal fibrosis
	Chronic vagal stimuli
	Tight esophageal longitudinal muscle
Structural changes in the diaphragm	Reduced matrix metalloproteinases
	Defective collagen formation
Structural changes in the crura	Dilatation of the myofibrillar spaces
	Swelling of sacrotubular structures
	Degeneration of myofibrils
	Disruption of the muscles
Decreased elastin in the ligaments	In phrenoesophageal ligament
	In gastrohepatic ligament

asymptomatic. In the more symptomatic group, complaints are mostly **mechanical symptoms** due to gastroesophageal obstruction, gastroesophageal reflux, strangulation and incarceration (Table 13.3). While in the cases with slipped fundoplication reflux symptoms are the main components of the clinical picture, obstructive symptoms including anorexia, early satiety, dysphagia, postprandial bloating, regurgitation and weight loss become more prominent in the cases with intact fundoplication. Incarceration and partial strangulation of displaced abdominal organs may cause chest or abdominal pain in addition to other specific symptomology depending on the herniated structures. Venous congestion of the mucosa due to chronic external pressure may result in gastric ulceration (***Cameron's ulcer***) and postprandial pain [19] (Fig. 13.1).

Cameron's ulcer may cause occult bleeding and iron deficiency anemia both resolve typically after herniorraphy. **Respiratory tract symptoms** secondary to chronic aspiration or intrathoracic displacement of the abdominal organs can also be seen and may include postprandial dyspnea, chronic cough, asthma, otitis media, sleep apnea, globus sensation, hoarseness, recurrent upper respiratory tract infections and recurrent pulmonary infections. In addition, patients may present with urgent signs and symptoms of acute conditions such as gastric volvulus, colopleural fistula or gastropericardial fistula [21–23].

Gastropericardial fistula may appear as a rare complication of penetrating peptic or neoplastic ulcers of the stomach within the recurrent hiatal hernia. Diagnosis should be suspected when a patient with an history of hiatal hernia repair present with chest/shoulder pain, dyspnea, atrial fibrillation, pericardial tamponade, pyrexia and upper gastrointestinal symptoms [23, 24]. Dyspnea and coughing with purulent

Table 13.3 The most common chief complaints of the patients with recurrent hiatal hernia [18]

	Incidence (%)
Dysphagia	26
Regurgitation	24
Heartburn	18
Nausea	10
Chest pain	6
Epigastric pain	6
Dyspnea	6
Anemia	4
Nocturnal choking	2

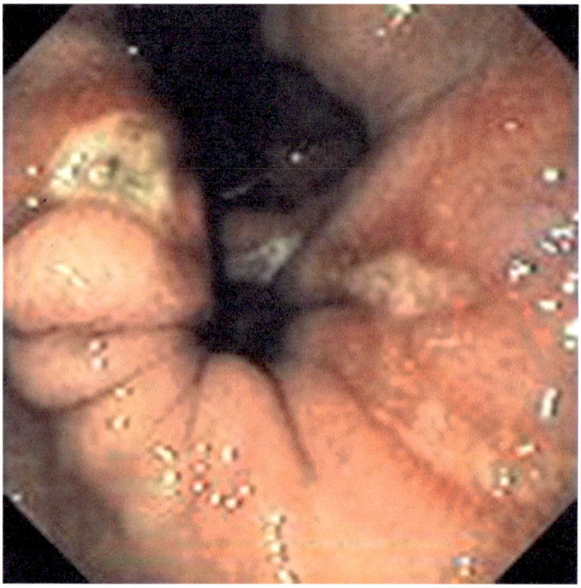

Fig. 13.1 Gastric ulcers distal to hiatal hernia at the points of diaphragmatic impingement on the stomach (–Cameron's ulcer) [20]

sputum discharge accompanied by with pyrexia, and sepsis should raise suspicion of a ***colopleural fistula*** especially in the patients with history of mesh repair of an hiatal hernia [22, 25]. Hemoptysis may add to these symptoms if the recurrence is complicated with ***gastrobronchial fistula*** [26].The classic presentation for acute ***gastric volvulus*** is severe epigastric pain, retching without vomiting and inability to pass a nasogastric tube (***Borchardt's triad***).

Symptom assessment should be standardized by using questionnaires both for follow-up and the quality of life measurement purposes [27–29]. However, it should be remembered that the positive predictive value of the symptoms is limited and the preoperative assessment should be supported by other methods [30].

In addition to symptomology, patient's past medical history should be questioned for the presence of chronic immunosuppression, ongoing steroid treatment, diabetes, morbid obesity and smoking as the other factors that may adversely influence the wound healing and increase the probability of a re-recurrence. Obesity in particular is a risk factor for failed antireflux procedure [31]. Nicotine addiction should also be questioned preoperatively. Tobacco usage has a well-known relation with herniations and wound healing similar to its detrimental effect on the lungs which may appear as a systemic spillover reflected in the herniation sites namely ***metastatic emphysema*** [32].

Evaluation of the former surgery is also essential. If available, previous operative report should be reviewed—for information about the diameter of hiatal hernia, management of the sac, preservation of the vagus nerves, post-operative length of the abdominal esophagus, type of the fundoplication and use of a mesh—to get an opinion on the anatomy prior to the initial operation.

13.4 Radiologic Studies

Plain chest radiographs may reveal a mediastinal mass with or without an air-fluid level. In the latter case fundus air is absent. Although the mass is predominantly retrocardiac and located to the left of the spine it may be large enough to even mimic a cardiomegaly. In the absence of gas within the hernia sac plain chest radiograph has a limited value in the differential diagnosis (Fig. 13.2). However in the presence of these findings, particularly in elderly patients with multiple comorbidities which may lead to diagnostic uncertainty, surgeon must maintain high index of suspicion for the presence of recurrent hiatal hernia [21].

A barium swallow or videoesophageal study may be useful in demonstrating the position of the hernia, location of the gastroesophageal junction, esophageal motility and is the preferred examination for the investigation of hiatal hernia recurrence under elective conditions (Fig. 13.3). Radiologic diagnosis of a sliding hiatal hernia can be made if more than four mucosal folds are recognizable 2 cm above the diaphragm in an upper gastrointestinal barium swallow series in a prone oblique position. Esophagus may appear tortuous and may become aperistaltic above the hiatus suggesting supradiaphragmatically positioned esophagogastric junction.

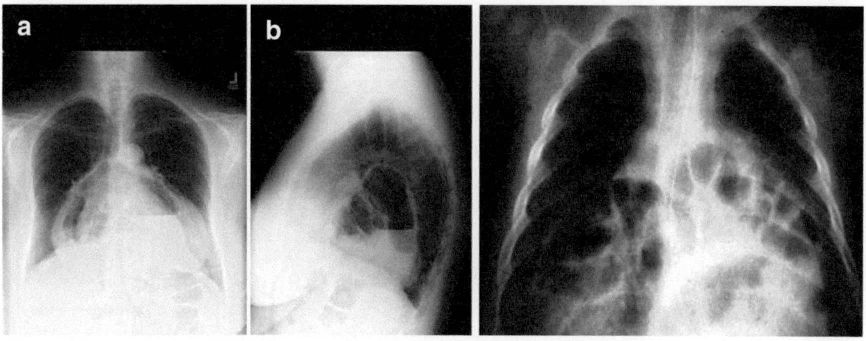

Fig. 13.2 Recurrent hiatal hernia on the PA (**a**) and lateral plain (**b**) chest radiographs with air-fluid levels (*on the left*), and with bowel gas in the mediastinum (*on the right*)

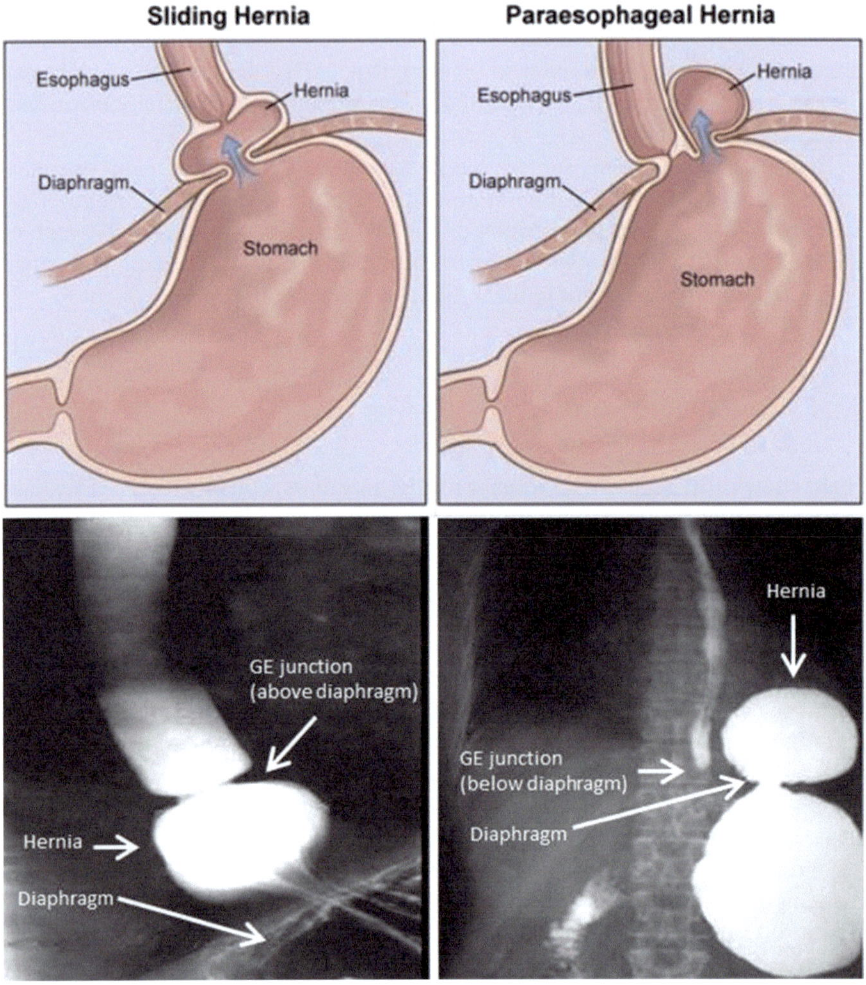

Fig. 13.3 Hiatal hernia on barium swallow

Under subacute conditions barium swallow may reveal complications like gastric volvulus (Fig. 13.4). On a dynamic study if the hernia is not reducible with the patient in an erect position and persistent within the thorax then it is considered to be an *incarcerated diaphragmatic hernia* [30].

Gastric emptying study should also be obtained in patients who had retained barium in the stomach 2 h after the end of barium swallow and on those who had food in the stomach during gastroscopy after overnight fasting [27].

Computerized tomography (CT) is not routinely used. But it may be useful in the elective cases without an air-fluid level in direct radiographs or with a neoplasia which requires staging and in urgent cases in which a barium swallow study is

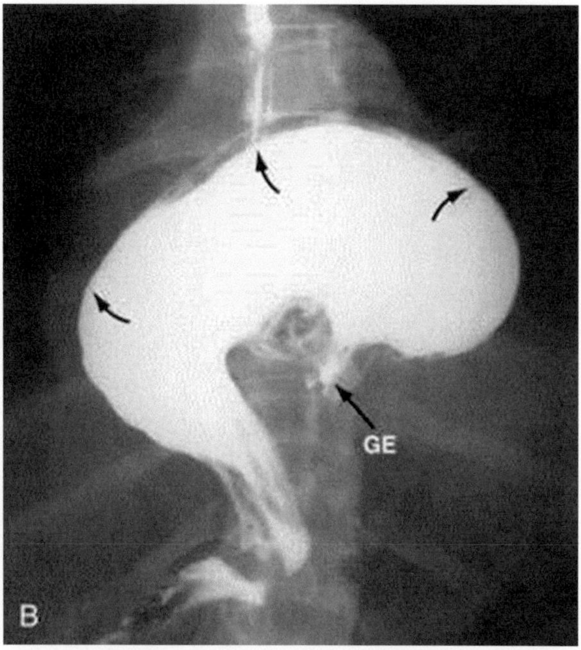

Fig. 13.4 Gastic volvulus. Note the supradiaphragmatic position of the stomach

contraindicated. Presence of an hernia sac in CT examination which is greater than 2 cm is radiologically accepted as a recurrent hiatal hernia (Fig. 13.5). In urgent cases, CT should be preferred to determine the size of the hernia, width of the hiatal defect, presence of the other intra-abdominal organs in the mediastinum and to rule out complications such as gastric volvulus or hollow organ perforation. Pneumatosis of the gastric wall, free gas and fluid outside the gastric wall within the hernia sac, and lack of contrast enhancement of the gastric wall are the CT findings suggestive of a gastric necrosis [30].

13.5 Upper Gastrointestinal Endoscopy

Endoscopy should be performed in all patients for evaluation of the esophageal and gastric mucosa for inflammation, ulcers, Barrett's esophagus, strictures and complications like mesh penetration. In addition endoscopy may play a therapeutic role in the cases complicated with gastric volvulus. Though often it is not possible to pass the endoscope into the duodenum the viability of the gastric mucosa can be assessed with upper endoscopy. Insufflation of the stomach can at times lead to unfolding of the volvulus and thus be therapeutic. A well-perfused stomach decompressed with an nasogastric tube can enable consideration of operative intervention on a

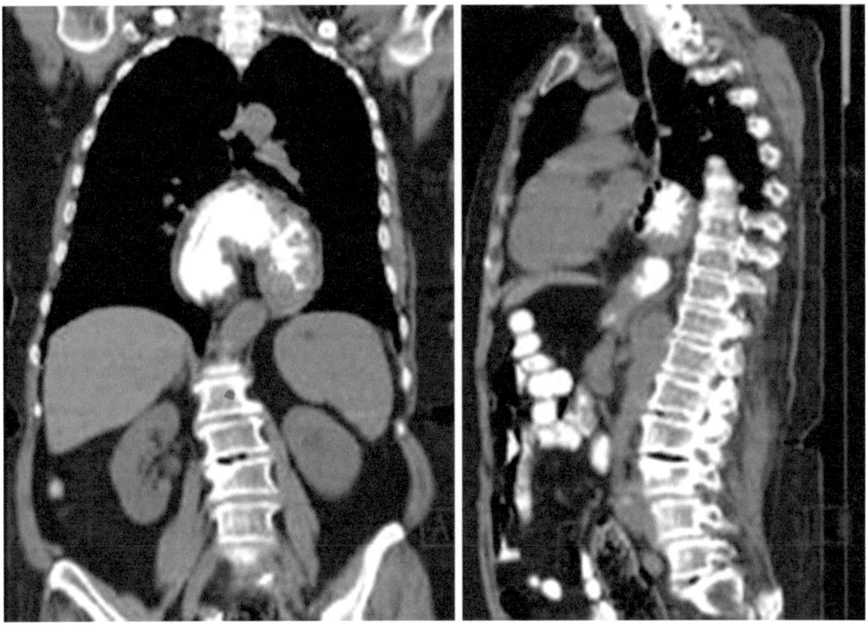

Fig. 13.5 CT appearance of a recurrent hiatal hernia

semi-urgent basis in daylight time. Intraoperative access to endoscopy during surgical treatment of recurrent hiatal hernia is highly advisable [10, 11, 18].

13.6 High Resolution Manometry

Manometric study indicated in the patients with an esophageal dysmotility during radiologic examination. Esophageal dysmotility may be in the form of ineffective esophageal motility, diffuse esophageal spasm, nutcracker esophagus, lower esophageal sphincter hypotension, lower esophageal sphincter hypertension or non-specific motor disorders and could account for the recurrent clinical picture (Table 13.4) [18]. It should be noted however; in the patients with large recurrent hernias catheter placement below the lower esophageal sphincter can be difficult.

13.7 Esophageal pH Monitoring

Determination of the esophageal pH changes using wireless Bravo capsule sensor is indicated in patients with heartburn or regurgitation as the chief complaint and in those with small recurrent hiatal hernia (<4 cm) to assess the functional integrity of the wrap.

Table 13.4 Manometric findings in esophageal dysmotility (LES_p = LES pressure)

Abnormality	Manometric finding
LES hypotension	$LES_p < 10$ mmHg
LES hypertension	$LES_p > 40$ mmHg
Nutcracker esophagus	Contractions of increased amplitude (>180 mmHg)
	Contractions of increased duration (>8 s)
Diffuse esophageal spasm	Increased number of swallows resulting in simultaneous contractions (>20%)
Ineffective motility	Contractions of decreased amplitude (<30 mmHg) in distal esophagus with >30% of wet swallows

13.8 Assessment Under Urgent Conditions

Although rare, recurrent hiatal hernias may present with acute complications that require urgent surgical management. These include acute gastric volvulus, organ perforation or penetration of the hollow organs in the sac to adjacent organs resulting in fistula. These conditions are with a significant mortality likely to the fact that they present in elderly patients with significant comorbidity and high perioperative risk due to their limited physiological reserve and do not tolerate any delay in diagnosis.

The key to the management is early recognition. Risk should be graded according to the American Society of Anesthesiologists (ASA) classification. Fluid and electrolyte deficiencies are assessed by determination of the serum levels. Blood gases and lactate levels are checked to detect acid-base imbalances. Presence of gastric necrosis, organ perforation, mediastinitis and other indications for preoperative initiation of antibiotics has to be ruled out. Tissue oxygenation should be assessed by pulse oximetry to initiate oxygen for the patients with low pO_2 levels. Early CT of the chest and abdomen is performed while the patient is in the emergency department. A decision is be made regarding the need for immediate operative intervention, endoscopy, or nasogastric tube (NGT) decompression.

Impossibility of passage of an NGT beyond the gastroesophageal junction should raise suspicion of organo-axial gastric volvulus. The role of the endoscopy as an assessment tool is described above.

Since large incarcerated paraesophageal hernias can cause cardiac compression, compromising cardiac output or arrhythmias, early anesthetic and intensive care involvement is critical in unwell patients. This may include arterial and central venous access for invasive monitoring, targeted fluid resuscitation and inotropic support [38].

Another urgent condition is the recurrent hernia that may be seen during pregnancy. Although it is a rare, intractable nausea, vomiting appearing as late onset hyperemesis gravidarum—after 20th week of gestation—should raise suspicion of a recurrent hiatal hernia, particularly in the presence of a mediastinal shift, dyspnea and history of an hiatal hernia repair [33–35].

13.9 Decision Making

Despite completion of a thorough preoperative workup of the patient in order to justify a reoperative attempt, the decision for reoperation must still be highly scrutinized by both the patient and the surgeon. Initial data in the literature indicates to an increased risk of complications for patients undergoing redo-laparoscopic operations emphasizing the possibility of blood loss, perforation of the esophagus, perforation of the stomach—occasionally requiring Roux-en-Y reconstruction—and injury to adjacent organs [36, 37].

More recent data however, possibly due to the evolution of the laparoscopic technology and use of the robotic surgery, revealed similar outcomes in the redo-laparoscopic surgery patients versus initial-surgery group with the exception of increased operative time due to re-identifying the relevant operative planes and blood loss which do not require transfusion [18, 28].

In this regard, a great amount of time and detail must be undertaken in educating the patient with regard to the proposed reoperative strategy and its associated risks emphasizing the importance of choosing a procedure with benefits outweighing the associated risks. This becomes more important particularly in acute and/or complicated cases in which exact management strategy may not be known until the pathology is properly assessed and require consent of the patient for all possibilities to repair the problem, including on-table endoscopy, laparoscopy, laparotomy, thoracotomy, feeding jejunostomy or gastrostomy.

Current Knowledge and Future Directions

- Recurrent hiatal hernia is recognized as the most common cause of the failure of an antireflux procedure with an incidence of approximately 50%
- Failed fundoplication may be classified as *slipped*, *malpositioned* or *loose* and may or may not be together with an hiatal hernia.
- A barium swallow or videoesophageal study may be useful in demonstrating the position of the hernia, location of the gastroesophageal junction, esophageal motility and is the preferred examination for the investigation of hiatal hernia recurrence under elective conditions
- Upper gastrointestinal endoscopy should be performed in all patients for evaluation of the esophageal and gastric mucosa for inflammation, ulcers, Barrett's esophagus, strictures and complications like mesh penetration.
- For reoperative procedures, there is an increased risk of complications including blood loss, perforation of the esophagus or stomach, and gastrointestinal leak necessitating repeat intervention.
- In the hands of experienced surgeons, outcomes of reoperative procedures are excellent.

References

1. Zaman JA, Lidor AO. An optimal approach to symptomatic paraesophageal hernia repair: important technical considerations. Curr Gastroenterol Rep. 2016;18:53. https://doi.org/10.1007/s11894-016-0529-6.
2. Mehta S, Boddy A, Rhodes M. Review of outcome after laparoscopic paraesophageal hiatal hernia repair. Surg Laparosc Endosc Percutan Tech. 2006;16:301–6.
3. Nason KS, Luketich JD, Qureshi I, et al. Laparoscopic repair of giant paraesophageal hernia results in long-term patient satisfaction and a durable repair. J Gastrointest Surg. 2008;12:2066–75.
4. Rosemurgy AS, Arnaoutakis DJ, Thometz DP, Binitie O, Giarelli NB, Bloomston M, Goldin SG, Albrink MH. Reoperative fundoplications are effective treatment for dysphagia and recurrent gastroesophageal reflux. Am Surg. 2004;70:1061–7.
5. Musunuru S, Gould JC. Perioperative outcomes of surgical procedures for symptomatic fundoplication failure: a retrospective case-control study. Surg Endosc. 2012;26:838–42.
6. Suppiah A, Sirimanna P, Vivian SJ, O'Donnell H, Lee G, Falk GL. Temporal patterns of hiatus hernia recurrence and hiatal failure: quality of life and recurrence after revision surgery. Dis Esophagus. 2017;30:1–8. https://doi.org/10.1093/dote/dow035.
7. Stylopoulos N, Rattner DW. The history of hiatal hernia surgery: from Bowditch to laparoscopy. Ann Surg. 2005;241:185–93.
8. Pandolfino JE, El-Serag HB, Zhang Q, Shah N, Ghosh SK, Kahrilas PJ. Obesity: a challenge to esophagogastric junction integrity. Gastroenterology. 2006;130:639–49.
9. Christensen J, Miftakhov R. Hiatus hernia: a review of evidence for its origin in esophageal longitudinal muscle dysfunction. Am J Med. 2000;108:3S–7S.
10. Curci JA, Melman LM, Thompson RW, Soper NJ, Matthews BD. Elastic fiber depletion in the supporting ligaments of the gastroesophageal junction: a structural basis for the development of hiatal hernia. J Am Coll Surg. 2008;207:191–6.
11. Weber C, Davis CS, Shankaran V, Fisichella PM. Hiatal hernias: a review of the pathophysiologic theories and implication for research. Surg Endosc. 2011;25:3149–53. https://doi.org/10.1007/s00464-011-1725-y.
12. Akimoto S, Nandipati KC, Kapoor H, Yamamoto SR, Pallati PK, Mittal SK. Association of body mass index (BMI) with patterns of fundoplication failure: insights gained. J Gastrointest Surg. 2015;19:1943–8.
13. Andolfi C, Jalilvand A, Plana A, Fisichell PM. Surgical management of paraesophageal hernias: a review. J Laparoendosc Adv Surg Tech. 2016;26:778–83. https://doi.org/10.1089/lap.2016.0332.
14. Tsang T, Walker R, Yu JD. Endoscopic reduction of gastric volvulus: the alpha-loop maneuver. Gastrointest Endosc. 1995;42:244–8.
15. Ortiz C, Gomez MA. Endoscopic treatment of gastric volvulus. Rev Col Gastroenterol. 2011;26:54–7.
16. Carrott PW, Hong J, Kuppusamy M, Koehler RP, Low DE. Clinical ramifications of giant paraesophageal hernias are underappreciated making the case for routine surgical repair. Ann Thorac Surg. 2012;94:421–6.
17. Carrott PW, Hong J, Kuppusamy M, Kirtland S, Koehler RP, Low DE. Repair of giant paraesophageal hernias routinely produces improvement in respiratory function. J Thorac Cardiovasc Surg. 2012;143:398–404.
18. Banki F, Kausnhik C, Roife D, Chawla M, Casimir R, Miller CC. Laparoscopic reoperative antireflux surgery: a safe procedure with high patient satisfaction and low morbidity. Am J Surg. 2016;212:1115–20.
19. Cameron AJ, Higgins JA. Linear gastric erosions. A lesion associated with large diaphragmatic hernia and chronic blood loss anemia. Gastroenterology. 1986;91:338–42.
20. http://www.endoatlas.com/st_ul_14.html.

21. Light D, Links D, Griffin M. The threatened stomach: management of the acute gastric volvulus. Surg Endosc. 2016;30:1847–52.
22. Komatsu T, Henteleff H. Colopleural fistula with atypical presentation as a complication of diaphragmatic hernia repair. Ann Thorac Surg. 2010;90(2):662–3.
23. Azzu V. Gastropericardial fistula: getting to the heart of matter. BMC Gastroenterol 2016;16:96. https://doi.org/10.1186/s12876-016-0510-8. URL: https://bmcgastroenterol.biomedcentral.com/articles/10.1186/s12876-016-0510-8. Accessed 21 Mar 2017.
24. Murthy S, Looney J, Jaklitsch MT. Gastropericardial fistula after laparoscopic surgery for reflux disease. N Engl J Med. 2002;346(5):328–32.
25. Peters van Ton AM, Diederik AL, Tjan DH. Colopleural fistula after hiatal hernia repair. BMJ Case Rep. 2016. https://doi.org/10.1136/bcr-2016-216814. URL: http://casereports.bmj.com/content/2016/bcr-2016-216814.long. Accessed 21 Mar 2017.
26. Bavry AA, Solorzano CC, Hocking MP. Unusual presentation of hemoptysis in a 78-year-old with previous Nissen fundoplication. Am Surg. 1998;64:1223–5.
27. Velanovich V. The development of the GERD-HRQL symptom severity instrument. Dis Esophagus. 2007;20:130–4.
28. Taghavi SA, Ghasedi M, Saberi-Firoozi M, et al. Symptom association probability and symptom sensitivity index: preferable but still suboptimal predictors of response to high dose omeprazole. Gut. 2005;54:1067–71.
29. Wennergren J, Levy S, Bower C, Miller M, Borman D, Davenport D, Plymale M, Roth JS. Revisional paraesophageal hernia repair outcomes compare favorably to initial operations. Surg Endosc. 2016;30:3854–60.
30. Lidor AO, Kawaji Q, Stem M, Fleming R, Schweitzer MA, Steele KE, Marohn MR. Defining recurrence after paraesophageal hernia repair: correlating symptoms and radiographic findings. Surgery. 2013;154:171–8.
31. Morgenthal CB, Lin E, Shane MD, et al. Who will fail laparoscopic Nissen fundoplication? Preoperative prediction of long-term outcomes. Surg Endosc. 2007;21:1978–84.
32. Cannon DJ, Read RC. Metastatic emphysema: a mechanism for acquiring inguinal herniation. Ann Surg. 1981;194:270–8.
33. Paterson WG, Goyal RK, Habib FI. Esophageal motility disorders. GI Motility Online. 2006. https://doi.org/10.1038/gimo20. https://www.nature.com/gimo/contents/pt1/fig_tab/gimo20_T3.html.
34. Schwentner L, Wulff C, Kreienberg R, Herr D. Exacerbation of a maternal hiatus hernia in early pregnancy presenting with symptoms of hyperemesis gravidarum: case report and review of the literature. Arch Gynecol Obstet. 2011;283:409–14. https://doi.org/10.1007/s00404-010-1719-3.
35. Lococo F, Cesario A, Meacci E, Granone P. Intrathoracic gastric perforation: a late complication of an unknown postpartum recurrent hiatal hernia. Interact Cardiovasc Thorac Surg. 2012;15:317–8. https://doi.org/10.1093/icvts/ivs209.
36. Eglinton T, Coulter GN, Bagshaw P, Cross L. Diaphragmatic hernias complicating pregnancy. ANZ J Surg. 2006;76:553–7.
37. Van Beek DB, Auyang ED, Soper NJ. A comprehensive review of laparoscopic redo fundoplication. Surg Endosc. 2011;25:706–12.
38. Juhasz A, Sundaram A, Hoshino M, Lee TH, Mittal SK. Outcomes of surgical management of symptomatic large recurrent hiatus hernia. Surg Endosc. 2012;26:1501–8.

Chapter 14
Recurrent GERD After a Fundoplication: Failure or Wrong Procedure

S. Mittal

Anti-reflux surgery in form of fundoplication is the gold standard for definitive treatment of gastro-esophageal reflux disease (GERD). Fundoplication is created by wrapping the gastric fundus around the distal 2–3 cm of esophagus, which lies tension free below the hiatus. With advent of minimally invasive techniques, there was greater patient and referring physician acceptability leading to an explosive increase in laparoscopic fundoplications being performed. Fundoplication is a procedure performed to improve quality of life and requires in-depth patient assessment and precise technical expertise to achieve optimal results. Excellent long-term satisfaction has been reported by several centers of expertise with greater than 95% patients reporting excellent satisfaction up to 10–20 years [1, 2].

A subset of patients reports either recurrent or new onset undesirable symptoms—either can be termed a failure of outcome. With the dramatic increase in number of procedures being performed, there has been a corresponding increase in number of patients with failed fundoplication. Surgeon's inexperience with technique or poor patient selection is likely to result in dissatisfied patients—resulting in failed fundoplication. In our experience, these two go hand-in-hand and with experience surgeons do a better job at patient selection.

Essentially a poor outcome or recurrent symptoms after a period of symptom control can be a result of poor patient selection, improper surgical technique, inadequate patient counseling or fundoplication disruption over time. We have discussed each of these in the following sections.

S. Mittal
Norton Thoracic Insitute, Phoenix, AZ, USA
e-mail: sumeetMittal@creighton.edu

M.A. Memon (ed.), *Hiatal Hernia Surgery*,
https://doi.org/10.1007/978-3-319-64003-7_14

14.1 What Is a Failed Fundoplication?

While experts may argue as to the definition and what comprises a failure; from a patient's perspective failure to provide durable symptom control and/or occurrence of undesirable symptoms is a failure. While being of paramount importance, patient symptoms alone are poor indicators of "recurrent GERD". Not infrequently profound esophageal dysmotility with or without tight fundoplication present with "recurrent regurgitation" and may be mistaken for recurrent GERD while the problem is poor esophageal emptying rather than an incompetent EGJ complex.

14.2 How to Evaluate a Dissatisfied ("Failed") Fundoplication Patient?

Evaluation for potential surgical intervention should be thorough and systematic in a patient presenting with recurrent symptoms or undesirable symptoms after previous anti-reflux surgery.

14.2.1 Patient History

Often in our clinic the first patient visit is a long 45–60 min patient interview. The reason is that not only does the surgeon needs to figure out how to best alleviate current symptoms but also understand underlying pathophysiology prior to first procedure. In our opinion the key elements of information which should be gathered includes:

(a) *Symptoms prior to first surgery and response to medications*

While the patient may be in a big rush and filled with anxiety to discuss present symptoms, it is imperative that we carefully elucidate original symptoms. If patient symptoms were of heartburn and regurgitation it is important to seek response (at least initially) to acid suppression therapy. Complete lack of response to acid suppression therapy is usually a red flag that the patient symptoms were probably not likely due to GERD. Duration of symptoms and progression along with associated symptoms such as dysphagia, cough etc. should also be sought after.

(b) *Work up done prior to surgery and results*

Efforts to get details of pre-operative work-up done and results of the tests should be sought after. Usually one can elicit from the patient themselves which tests were done and where (most patients are unlikely to forget having a manometry or pH done). It is important to personally review these test results to confirm that the patient had reflux and make some degree of assessment of baseline esophago-gastric motility. If the barium swallow reports poor clearance or a dilated esophagus then it is safe to assume severe underlying esophageal dysmotility. Similarly an EGD report with documented food in stomach would indicate underlying gastroparesis. Absence of an elevated 24 h pH score and lack of classical symptoms with poor response to medications in all likelihood indicates absence of GERD in the first place.

(c) *Symptoms immediately after surgery*

After getting the information in regards to pre-operative symptoms and tests, we like to enquire about the immediate postoperative period. Some degree of dysphagia and gas-bloat is near universal. Almost all patients report a great degree of improvement in heartburn and regurgitation regardless of how poorly the surgery might have been done provided the initial diagnosis of GERD was correct. This is because even transient reduction of HH and creation of any degree of fundoplication results in a greater competence of GEJ complex. Initial symptoms of dysphagia are managed with assurance and continued liquid diet till symptoms improves which is about 4–6 weeks. Only in cases with complete dysphagia i.e. unable to tolerate even their own saliva and clear liquids do we recommend doing a barium or endoscopy to rule out a slipped fundoplication or rarely a twisted fundoplication. While gentle dilation at this time may help symptoms transiently we prefer to wait for 4–6 weeks before endoscopic dilation for dysphagia. Similarly early postoperative bloating is self-limiting in severity and duration. However, severe and persistent bloating should raise concern for either missed or (occasionally) developing gastroparesis. Persistence of cough and other extra-esophageal symptoms could indicate that the symptoms were never associated with GERD even though pathological GERD may have been objectively documented pre-operatively.

(d) *Occurrence of current symptoms and response to medications*

After the above information we start discussing patient's present symptoms and duration of symptoms. For obstructive symptoms i.e. dysphagia it is important to note whether the problem persisted after the first surgery or did it develop de novo after a dysphagia free interval. Similarly whether the heartburn and regurgitation symptoms resolved and to what degree and if there was an inciting event such as severe gaging, retching or vomiting which lead to recurrence. Additionally it is imperative to ask whether the present symptoms are similar to those pre-operatively and how does the response to medications compare to preoperative response. If predominant symptoms were extra-esophageal and persisted after surgery one must take in to consideration that the symptoms are not related to GERD even though pathological GERD was present pre-operatively and classical symptoms (if any) have resolved. On the flip side if heartburn and regurgitation recurred after a bout of retching and respond to an extent to acid suppression then it is most likely recurrent GERD.

14.2.2 Diagnostic Tests

(a) *Upper Gastrointestinal Endoscopy (EGD)*

All patients should undergo upper gastrointestinal endoscopy by the operating surgeon. Vast majority of gastroenterologists and for that matter most surgeons are inherently unfamiliar with post-fundoplication anatomy and descriptive terms [3]. Upper endoscopy is also used to look for mesh/foreign body erosion and Barrett's esophagus (and degree of dysplasia). An intact symmetrical fundoplication on retroflex view goes a long way to argue against recurrent GERD. Gastric bezoar point to delayed gastric emptying while phlegm/saliva in the esophagus towards significant esophageal dysmotility. Endoscopic assessment of failed fundoplication is shown in Fig. 14.1.

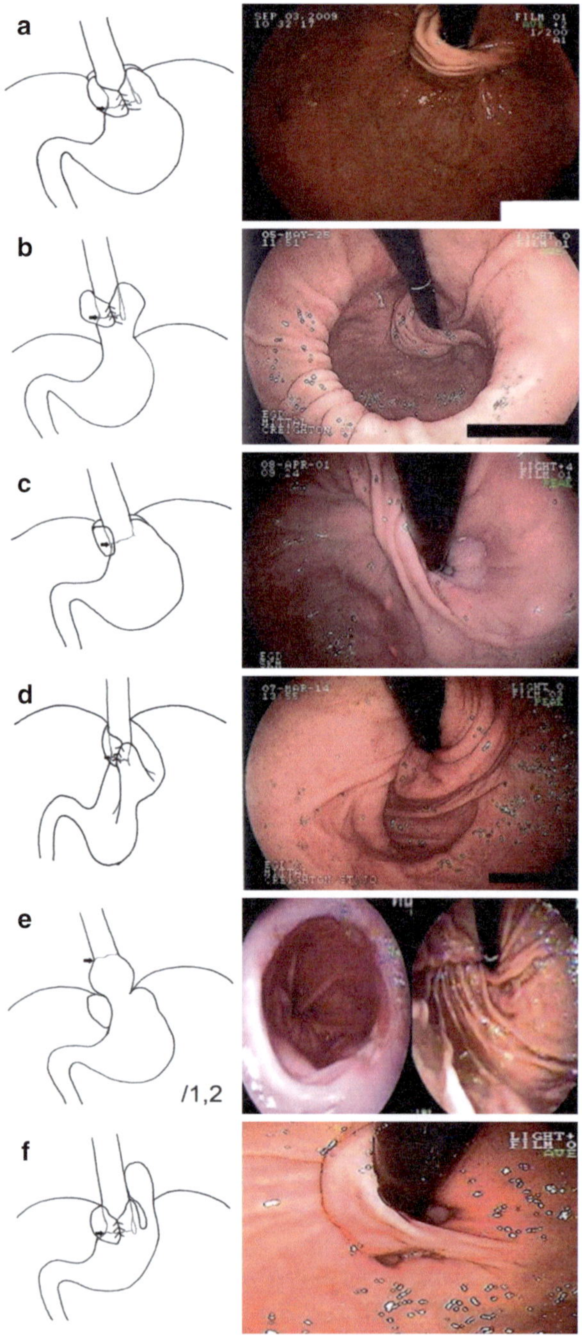

Fig. 14.1 Endoscopic evaluation of postfundoplicational alterations. (**a**) Properly positioned infradiaphragmatic fundoplication. (**b**) Intrathoracic fundoplication. (**c**) Disrupted infradiaphragmatic fundoplication. (**d**) Twisted infradiaphragmatic fundoplication. (**e**) Slipped fundoplication. (**f**) Paraesophageal hernia with a properly positioned fundoplication [8]

(b) *Barium esophagram*

A contrast esophagram is perhaps the most important dynamic test to assess benign esophageal disease. We recommend obtaining a video esophagram that can be reviewed in real time in case the surgeon cannot be present during the study. Esophageal bolus transit and clearance is best assessed with this dynamic study. Lateral views clearly delineate the location of the GEJ, fundoplication and their relation to the hiatus.

(c) *Manometry*

High resolution manometry is routinely done to assess esophageal motility. It is also useful to assess GEJ and fundoplication configuration and distinct patterns have been described in literature. Masato et al. [4]. Figure 14.2.

a

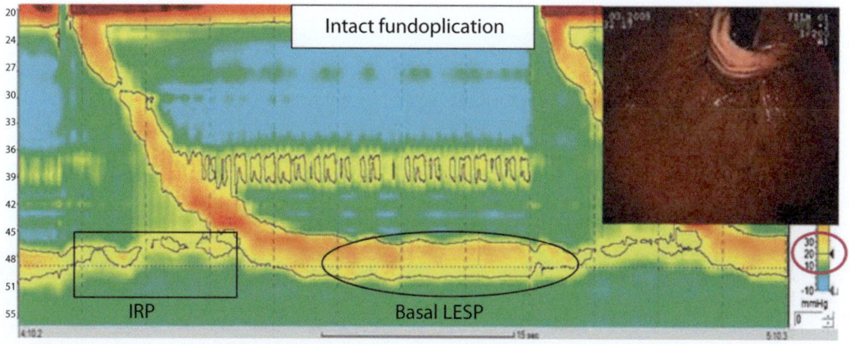

Fig. 14.2 (**a**) The HRM pressure topography of a patient with intact fundoplication. Compared to a healthy volunteer, the basal LES pressure is higher, but there is good LES relaxation during deglutition as the IRP is within normal limits. LES lower esophageal sphincter, IRP integrated relaxation pressure. Endoscopic picture reprinted from [4]. (**b**) Disrupted fundoplication. There is good relaxation with deglutition; however, the basal LES pressure is lower than in an intact fundoplication. LES lower esophageal sphincter. (**c**) The HPZ pressure pattern of a patient with a twisted fundoplication is shown in (**c**). One can see the high contractions and pressures in distal esophagus with high DCI and is indicative of outflow obstruction. These patients usually present with dysphagia or chest pain rather than reflux symptoms. LES lower esophageal sphincter, IRP integrated relaxation pressure, DCI distal contractile integral. (**d**) The HPZ pressure topography of an intact intra-thoracic fundoplication. In this patient, the HPZ is split into two: the distal HPZ represents the crus as the pattern indicates. The fundoplication is represented by the proximal HPZ. There is adequate pressure in the fundoplication with good relaxation as measured by a normal IRP. Such patients usually present with post-prandial chest/epigastric discomfort due to distention of herniated stomach. *HPZ* high pressure zone, *IRP* integrated relaxation pressure. (**e**) HRZ patterns in a patient with disrupted intra-thoracic fundoplication. The distal HPZ represents the crus. The proximal HPZ represents the area of the disrupted fundoplication. The basal LES pressure is low and there is a normal IRP. The low LES pressure indicates a disrupted fundoplication. *HPZ* high pressure zone, *IRP* integrated relaxation pressure, *LES* lower esophageal sphincter. Endoscopic picture reprinted from [4], with permission from Springer. (**f**) The HRZ patterns in a patient with slipped fundoplication. The proximal HPZ is the native LES and has low basal LES pressure with complete relaxation (normal IRP). The fundoplication is at the level of the crus. The diaphragmatic *HPZ* overlaps the fundoplication. *HPZ* high pressure zone, *LES* lower esophageal sphincter, *IRP* integrated relaxation pressure. Endoscopic pictures reprinted from [5], with permission from Springer. (**g**) Secondary achalasia is shown in **g**. These patients have aperistaltic esophageal body contractions. There is only a single HPZ pressure topography, but the LES pressure and the IRP are high. *HPZ* high pressure zone, *LES* lower esophageal sphincter, *IRP* integrated relaxation pressure. From Masato et al. [4]

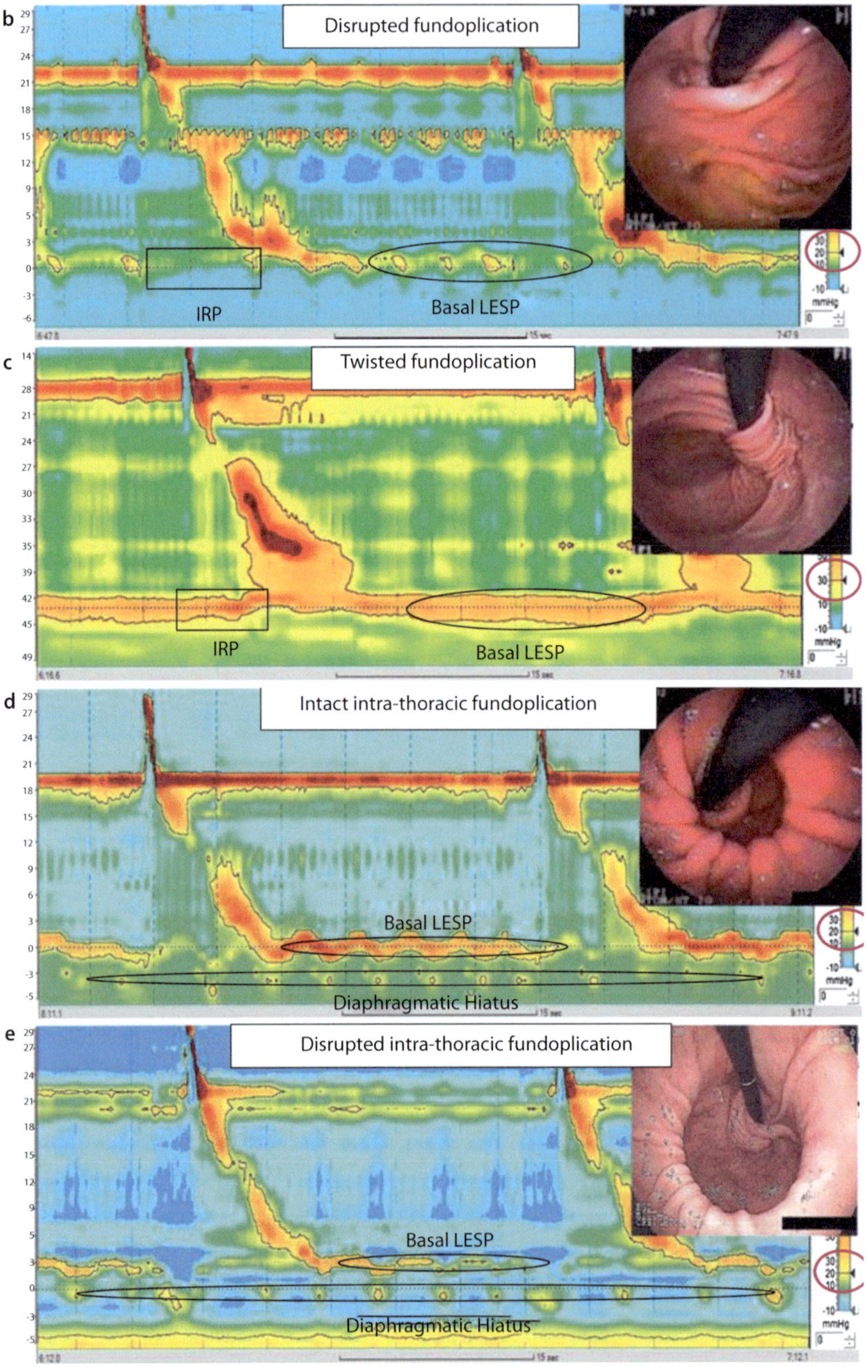

Fig. 14.2 (continued)

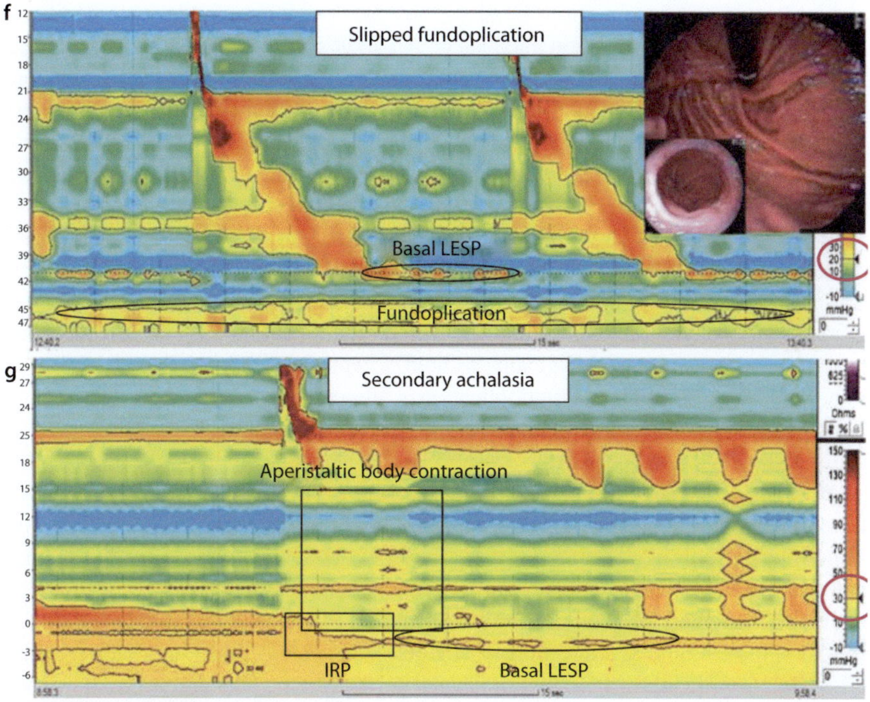

Fig. 14.2 (continued)

(d) *Prolonged pH monitoring*

Either 24 h catheter based or 48 h Bravo pH monitoring off acid suppression therapy is the gold standard to assess for extent of gastro-esophageal reflux. In our experience impedance reflux testing on therapy has not been very useful.

(e) *Gastric Emptying Study (GES)*

Nuclear medicine GES is useful to assess presence and degree of delayed gastric emptying and will help direct the need for gastric drainage procedure. A 4 h study is preferable and moderate to severe delayed GE should be addressed with either a pyloroplasty or anterectomy at the time of redo surgery.

14.3 How to Classify Failed Fundoplication?

Failed fundoplication have most commonly classified anatomically based on recurrence of hiatus hernia, relative location of the fundoplication to lower esophagus and geometry of the fundoplication. Jobe et al. [6] described in detail endoscopic characteristics of technically sound fundoplication and laid out the criteria for endoscopic assessment. However, majority of endoscopic assessment done in the community do not describe the fundoplication adequately. An audit of reported endoscopic findings by community gastroenterologists by Juhasz et al. [3] revealed a shockingly low concordance with subsequent findings of an experienced foregut surgeon. Surprisingly they found that nearly a 1/3rd of the endoscopic reports did not even mention a previous fundoplication while majority of the reports simply stated, "fundoplication changes noted" without any specific description. Proper and uniform endoscopic assessment of fundoplication is an import aspect in assessing causes of failure and devising a management strategy. Various terminologies have been used to describe failed fundoplication anatomy. Most commonly terms such as recurrent hiatus hernia, slipped, intra-thoracic, disrupted, twisted and telescopic fundoplication have been used. They have also been used interchangeably without accepted definitions. For example one may classify an intra-thoracic fundoplication is "slipped into the chest" or "telescoping in to the chest" while a fundoplication at the hiatus with GEJ above the hiatus may be called " slipped below the GJ" or recurrent HH" or "misplaced fundoplication".

Horagan et al. [7] were the first to propose an anatomic classification for failed fundoplication. They classified failed fundoplication into type IA (both EGJ and Fundoplication above the hiatus), type 1B (GEJ above hiatus with fundoplication below the hiatus, type II (only a portion of fundus/ greater curvature herniated above the hiatus) and type III (body of the stomach used to create the wrap rather than the fundus) (Table 14.1). More recently a standardized system based on location of the GEJ relative to the hiatus, the fundoplication relative to the GEJ and geometry of the fundoplication has been proposed by Mittal et al. [8] (Table 14.2). Each of the component E, S, F and P are given a 'suffix' and final description is given as $E_xS_xF_xP_x$.

While not discussed in literature till now a failed fundoplication may be better classified based on the underlying physiological derangements. Normal gastrointestinal function requires the ante-grade esophageal clearance thru the gastroesophageal junction (GEJ) and gastric clearance thru the pylorus along with a competent lower esophageal junction (LES) to prevent backflow. Furthermore, some degree of GEJ complex incompetence (permissiveness) is desirable to allow for gastric venting i.e. belching.

Poor esophageal emptying due to either poor motility and/or non-compliant lower esophageal sphincter- fundoplication (LES-F) complex will manifest with dysphagia and bland regurgitation. Not infrequently, in patients with poor motility, there may be aspiration associated cough or throat clearance. The patient or an inexperienced physician may confuse these symptoms as recurrent reflux, especially if regurgitation and cough are more prominent. On the other hand a non-functioning LES-F complex with poor competence allowing abnormal backflow of gastric contents will present with true recurrent GERD. Underlying delayed gastric emptying either pre-existing or due to vagal injury will present with bloating, nausea and

Table 14.1 Classification of failed fundoplication (by Horgan et al. [7])

Type of failure	Description
Type Ia	Both GEJ and fundoplication herniated above the hiatus
Type Ib	GEJ above the hiatus and fundoplication at the hiatus
Type II	Herniated stomach/greater curvature with GEJ and fundoplication below the hiatus
Type III	Wrong part (body) of the stomach used for fundoplication

Table 14.2 Endoscopic classification of failed fundoplication (by Mittal et al. [8])

Classification of the endoscopic findings of fundoplication	
Type of failure	Description
"E" component	Distance of GEJ to the level of crura component
E_0	GEJ is located intra-abdominally, at or under the level of crura
E_1	GEJ is located less than 2 cm above the level of crura
E_2	GEJ is located more than 2 cm above the level of crura
"S" component	Amount of gastric tissue above the fundoplication and below the GEJ
S_0	Fundoplication is around the distal esophagus
S_1	Less than 2 cm gastric tissue above the fundoplication
S_2	More than 2 cm gastric tissue above the fundoplication
"F" component	Description of the fundoplication
F_0	Intact fundoplication (competent, symmetrical)
F_{1a}	Partially disrupted fundoplication
F_{1b}	Completely disrupted fundoplication
F_{2a}	Twisted fundoplication
F_{2b}	Two-compartment stomach
"P" component	Present of paraesophageal hernia (verified by endoscopy or esophagogram)
P_0	No PEH
P_1	Recurrent PEH

epigastric pain, which may again be interpreted as recurrent GERD by patients and physicians alike. Not infrequently these symptoms become more prominent once reflux symptoms are addressed specially in patients with underlying Irritable Bowel Syndrome (IBS). There is a significant overlap in the clinical spectrum of GERD and IBS. Careful assessment of each dissatisfied post-fundoplication patient is essential to identify the underlying physiological derangement and one must be aware that more than one derangement may co-exist.

In the dissatisfied post-fundoplication patient, the anatomical and physiological findings should be concordant with symptomatology before surgical re-intervention is attempted. In our experience, patients with functional complaints without supportive objective findings may present with "failed fundoplication" and as "dissatisfied patients" and are best addressed with reassurance and counseling rather than surgical re-intervention.

14.4 Causes of Failed Fundoplication

14.4.1 Poor Patient Selection

Objective evidence of the presence of pathological reflux is important before a surgical fundoplication. Campos et al. showed that a good response to acid-suppression therapy, abnormal preoperative 24-h pH score and typical symptoms were good predictors of success of fundoplication [9]. While logical, it is surprising that it is not uncommon for patients with failed fundoplication to not have had an adequate documentation of disease prior to surgery. In these patients, it is hazardous to guess whether the surgery has failed or the disease never existed.

In our opinion, 'objective' evidence of GERD are: a classical history of heartburn or regurgitation with a very good response to acid suppressive therapy or grade B or greater reflux esophagitis noted on endoscopy. In absence of these, an elevated 24-h pH score as measured by prolonged monitoring off acid suppression is considered gold standard test.

In addition to above clinical scenario, esophago-gastric motility assessment should be done prior to surgery. High-resolution manometry and video esophagram are used to assess esophageal function and a gastric emptying study is used as indicated by patient symptoms to assess gastric motility. Additionally we strongly advocate that the operating surgeon performs an endoscopic assessment preferably pre-operatively and if not possible in the operative room prior to surgery.

Common foregut symptoms of heartburn, regurgitation and dysphagia span the gamut of underlying esophageal disorders from GERD to Achalasia and not infrequently are simply functional. Included in these are scleroderma patients who often present with severe reflux. Precise diagnosis is needed to direct appropriate surgical procedure. Patients with scleroderma and primary aperistalsis (non – Achalasia) may be better managed with primary laparoscopic Roux-en-Y gastric bypass (LRYGB) rather than a partial fundoplication.

14.4.2 Improper Surgical Technique

Multitude of fundoplication configurations both via thoracic and abdominal cavity have been described ranging from partial anterior or posterior to a complete fundoplication. All types of fundoplications require obtaining an adequate intra-abdominal length of the esophagus around which the fundus is wrapped such that the entire complex lays tension free below a closed hiatus.

The surgical technique needs to sufficiently mobilize the mediastinal esophagus to achieve adequate infra-diaphragmatic esophageal length. The crus pillars need to be approximated to close the hiatus with or without mesh reinforcement. Finally, the fundus (part of the stomach above an imaginary horizontal plane from the GEJ) is wrapped and anchored around the distal esophagus. Inadequate esophageal length will result in the positioning of fundoplication around the proximal stomach resulting in a "slipped wrap". Inadequate integrity of crus closure will result in re-herniation of the GEJ above the hiatus with (herniated) or without (slipped) fundoplication. Using the body of the stomach rather than fundus to create the 'fundoplication' usually results in a twisted fundoplication. We routinely perform and strongly recommend that an intra-operative endoscopy should be done to assess fundoplication prior to finishing the procedure.

Inadequate attention to these essential surgical steps will increase the likelihood of "failed fundoplication".

14.4.3 Inadequate Patient Counseling

A correctly created fundoplication increases barrier pressure and decreases the compliance (i.e., permissiveness) of the GEJ compared to the non-operative state. This requires patients to eat slowly and to chew the food bolus thoroughly, otherwise they risk experiencing dysphagia. Additionally, given the inherent loss of transient lower esophageal sphincter relaxations (TLESRs) after the fundoplication, patients may not be able to belch easily, and must avoid carbonated beverages especially in the immediate post-operative period. It is imperative that the patients be counseled to be cautious and expect these symptoms in the early post-operative period. These tend to resolve to a great extent in the first few weeks following fundoplication.

Retching, gagging and vomiting increase the likelihood of wrap herniation or disruption, resulting in recurrent GERD. This is a life-time caution that the patients must be aware of and take precautions against and, have easy and ready access to anti-emetics. We have also encountered some patients who gag themselves during vigorous tongue cleansing and this increases failure. Simple counselling to avoid this has helped tremendously [10].

Additionally, it has been proposed that heavy lifting should be avoided in the early post-operative period to allow for healing of apposed tissues. Comprehensive patient counseling should improve patient compliance with post-operative care and help reduce failure rates.

14.4.4 Fundoplication/Hiatus Disruption

Crus closure and fundoplication are secured with sutures. Natural forces and tissue characteristics may slowly or abruptly disrupt these anchoring sutures and the scarring, resulting in recurrent hiatus hernia and or disrupted fundoplication. Use of synthetic mesh has been shown to decrease recurrence of hiatus hernia but is also associated with increased incidence of severe complications [11, 12]. On the other hand, bio-prosthesis, though safer, have been shown to decrease only short term recurrence without affecting long term recurrence rate [13]. Improved understanding of factors leading to recurrent hiatus hernia and development of better surgical techniques/tools including mesh is needed to decrease these causes of failure.

14.4.5 Patient Body Habitus

Obesity is a risk factor for GERD and prevalence of obesity has dramatically increased in the Western world especially in the US. Perez et al. [14] were the first to report that morbid obesity is associated with poor outcomes after primary anti-reflux surgery. However, others [5] have argued that obesity does not affect outcomes. However, most surgeons agree that fundoplication may not be the best procedure for reflux control in morbidly obese patients. Laparoscopic Roux en Y Gastric Bypass (LRYGB) is an excellent anti-reflux operation that additionally provides for significant weight loss and it's associated salutatory effects on health. Most surgeons would steer morbidly obese patients (BMI > 35 kg/m^2) towards a LRYGB as primary intervention. While BMI > 35 kg/m^2 has been used as a cut of to direct towards bariatric procedure a study by Akimoto et al. [15] showed that patients with BMI > 30 kg/m^2 have similar patterns of failure after fundoplication as those with BMI > 35 kg/m^2 and these are distinct from failure patterns in patients with BMI < 30 kg/m^2. Performing a fundoplication in a morbidly obese patient can be judged partly a wrong patient choice and partly a wrong procedure choice, but occasionally it has to be considered in severely symptomatic patients (especially with volume regurgitation and pulmonary disease) if insurance denies coverage for bariatric procedure.

14.5 Conclusions

Recurrent GERD after fundoplication is a complex situation and requires exclusion of other diagnoses which may mimic GERD symptoms (delayed gastric emptying or post fundoplication achalasia) as well as separating the real symptoms from functional ones. Not infrequently, an anatomically distorted fundoplication will not have any associated symptoms and these should not undergo redo surgery. In cases with objective recurrence of the disease, many underlying factors—both patient and technical, may be responsible and must be explored to avoid failure of redo surgery. In certain situations such as missed short esophagus or failure to create a symmetrical fundoplication, there is technical inadequacy or surgical inexperience. However, non-identification of severe dysmotility or even achalasia and delayed gastric emptying, and proceeding with fundoplication should be diligently avoided.

What Is the Current Knowledge and What Future Direction Is Required

- Laparoscopic anti-reflux surgery in form of hiatus hernia repair and fundoplication is the gold standard for definitive management of pathological GERD. Excellent patient centered outcomes have been reported with greater than 90% patient satisfaction at 10 years.
- A subset of patients require re-operative intervention for failed fundoplication which is technically more difficult and associated with increased peri-operative morbidity along with lesser patient oriented outcomes compared to primary fundoplication.

- A uniformly accepted and widely endorsed definition of what constitutes a failed fundoplication is needed which may help tailor the subsequent treatment strategies.
- Understanding the causes of failure need to be elucidated and best strategies to minimize these undertaken.
- Additionally, surgical outcomes of community centers (where majority of the procedures are done) are less than stellar and have scared patients and referring physicians alike resulting in significant decline in use of the procedure.
- Future undertakings need to critically assess learning curve for laparoscopic anti-reflux surgery and incorporating appropriate curricula for training surgeons to work-up patients prior to surgical intervention.

References

1. Zaninotto G, Portale G, Costantini M, Rizzetto C, Guirroli E, Ceolin M, et al. Long-term results (6–10 years) of laparoscopic fundoplication. J Gastrointest Surg. 2007;11(9):1138–45.
2. Robinson B, Dunst CM, Cassera MA, Reavis KM, Sharata A, Swanstrom LL. 20 years later: laparoscopic fundoplication durability. Surg Endosc. 2015;29(9):2520–4.
3. Juhasz A, Sundaram A, Hoshino M, Lee TH, Filipi CJ, Mittal SK. Endoscopic assessment of failed fundoplication: a case for standardization. Surg Endosc. 2011;25(12):3761–6.
4. Masato H, Srinivasan A, Mittal SK. High resolution manometry patterns of lower esophageal sphincter complex in symptomatic post-fundoplication patients. J Gastrointest Surg. 2012;16(4):705–14.
5. D'Alessio MJ, Arnaoutakis D, Giarelli N, Villadolid DVm Rosemurgy AS. Obesity is not a contra-indication to laparoscopic Nissen fundoplication. J Gastrointest Surg. 2005;9:949–54.
6. Jobe BA, Kahrilas PJ, Vernon AH, Sandone C, Gopal DV, Swanstrom LL, et al. Endoscopic appraisal of the gastroesophageal valve after antireflux surgery. Am J Gastroenterol. 2004 Feb;99(2):233–43.
7. Horgan S, Pohl D, Bogetti D, Eubanks T, Peligrini C. Failed anti-reflux surgery: what have be we learned from reoperations? Arch Surg. 1999;134(8):809–15.
8. Mittal SK, Juhasz A, Ramanan B, Hoshino M, Lee TH, Filipi CJ. A proposed classification for uniform endoscopic description of surgical fundoplication. Surg Endosc. 2014;28(4):1103–9.
9. Campos G, Peters JH, TR DM, Öberg S, Crookes PF, Tan S, et al. Multivariate analysis of factors predicting outcome after laparoscopic Nissen fundoplication. J Gastrointest Surg. 1999;3(3):292–300.
10. Iqbal A, Kakarlapudi GV, Awad ZT, Haynatzki G, Turaga KK, Karu A, et al. Assessment of diaphragmatic stressors as risk factors for symptomatic failure of laparoscopic Nissen fundoplication. J Gastrointest Surg. 2006;10(1):12–21.
11. Nandipati K, Bye M, Yamamoto SR, Pallati P, Lee T, Mittal SK. Reoperative intervention in patients with mesh at the hiatus is associated with high incidence of esophageal resection—a single-center experience. J Gastrointest Surg. 2013;17(12):2039–44.
12. Stadlhuber RJ, Sherif AE, Mittal SK, Fitzgibbons RJ, Brunt LM, Hunter JG, et al. Mesh complications after prosthetic reinforcement of hiatal closure: a 28-case series. Surg Endosc. 2009;23(6):1219–26.
13. Frantzides CT, Carlson MA, Loizides S, Papafili A, Luu M, Roberts J, et al. Hiatal hernia repair with mesh: a survey of SAGES members. Surg Endosc. 2010;24(5):1017–24.

14. Perez AR, Moincure AC, Rattner DW. Obesity adversely affects the outcome of anti-reflux operations. Surg Endosc. 2001;15:986–9.
15. Akimoto A, Nandipati KC, Kapoor H, Yamamoto SR, Pallati PK, Mittal SK. Association of Body Mass Index (BMI) with patterns of fundoplication failure: insights gained. J Gastrointest Surg. 2015;19(11):1943–8.

Chapter 15
Management of Recurrent Paraesophageal Hernia

John H. Rodriguez and Jeffrey Ponsky

15.1 Introduction

Laparoscopy has become the standard approach for management of most benign foregut disease including antireflux and hiatal hernia repair. Anatomic recurrence after repair of paraesophageal hernias is high, however, the clinical significance of such findings seems to be less relevant [1]. Reoperative foregut surgery has a significantly higher morbidity and mortality than their primary counterparts. Fortunately, recurrence leading to reintervention is far less common, with a 10 year cumulative risk close to 7% [2].

The risk of recurrence is likely multifactorial, and many different factors have been investigated. The best results are typically achieved during initial intervention. Despite some controversies, complete mediastinal dissection and sac reduction, adequate esophageal length, crural closure, and a well constructed fundoplication, constitute some of the surgical principles to be followed at the time of paraesophageal hernia repair [1]. Recently, the role of preoperative body mass index has been taken into consideration as one of the most important factors that predict recurrence after repair [3].

The goal of this chapter is to review the clinical presentation, preoperative evaluation, and surgical planning relevant to repair of recurrent paraesophageal hernias.

J.H. Rodriguez, M.D. • J. Ponsky, M.D. (✉)
Section of Surgical Endoscopy, Cleveland Clinic, Cleveland, OH, USA

Lerner College of Medicine, Cleveland Clinic, Cleveland, OH, USA
e-mail: JPonsky@yahoo.com

M.A. Memon (ed.), *Hiatal Hernia Surgery*,
https://doi.org/10.1007/978-3-319-64003-7_15

15.2 Clinical Presentation

Primary paraesophageal hernias are typically found incidentally on imaging studies. The same is true for recurrent hernias. Symptoms related to a recurrence may differ from those present during initial presentation. Clinical features can be grouped into reflux type or obstructive type symptoms. Proper history taking is crucial in understanding the correlation between symptoms and hernia recurrence. Patients presenting with gastroesophageal reflux disease should be evaluated and treated no different than during initial presentation. Antireflux lifestyle modifications and antisecretory medication should be the first steps in management, as these patient rarely require additional surgical intervention.

Obstructive type symptoms such as dysphagia, epigastric pain, early satiety, nausea, or vomiting, tend to be more bothersome and require additional investigation. The etiology of such symptoms can be multifactorial so imaging and functional studies may be needed to uncover the underlying precipitating factor. In most cases, every effort should be made towards medical optimization of the patient before considering reintervention.

Vagal nerve injury is a feared complication after foregut surgery. This sequela has been described in up to 10% of patients [4] following surgical foregut intervention. Symptoms resulting from vagal nerve injury are typically related to alterations in gut physiology and may include diarrhea, gas bloat syndrome, nausea, and vomiting [5]. Resulting delayed gastric emptying can be extremely debilitating and may have severe consequences such as malnutrition and adult failure to thrive.

15.3 Evaluation

Evaluation of patients presenting with a recurrent paraesophageal hernia is commonly triggered by symptoms. A combination of anatomic and functional studies are needed to better understand the underlying mechanism responsible for symptoms. Anatomic recurrence in an otherwise asymptomatic patient requires no further workup. Patients should be counseled on the importance of such finding and warning signs that may develop in the future.

As previously mentioned, careful history taking can help distinguish the etiology of symptoms and guide relevant workup. Physical examination can help assess nutritional status both in cases of malnutrition and morbid obesity. An accurate height and weight should be obtained in every patient to document body mass index.

A clear anatomic understanding can be achieved with a combination of imaging, endoscopy, and review of operative reports. Upper gastrointestinal contrast study is likely the most relevant radiologic exam in clinical practice and should be obtained in every case. It requires careful interpretation, but will help the surgeon understand the size of a recurrence, presence of a fundoplication, and location of the gastroesophageal junction. With careful review, the study can also provide hints into functional disorders such as reflux, pseudoachalasia from a tight fundoplication or hiatal closure, and poor esophageal peristalsis.

Computed tomography can be helpful in evaluating large recurrences or in patients presenting with acute complications. It is not a routine study in our practice, but it is a common source for diagnosis of incidental anatomic recurrence.

Endoscopy is a very useful tool that can complement imaging studies. It should be performed by a proceduralist that is familiar with post surgical anatomy. The mucosa of the esophagus, stomach, and duodenum should be carefully inspected. The gastroesophageal transition zone should be examined and measured using the incisors as a reference point. It's relation with the diaphragmatic pinch should be documented as well, as it is a good estimator of the size of a recurrence. The endoscopist should carefully examine the proximal stomach in retroflex position to try to identify any evidence of a fundoplication, and its overall appearance. Resistance to passing the scope can be seen in cases of tight fundoplication or hiatal closure. The indentation of a fundoplication and it's relationship to the gastroesophageal junction should also be noticed and documented. Gastric folds should not be seen proximal to a fundoplication, as it can be a sign of slippage or poor construction. The presence of food bezoars in the stomach should be a warning sign of post surgical gastroparesis and may require further evaluation.

Functional studies should be focused on expanding the knowledge of foregut physiology. The authors strongly recommend a 4 h solid protocol gastric emptying scintigraphy on every patient being considered for revisional foregut surgery. The presence of delayed gastric emptying should be documented prior to any intervention and may alter surgical planning. Post surgical gastroparesis may be the underlying etiology for symptoms that can be wrongfully attributed to a hernia recurrence.

High resolution esophageal manometry can be useful when the etiology of dysphagia is somewhat unclear. It can also help identify high pressure areas following antireflux surgery. Poorly constructed fundoplication can also result in unwanted pressurization of the gastroesophageal junction. Esophageal pH study should be obtained in cases where reflux is a cardinal sign, but is not necessary during other presentations.

15.4 Surgical Planning

Following proper surgical principles during initial repair of paraesophageal hernias is the most important factor to prevent symptomatic recurrences [1]. The difficulty of recurrent operations tends to increase with each additional operation due to adhesion formation and loss of tissue planes. The risk of injury to intra abdominal organs such as the stomach and esophagus has been described to be as high as 30% [6]. Therefore, surgeons attempting repair of recurrent hernia should be capable of confronting every possible scenario.

The decision to re-intervene in cases of recurrent paraesophageal hernias needs to be made with proper planning. Obtaining operative records is crucial in understanding and anticipating potential pitfalls. Relevant pieces of information can help predict critical steps and prepare the surgeon. Description of complete mediastinal dissection with reduction of the sac during the initial operation is key in anticipating the difficulty of this step. Normal anatomical planes are harder to find and risk of injury to the pleura can be significantly higher. Use of mesh during the previous operation to reinforce the hiatus tends to cause a more severe inflammatory reaction, especially in cases where biologic mesh was used. Description of a fundoplication should be carefully interpreted. Type of fundoplication, mobilization of the greater curvature, and pexy of the wrap to the crus are important details to obtain.

There are special situations to consider when planning recurrent cases. Gastric motility along with interpretation of symptoms can point towards poor gastric emptying as the possible etiology for recurrent foregut symptoms. Failure to address this will result in lower satisfaction and poor outcomes, In cases of small recurrences with significant symptoms secondary to poor gastric emptying (bloating, nausea, vomiting), the goal of therapy should be directed towards this and not necessarily on the recurrence. When the etiology is not completely clear, careful interpretation of preoperative imaging is necessary. Endoscopy with injection of Botulinum toxin in the pylorus may help temporarily alleviate symptoms in some patients. In these cases, improvement confirms the etiology and will help direct definitive therapy. A gastric drainage procedure such as a laparoscopic pyloroplasty or endoscopic per-oral pyloromyotomy (POP) should be considered as initial therapy and may potentially avoid any need for more proximal dissection. In more severe cases, near total gastrectomy with reconstruction may be necessary.

Morbid obesity is another major factor that should be taken into consideration at the time of revision. Patients with BMI > 35 kg/m^2 should be strongly considered for revision into bariatric anatomy [7]. Both roux en Y gastric bypass and sleeve gastrectomy are reasonable options. However, the higher incidence of GERD after sleeve gastrectomy should be considered. Gastric bypass is the best known surgical alternative for management of GERD [8], and should be considered as the best option in this patient population. Patients who are candidates for bariatric surgery should be enrolled in a multidisciplinary clinic. Proper preoperative evaluation including nutritional counseling, psychological evaluation, and medical optimization are key components to ensure the best possible postoperative outcome. Sleeve gastrectomy has also been evaluated as a combined operation during paraesophageal hernia repair [9]. It is technically easier than gastric bypass and follows the surgical principles of esophageal lengthening initially described by Collis [10]. Foregut anatomy after bariatric surgery has the potential benefit of reducing the risk of symptoms in case of a recurrence. Transhiatal migration of a gastric pouch or proximal sleeve does not commonly result in significant symptoms.

15.5 Technical Considerations

- *Surgical approach*: recurrent paraesophageal hernias can be operated through a transabdominal or transthoracic approach. This decision is based mostly on surgeon's preference and experience. Open vs. minimally invasive is another factor to consider. Laparoscopy has gained a leading role in management of benign foregut disease [11]. The authors prefer a transabdominal laparoscopic approach for all cases. Five laparoscopic trocars are placed in a gentle "U" configuration, and the Nathanson liver retractor is used when needed through a separate epigastric incision. The use of long laparoscopic instruments facilitates mediastinal dissection. This approach is highly successful even in cases of previous laparotomy or thoracotomy.

- *Management of the shortened esophagus*: inadequate intraabdominal esophageal length has been described as a predisposing factor for recurrence [12]. Adequate mediastinal dissection during the initial operation will significantly increase the difficulty of further mediastinal dissection during reoperation. Esophageal lengthening should be considered in recurrent cases, specially when adequate mobilization cannot be achieved. Laparoscopic Collis gastroplasty has been described as the treatment of choice for management of this challenging situation [13]. Bariatric surgery is another alternative that can help address this problem. Construction of a small tubular proximal gastric pouch, or tubularization of the stomach during sleeve gastrectomy, will achieve the same goal.
- *Management of previous fundoplication*: construction of a Nissen fundoplication has been advocated as a routine practice during initial repair of paraesophageal hernia repair [14]. The rationale for this practice is somewhat controversial. Many experts believe that transhiatal migration of a wrap is responsible for severe symptoms, and acute complications requiring emergent intervention [15]. In many cases, poor construction of a fundoplication is the main culprit for failure. Either wrap disruption, proximal migration of distal stomach (slippage), or transhiatal migration of an intact wrap can be encountered. It is our practice to completely undo a previous fundoplication during revisional surgery. In many instances, the fundus may become ischemic requiring resection. Reconstruction of fundoplication is feasible and can be done safely. Emphasis should be made on proper construction. Using the fundus and not body of the stomach is crucial, as well as positioning over the distal esophagus. When a bariatric operation is considered, it is necessary to completely take down a previous fundoplication to avoid "double stapling" of tissue when a pouch or sleeve is constructed.
- *Management of the crural defect*: many different techniques have been described for closing large or challenging hiatal defects. Many recurrent defects can be closed with either interrupted, figure-of-eight, or running non-absorbable suture. Using self-locking barbed suture can help maintain the tension as the defect is being approximated. Relaxing incisions on the diaphragm have been advocated to reapproximate large crural defects [16]. Mesh reinforcement has been shown to decrease the risk of recurrence in the early stages after repair [1] and should be considered. Bio-absorbable or biologic mesh is preferred due to the decreased risk of erosion into the esophagus. However, large series have been published using synthetic mesh with adequate safety [17]. Some large defects show a pattern characterized by elongation and bowing of the left crus with a relatively vertical right crus. In these cases, left cruroplasty can be performed to shorten the elongated muscle and facilitate symmetric closure.
- *Intraoperative endoscopy:* endoscopy during primary and revisional cases can be an invaluable tool in assisting the surgeon through challenging cases. Identification of anatomic landmarks such as the gastroesophageal junction can be facilitated by combined endoscopic and laparoscopic visualization. Endoscopy can also be

useful to identify the presence of a fundoplication and assist the surgeon during dissection. In cases where gastrectomy is performed, evaluation of anastomosis for bleeding or integrity can be easily performed.

- *Fluorescence imaging:* the use of fluorescence imaging has gained significant interest in modern day surgery. It may play a useful role during complex revisions, especially those requiring reconstruction. Intraoperative immunofluorescence can help assess viability and adequate perfusion of tissues prior to reconstruction. This may alter surgical conduct and help prevent potential complications secondary to tissue ischemia [18].

15.6 Post Operative Care

Patients undergoing revisional foregut procedures are at increased risk of gastrointestinal, pulmonary, and systemic complications. There is controversy on the role of post-operative imaging to routinely evaluate these patients with upper gastrointestinal contrast studies. However, radiologic documentation of an intact repair postoperatively is valuable and has become routine in our practice. Early recurrence will most likely need immediate reintervention and can be easily detected on imaging. Upper GI should also be considered in patients undergoing complex revisions requiring resection and anastomosis.

Diet can be started at the discretion of the surgeon and usually consists of a liquid consistency diet for 2 weeks. This is then advanced as tolerated by the patient. Patients undergoing fundoplication or reconstruction with gastrojejunal or esophagojejunal anastomoses can experience dysphagia early in the postoperative period. This needs to be taken into consideration during patient education so they can be guided towards the right choices. Progressive dysphagia can be a warning sign and should be investigated further with imaging or endoscopy.

Growing clinical experience with enhanced recovery pathways have proven beneficial for patients undergoing GI surgery. Use of non narcotic medications, early mobility, aggressive anti-nausea therapy, and early oral intake play a significant role in post-operative recovery.

15.7 Conclusion

Surgical management of recurrent paraesophageal hernia present unique technical challenges. Careful pre-operative evaluation and delineation of cardinal symptoms should guide the recognition of common pitfalls encountered during revisional surgery. As previously stated, surgical planning is crucial in optimizing results and minimizing complications. Surgeons performing these operations need to be prepared to manage technical barriers and should choose the best technical approach.

What Is the Current Knowledge and What Future Direction Is Required

- Radiologic recurrence rate after paraesophageal hernia repair is high, but indications leading to revisional surgery remain low
- Initial repair of paraesophageal hernia should focus on managing the technical aspects that help decrease the risk of a recurrence. These include complete mediastinal dissection and sac reduction, adequate esophageal length, crural closure, and a well constructed fundoplication
- Morbidly obese patients should be considered for combined bariatric surgery at the time of paraesophageal hernia repair if indicated. This should be done following bariatric principles to optimize results.
- Surgical management of paraesophageal hernia recurrence is technically challenging. Patients should undergo adequate preoperative workup including anatomic and functional studies.
- Use of preoperative and intraoperative endoscopy is an invaluable tool that should be considered by every surgeon performing revisional foregut surgery.
- Further studies are needed to clarify additional factors that lead to failure after paraesophageal hernia repair. Doing right the first time can avoid the need for reintervention.

Appendix

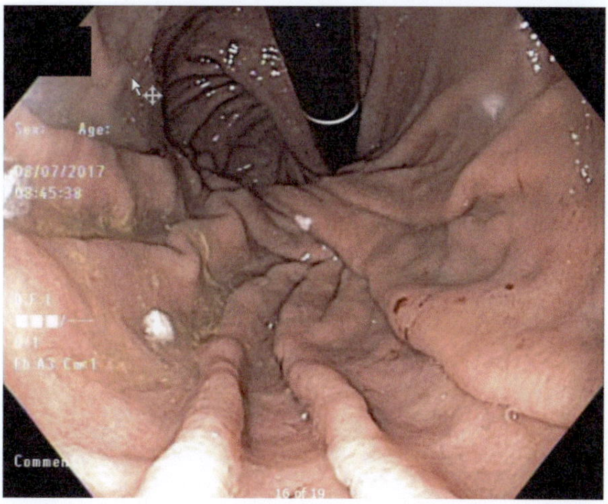

Fig. A.1 Endoscopic view of recurrent PEH with transhiatal wrap migration

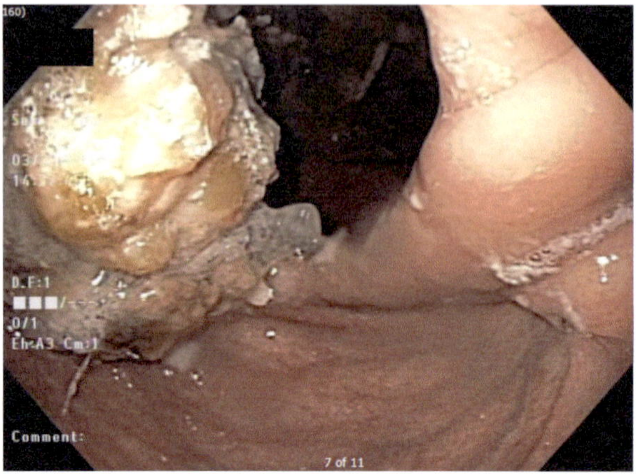

Fig. A.2 Gastric bezoar during EGD demonstrating post surgical gastroparesis

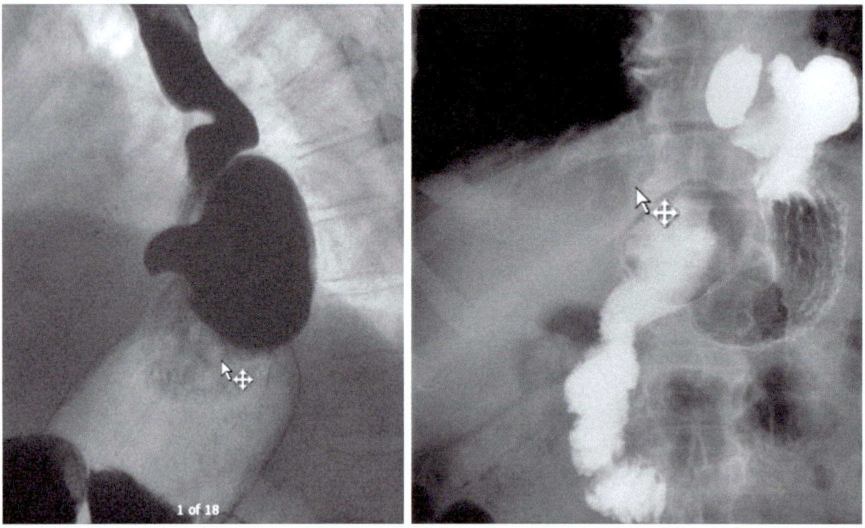

Fig. A.3 Upper GI showing transhiatal wrap migrationand recurrent PEH

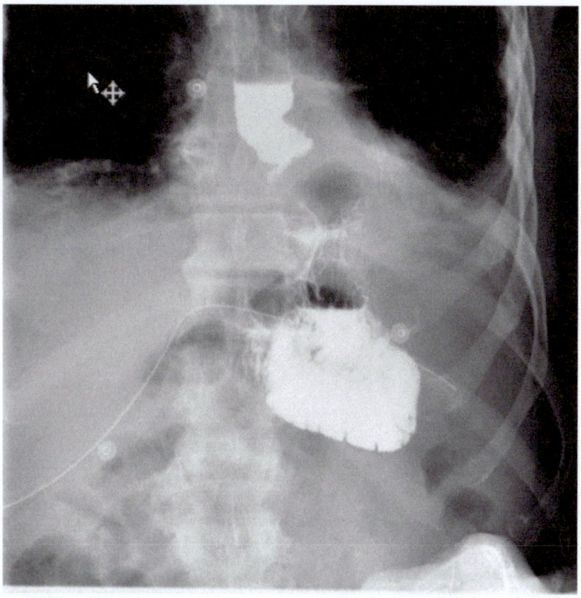

Fig. A.4 Upper GI on postoperative day one demonstrating sub diaphragmatic gastric pouch and Roux en Y gastrojejunostomy

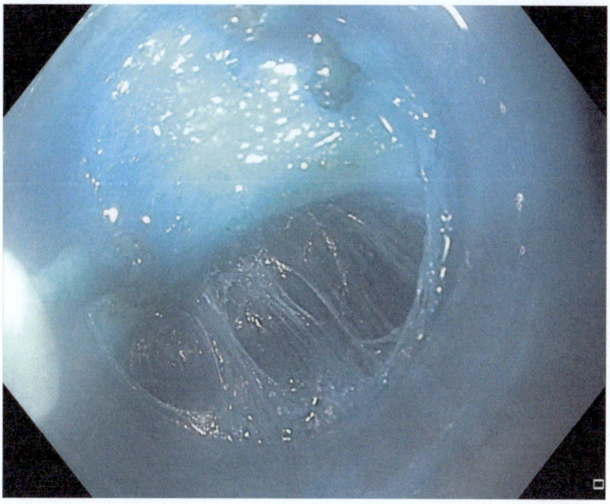

Fig. A.5 Endoscopic view of pyloric sphincter during per oral pyloromyotomy

References

1. Oelschlager BK, Petersen RP, Michael Brunt L, Soper NJ, Sheppard BC, Lee M, Rohrmann C, Swanstrom LL, Pellegrini CA. Laparoscopic paraesophageal hernia repair: defining long-term clinical and anatomic outcomes. J Gastrointest Surg. 2012;16(3):453–9. https://doi.org/10.1007/s11605-011-1743-z.
2. Zhou T, Harnsberger C, Broderick R, Fuchs H, Talamini M, Jacobsen G, Horgan S, Chang D, Sandler B. Reoperation rates after laparoscopic fundoplication. Surg Endosc. 2014;29(3):510–4. https://doi.org/10.1007/s00464-014-3660-1.
3. Akimoto S, Nandipati KC, Kapoor H, Yamamoto SR, Pallati PK, Mittal SK. Association of body mass index (BMI) with patterns of fundoplication failure: insights gained. J Gastrointest Surg. 2015;19(11):1943–8. https://doi.org/10.1007/s11605-015-2907-z.
4. Lindeboom MYA, Ringers J, van Rijn PJ, Neijenhuis P, Stokkel MP, Masclee AA. Gastric emptying and vagus nerve function after laparoscopic partial fundoplication. Ann Surg. 2004;240(5):785–90. https://doi.org/10.1097/01.sla.0000143124.30911.0f.
5. van Rijn S, Roebroek YG, Conchillo JM, Bouvy ND, Masclee AA. Effect of vagus nerve injury on the outcome of antireflux surgery: an extensive literature review. Dig Surg. 2016;33(3):230–9. https://doi.org/10.1159/000444147.
6. Juhasz A, Sundaram A, Hoshino M, Lee TH, Mittal SK. Outcomes of surgical management of symptomatic large recurrent hiatus hernia. Surg Endosc. 2011;26(6):1501–8. https://doi.org/10.1007/s00464-011-2072-8.
7. Salvador-Sanchis JL, Martinez-Ramos D, Herfarth A, Rivadulla-Serrano I, Ibañez-Belenguer M, Hoashi JS. Treatment of morbid obesity and hiatal paraesophageal hernia by laparoscopic Roux-en-Y gastric bypass. Obes Surg. 2008;20(6):801–3. https://doi.org/10.1007/s11695-008-9656-y.
8. El-Hadi M, Birch D, Gill R, Karmali S. The effect of bariatric surgery on gastroesophageal reflux disease. Can J Surg. 2014;57(2):139–44. https://doi.org/10.1503/cjs.030612.
9. Rodriguez JH, Kroh M, El-Hayek K, Timratana P, Chand B. Combined paraesophageal hernia repair and partial longitudinal gastrectomy in obese patients with symptomatic paraesophageal hernias. Surg Endosc. 2012;26(12):3382–90. https://doi.org/10.1007/s00464-012-2347-8.
10. Collis JL. An operation for hiatus hernia with short oesophagus. Thorax. 1957;12(3):181–8. https://doi.org/10.1136/thx.12.3.181.
11. Zehetner J, Demeester SR, Ayazi S, Kilday P, Augustin F, Hagen JA, Lipham JC, Sohn HJ, Demeester TR. Laparoscopic versus open repair of paraesophageal hernia: the second decade. J Am Coll Surg. 2011;212(5):813–20. https://doi.org/10.1016/j.jamcollsurg.2011.01.060. Epub 2011 Mar 23
12. Kunio NR, Dolan JP, Hunter JG. Short esophagus. Surg Clin N Am. 2015;95(3):641–52. https://doi.org/10.1016/j.suc.2015.02.015.
13. Swanstrom LL, Marcus DR, Galloway GQ. Laparoscopic collis gastroplasty is the treatment of choice for the shortened esophagus. Am J Surg. 1996;171(5):477–81. https://doi.org/10.1016/s0002-9610(96)00008-6.
14. Furnée EJ, Draaisma WA, Gooszen HG, Hazebroek EJ, Smout AJ, Broeders IA. Tailored or routine addition of an antireflux fundoplication in laparoscopic large hiatal hernia repair: a comparative cohort study. Am J Surg. 1996;171(5):477–81.
15. Singhal T, Balakrishnan S, Hussain A, Grandy-Smith S, Paix A, El-Hasani S. Management of complications after laparoscopic Nissen's fundoplication: a surgeon's perspective. Ann Surg Innov Res. 2009;3(1):1. https://doi.org/10.1186/1750-1164-3-1.
16. Horgan S, Eubanks TR, Jacobsen G, Omelanczuk P, Pellegrini CA. Repair of paraesophageal hernias. Am J Surg. 1999;177(5):354–8. https://doi.org/10.1016/s0002-9610(99)00061-6.
17. Targarona EM. Mesh in the hiatus. Arch Surg. 2004;139(12):1286.https://doi.org/10.1001/archsurg.139.12.1286.
18. Degett TH, Andersen HS, Gögenur I. Indocyanine green fluorescence angiography for intraoperative assessment of gastrointestinal anastomotic perfusion: a systematic review of clinical trials. Langenbeck's Arch Surg. 2016;401(6):767–75. https://doi.org/10.1007/s00423-016-1400-9.

Chapter 16
Revision Strategies for Recurrent Paraesophageal Hiatal Hernia

Jeffrey R. Watkins and Ralph W. Aye

16.1 Introduction

Laparoscopic re-operative paraesophageal hernia repair represents one of the most challenging problems facing modern foregut surgery. The incidence of hiatal hernia increases with advancing age and its overall estimated prevalence is as high as 50%, with larger paraesophageal hernias comprising approximately 5% of that number [1–3]. Thousands of primary laparoscopic paraesophageal hernia repairs are performed annually and will likely increase as the aging population continues to grow in number.

With the large number of primary repairs being performed, the number of revisional operations is increasing as well. What is surprising, however, is the high rate at which recurrence occurs. Regardless of the technique used, long-term data consistently show a radiographic recurrence rate of over 50% after operative repair [4, 5]. While only 3–6% of these recurrences require operative intervention in the short term, the high rate of anatomic failure is indeed worrisome [6, 7]. This underscores the need for experienced foregut surgeons at high volume centers to undertake the difficult endeavor of addressing the issue of recurrent paraesophageal hiatal hernias.

In this chapter, the following points will be addressed

- Causes of failure after primary paraesophageal hernia repair
- Identifying recurrence and the indications for reoperation
- Surgical strategies for re-operative paraesophageal hernias

J.R. Watkins, M.D. • R.W. Aye, M.D. (✉)
Swedish Thoracic and Esophageal Surgery,
1101 Madison Suite 900, Seattle, WA 98104, USA
e-mail: Ralph.aye@swedish.org

M.A. Memon (ed.), *Hiatal Hernia Surgery*,
https://doi.org/10.1007/978-3-319-64003-7_16

Table 16.1 Factors contributing to fundoplication failure

Tension	Radial
	Axial
Technical	Misplaced wrap
	Incomplete hiatal dissection
	Misidentified GEJ
	Loose sutures
	Improperly tied knots
	Poor tissue bites
	Surgeon experience
	Asymmetric fundoplication
	Tightness of fundoplication
	Tightness of crural closure
Patient factors	BMI >35
	Acid-suppression medication unresponsiveness
	Barrett's esophagus
	Atypical symptoms
	Psychiatric illness
	Short esophagus
	Post-operative diaphragmatic stressors

16.2 Causes of Failure

While the reasons for such a high recurrence rate of paraesophageal hernia are multifactorial, there are several factors that are generally recognized (Table 16.1). These likely not only caused the primary operation to fail, but will also lead to failure of the re-operation if they are not recognized and addressed. These can be broken down into physiologic factors and technical factors. The physiologic factors relate to the intrinsic and extrinsic forces exerted on the esophagus and gastroesophageal junction. Technical factors are related to intraoperative surgical decision-making and execution as well as post-operative care. Most of these factors can be addressed with careful planning and surgeon experience. It is important to identify causes of failure and properly address them in order to avoid repeating the same mistake that led to the initial recurrence.

16.2.1 Radial and Axial Tension

There are two major forces acting on the repair of the hiatal hernia that lead to disruption of the repair and ultimate failure: radial tension and axial tension (Fig. 16.1). Radial tension at the hiatus acts upon the diaphragm in a plane perpendicular to the esophagus. This tension results in the movement of crural fibers away from the

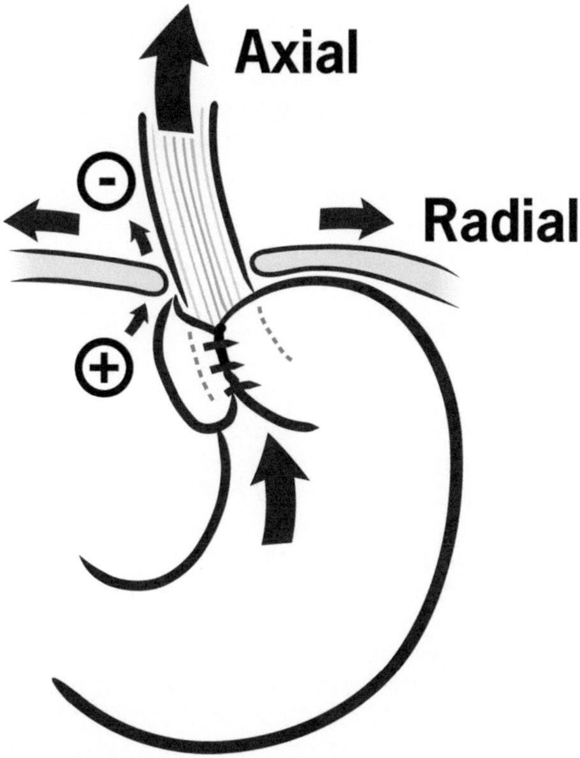

Fig. 16.1 Diagram of forces acting upon the esophagus and GEJ. Axial tension acts parallel to the esophagus and causes cephalad migration. Radial tension acts perpendicular to the esophagus but parallel to the diaphragm and results in widening of the crura

midline and a widening of the diaphragmatic hiatus. It is opposed by the phrenoesophageal ligament which helps keep the hiatus in place around the esophagus. The dynamic nature of the diaphragm and its constant motion over time causes stretching and even break down of a sutured crural repair with resultant failure and recurrence of the hernia. When the radial forces overcome the forces keeping the hiatus together, the hiatus loosens and allows herniation to occur. When repairing hiatal hernias, increased radial tension is manifested as difficulty re-approximating the left and right crural pillars.

Axial tension is related to the cephalad forces acting on the esophagus both intrinsically and extrinsically and is manifest as the tendency for the gastroesophageal junction (GEJ) to migrate upward into the mediastinum. There is a natural physiologic movement of the GEJ of up to 2.5 cm in non-hernia patients, with the phrenoesophageal membrane acting as an elastic recoil mechanism to return the GEJ to its proper anatomic configuration [8]. When the phrenoesophageal ligament becomes attenuated, the amount of recoil decreases and results in herniation [9]. Additional forces include negative intra-thoracic pressure, positive intra-abdominal pressure, contractile forces of the longitudinal esophageal musculature, and increased intra-gastric pressure. In addition, chronic displacement of the GE junction into the chest combined with fibrosis from recurrent esophagitis can make re-establishment of adequate intra-abdominal esophagus difficult (short esophagus), with resultant axial tension on the repair. After primary repair of a paraesophageal hernia, this axial tension acting on the esophagus continues unopposed and can result in disruption of the hiatal closure or any fixation sutures resulting in intrathoracic migration of the GEJ and fundoplication.

16.2.2 Technical Issues

There are several technical factors at the time of the index operation over which the surgeon has control and which can result in reduced likelihood of recurrence. A full mobilization of the distal esophagus up to or above the inferior pulmonary veins will improve intra-abdominal length and decrease axial tension on the short esophagus. Intra-operative endoscopy with endoscopic confirmation of the squamocolumnar junction will aid in correctly placing the wrap at and above the GE junction rather than too low.

The actual shaping of the fundoplication by utilizing the correct portion of the fundus and bringing it around the esophagus with the proper configuration is critical. If the gastric body rather than the fundus is used to construct the wrap, a type III failure may occur (Fig. 16.2). In order to avoid an overly tight wrap, the fundoplication is most often constructed over a bougie. Data suggests a decrease in postoperative dysphagia with the use of a bougie. There is however a real possibility of dilator perforation during insertion, which is estimated at 1% [10, 11]. In addition, standardization of crural closure has been elusive, and an overly tight cruroplasty may lead to postoperative dysphagia and need for dilation or revision, whereas overly loose closure can be a factor in recurrent herniation.

16.2.3 Patient Factors

There are several factors relating to the patients that can affect the rate of recurrence. Paraesophageal hernias occur mainly in the aging population, which is likely related to attenuation of the phrenoesophageal membrane (and perhaps other connective tissue involving the repair) and subsequent recurrence [9]. Factors that put patients at a higher risk of failure are pre-operative (body mass index) BMI >35, unresponsiveness to acid-reducing medications, atypical symptoms, and psychiatric illness [12]. While there is no absolute BMI cutoff beyond which a repair should not be performed, dietary counseling and referral to a bariatric surgeon should be considered for any patients with BMI >35. Post-operatively, tight nausea control should be implemented in order to avoid retching, which can increase intra-abdominal pressure and is a primary factor associated with recurrence. In addition, patients should be counseled to avoid any inordinate heavy lifting, straining or strenuous exercise which could lead to increased intra-abdominal pressure and resultant recurrence.

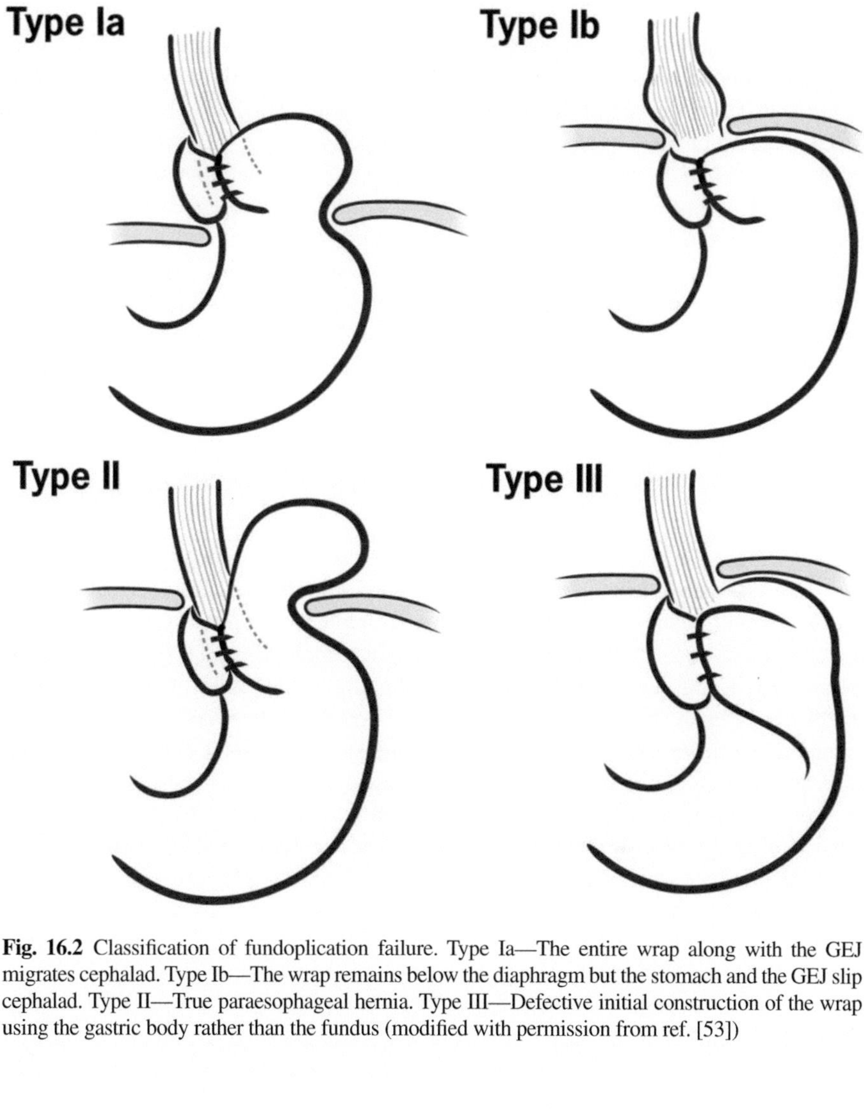

Fig. 16.2 Classification of fundoplication failure. Type Ia—The entire wrap along with the GEJ migrates cephalad. Type Ib—The wrap remains below the diaphragm but the stomach and the GEJ slip cephalad. Type II—True paraesophageal hernia. Type III—Defective initial construction of the wrap using the gastric body rather than the fundus (modified with permission from ref. [53])

16.2.4 Classification of Failures

Anatomic failure can be classified based on the type of failure and it is helpful to identify the type of failure as an indicator of the underlying cause (Fig. 16.2). Increased radial and axial tension can lead to a Type IA failure and is seen when the entire wrap along with the gastroesophageal junction migrates cephalad resulting in an intra-thoracic fundoplication. This is the most common type of failure. A variation on this problem is the so-called slipped Nissen, or Type IB failure in which the wrap remains below the diaphragm but the stomach and the gastroesophageal junction slip upward through the wrap resulting in the GEJ residing within the mediastinum. This failure may occur due to misjudging the location of the true GEJ with the wrap placed low around the cardia instead of the fundus, from increased axial tension due to unrecognized short esophagus, or as a result of chronic stress on the GEJ from intra-gastric pressure. When in doubt, poor placement can be avoided by intraoperative endoscopy and identification of the true junction. Type II failure is analogous to the true paraesophageal hernia. Breakdown of the crural repair sutures with an intact wrap and normally located GEJ can result in intra-thoracic stomach with dysphagia, pain, or potential gastric volvulus despite an appropriately placed wrap. Finally, a defective initial construction of the wrap results in a Type III failure as described above, caused by utilizing the mid-body of the stomach to fashion the wrap rather than the fundus.

16.3 Identifying Recurrence After Hiatal Hernia Repair

Identifying and defining symptoms is one of the most important steps in treating recurrent hernias. Many patients experience new symptoms after an otherwise satisfactory primary hernia repair, such as gas-bloat, hyper-flatulence, or mild dysphagia even in the absence of documented anatomical defects or technical errors. Without investigations it may be difficult to determine which symptoms are due to the physiologic effects of the wrap versus the effects of a recurrence. It is imperative then to obtain a good symptomatic history detailing exactly when the symptoms started, progression, and temporal relation to oral intake. Symptomatic management is the first step in the early postoperative period unless there is strong reason to suspect disorder of the repair. For persistent, progressive, or atypical symptoms, objective studies will be needed to determine the presence and correlation of anatomic defects with symptoms.

The most common post-operative symptoms related to recurrence are heartburn, regurgitation, dysphagia, and pain [13]. Any of these may be the result of the repair itself. For example, the sensation of heartburn may be caused by esophageal distension or spasm secondary to the effect of the wrap rather than failure of the repair. However, if any of these symptoms persist beyond the first 3 months, a focused workup should be implemented in order to identify any possible recurrence and assist therapeutic decision-making.

It is reasonable to start with two-phase esophagography. This test will help elucidate esophageal and gastric anatomy including an obstructing repair, anatomic recurrence and its classification, intra-thoracic wrap migration, and strictures or other anatomic abnormalities and is the most sensitive test for recurrent herniation (Fig. 16.3) [14]. It can also provide useful information on the basic function of the gastroesophageal junction and valve, visualizing both transit and reflux, though it is less reliable with regard to recurrent reflux. The pylorus can be examined as well in order better identify vagal injury and resultant hypertonicity of the sphincter mechanism. Anatomic recurrence is commonly defined as 2 or more cm of stomach and/or GEJ above the diaphragmatic crura although several variations of the diagnostic criteria exist [15].

Endoscopy is important in the workup in order to visualize any intra-luminal abnormalities. Erosions, esophagitis, or gastritis can be identified and help reinforce the diagnoses of reflux and recurrence. A recurrent hiatal hernia can be seen and the configuration of the gastroesophageal flap valve based on the Hill system can be graded (Fig. 16.4). The presence of a stricture or narrowing may prompt additional manometric evaluation. Rarely, erosion of suture or mesh into the lumen will be detected.

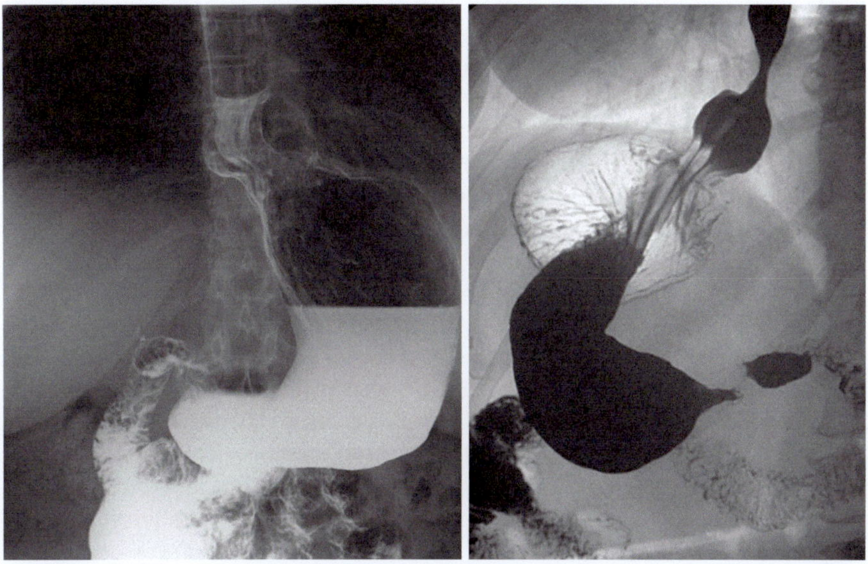

Fig. 16.3 Images from video contrast esophagograms demonstrating fundoplication failure. Type Ia failure is shown on the *left*, with both the intact wrap and GEJ herniated above the level of the diaphragm. A type Ib failure is seen in the *right image* with only the GEJ herniating above the level of the diaphragm while the majority of the fundus remains intra-abdominal

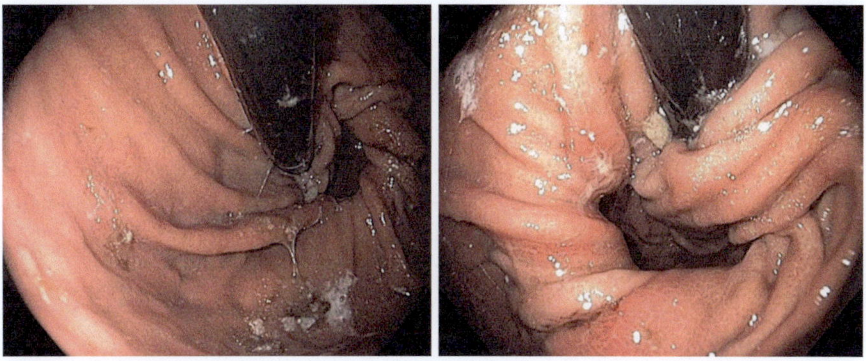

Fig. 16.4 Endoscopic view of Type II or true paraesophageal hernia failure. Note the GEJ is below the diaphragm but the fundus has herniated cephalad creating a characteristic endoscopic view

Manometry is not an essential part of the evaluation of recurrent PEH, but may prove useful in certain circumstances. If pre-operative manometry is available and the patient denies any new dysphagia, then repeat manometric evaluation is unlikely to add any additional usefulness. However, if the patient has new-onset dysphagia or there is uncertainty surrounding the patient's esophageal motility, then manometry should be performed to rule out any esophageal motility disorders of the esophageal body or the reconstructed GEJ, to help determine optimal reconstruction.

Objective evaluation of reflux in the form of 24-h pH monitoring is vital to identify the presence of acid reflux, especially if anatomic recurrence is subtle or absent and the etiology of symptoms is unclear. In the case of large recurrent anatomic defects clearly attributable to the patient's symptoms, pH monitoring is less helpful as re-operation is likely regardless of the pH study outcome. Any patients with symptoms of reflux and a positive DeMeester score in the setting of anatomic recurrence should be considered for revisional surgery.

If there is concern for vagus nerve injury or impaired gastric motility, a gastric emptying study is helpful in determining gastric function. The incidence of gastroparesis requiring a gastric emptying procedure can be as high as 12% after re-operation and increases with each subsequent recurrence [16]. A patient who gives a history of nausea or extended bloating after meals should make the surgeon suspicious for gastric emptying issues. If a gastric emptying test shows delayed gastric emptying, careful consideration must be given to the management of abnormal gastric emptying in the setting of previous hernia repair. If on endoscopy the pylorus is dysfunctional, a trial of endoscopic botulinum toxin may improve emptying and signal a good chance of success for pylorplasty or pyloromyotomy at the time of reoperation [17]. If the sphincter mechanism is functional without increased tone or obstruction, however, then pro-motility agents may be attempted.

16.3.1 When to Operate

The indications for re-operation are similar to those for primary operation: symptoms from herniation such as obstruction/risk of incarceration, dysphagia, anemia, and dyspnea; or symptoms of inadequately controlled reflux. The operative risks and the predictability of success are a bit more problematic and there should be a higher threshold for recommending re-operation, particularly in the elderly. As with primary surgery, it is vital to determine the goals of the operation relative to the patient's symptoms and objective findings and to weigh the risks against the realistic expectation of benefit. In some cases continued medical management may be the better alternative until the situation progresses.

16.4 Surgical Strategies

Although once the mainstay of re-operative hiatal hernia repair, the open approach has been largely supplanted by laparoscopic paraesophageal hernia repair over the last 20 years. Compared to the open trans-abdominal and trans-thoracic approaches,

Table 16.2 Key operative steps in the management of recurrent paraesophageal hernia repair

Step	Details
1. Anesthesia/preparation	Pre-operative antibiotics, VTE prophylaxis, placement of urinary catheter
2. Entry/insufflation	Veress, direct optical, or open entry per surgeon preference. Preliminary placement of liver retractor with re-adjustment after adhesiolysis
3. Adhesiolysis	Establish plane between caudate lobe and pre-aortic fascia continuing on to right crus
4. Hiatal dissection	Proceed from anterior rim freeing up left and right rim of hiatus and stomach from retroperitoneum
5. Identification/preservation of vagus nerves	Nerves are at risk due to displacement at hiatus, must take care dissecting the 12 and 6–7 o'clock positions. Identify nerves on proximal esophagus more easily and follow distally
6. Takedown of previous fundoplication	Divide previous fundus, take down both anterior and posterior wings of fundus and remaining attachments must be divided. Restore normal anatomy and investigate for injury
7. Crural closure	Determine amount of tension on crus and close primarily with mesh overlay. May choose to perform diaphragmatic relaxing incision with PTFE bridge
8. Intraoperative endoscopy	Identify true GEJ by applying pressure with blunt grasper and correlating with intra-luminal findings. Check for injury using insufflation and leak test
9. Evaluation of esophageal length	Complete hiatal mobilization and retract GEJ anterior towards hiatus and measure intra-abdominal length. Utilize lengthening procedure or Hill fixation sutures if less than 2.5 cm
10. Fundoplication	Perform full or partial fundoplication depending on surgeon preference with or without gastropexy

laparoscopy has been shown to decrease hospital length of stay, postoperative pain, and respiratory complications while offering similar outcomes [18, 19]. In experienced hands, the laparoscopic approach is safe even in the setting of previous laparoscopy or even laparotomy with low conversion rates of around 7% [20, 21]. It has been shown that results with reoperation are superior in experienced centers, however, and typically these operations should be performed only by surgeons experienced in re-operative repair [22]. If there is concern for ischemia, perforation or gross spillage, however, an open approach may be warranted [23]. Important key steps relating to re-operative paraesophageal hernia repair will be discussed in this section (Table 16.2).

16.4.1 Preparation

It is important to communicate with anesthesia regarding the preparation of the patient for the operating room, including the expected duration of the case and the potential for higher than usual blood loss or the need to convert to open surgery. Pre-operative antibiotics are given, particularly given the higher risk of enterotomy, along with subcutaneous heparin for venous thromboembolus prophylaxis [24]. A urinary catheter is used routinely for urine output monitoring given the unknown expected length of re-operations. If the patient has any other concerning comorbidities or invasive hemodynamic monitoring is desired, a radial arterial line may be placed.

16.4.2 Exposure/Dissect3ion

Once the patient is positioned, the abdomen is entered and insufflated. If there are concerns about extensive adhesions, an open entry approach can be performed. There is little difference, however, between the safety of entry method even in the setting of a re-operation. A veress needle or direct optical entry can be used for insufflation without any difference in rate of complications [25]. We have found left subcostal veress needle insertion followed by optical entry to be highly reliable and safe even following prior upper laparotomy for peritonitis. In the presence of extensive adhesions, a second port is placed wherever access can be obtained following initial entry and adhesions are progressively divided until further ports can be placed.

Once the abdomen is insufflated, a liver retractor is preliminarily put into place. It will likely need to be adjusted once typical adhesions between stomach and liver are divided. General adhesiolysis is performed to free the working space in the upper abdomen, making sure to avoid any bowel or other intra-abdominal viscera. If bowel is injured during the taking down of adhesions, a repair with interrupted 3-0 silk suture or a two-layer closure with inner absorbable suture is appropriate. Once all gross adhesions are divided, the dissection of the hiatus is started inferiorly between the stomach and the left lobe of the liver. Care must be taken to avoid starting or extending so inferiorly that the hepatic artery or bile duct structures are at risk. The initial goal should be establishing a plane between the caudate lobe and the left aspect of the pre-aortic fascia/left crus, as this plane will take one safely upward to the right aspect of the hiatus and right lateral crus (Fig. 16.5). There are usually adhesions from the previous surgery around this area and it is important to free up the plane from medial to the caudate lobe to the point that the inferior vena cava can be visualized and pro-

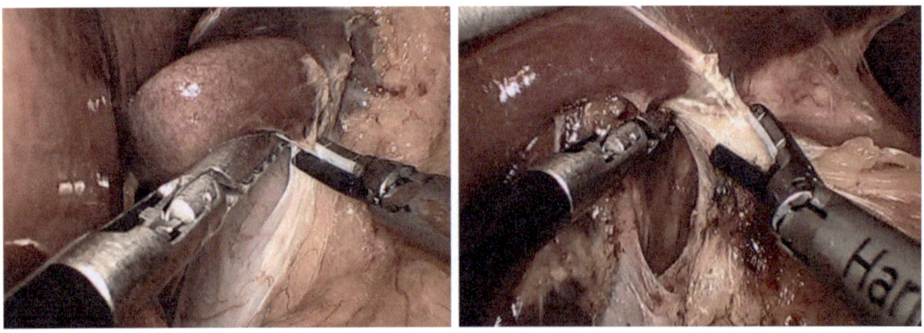

Fig. 16.5 Establishing the plane between the caudate lobe and the stomach and pre-aortic fascia. The inferior vena cava must be visualized and protected, being careful not to injure the vessel. Once this plane is freed, the right crus is identified and the hiatal dissection begun

tected, being careful not to injure the vessel. Once this plane is freed, the right crus can be identified and the hiatal dissection begun.

From this point the dissection is performed from the aspect which is most clear and expedient, and this will continue to change throughout the dissection. Typically we begin along the anterior rim of the hiatus defining the plane between the crus and the edge of the stomach. The left anterior aspect of this dissection can be difficult and it is often helpful at this point to move to the left posterior aspect of the dissection, freeing the stomach from the retroperitoneum and working posteriorly and medially as far as possible. This will gain access to the posterior-left aspect of the hiatus which can then be followed anteriorly. The right posterior dissection can be particularly challenging if the stomach is densely adherent to the pre-aortic fascia and the plane of dissection is not clear. This may require bold dissection with the risk of enterotomy.

One of the most important points in redo hiatal hernia surgery is identification and preservation of the vagus nerves. Because of adhesions, the location of the nerves often deviates from normal anatomy. Particular care must be taken when dissecting at the 12 o'clock and the 6–7 o'clock positions around the hiatus. The anterior vagus nerve may be adhered anteriorly to the pericardium and can be inadvertently damaged while taking down the hernia sac. It is also at risk in the region of the GEJ. The posterior vagus nerve can be adhered posteriorly along the aorta to the decussation of the left and right crura and can be easily injured while dissecting the esophagus posteriorly. During re-do operations, scar tissue and adhesions around the hiatus and prior fundoplication make vagal identification difficult, and the nerves are best identified proximally along the esophagus in the mediastinum and followed distally towards the fundoplication.

Once the hiatus has been freed and vagus nerves are identified and preserved, the previous fundoplication can be taken down. It is important to restore the stomach and especially the fundus to its normal anatomic state in order to correctly identify landmarks and fashion a new fundoplication. Failure to completely un-do the prior fundoplication will likely result in another incorrectly performed fundoplication and high likelihood of failure. Once the hernia is reduced and the fundoplication can be visualized, it is helpful to slide a grasper into the inferior portion

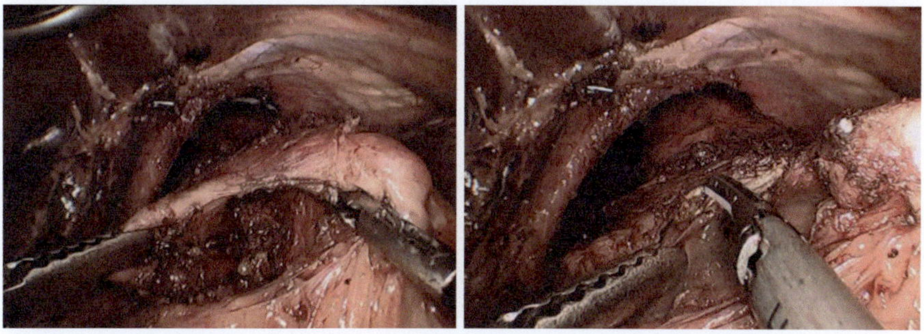

Fig. 16.6 A previous fundoplication is identified anteriorly (*left*) where the anterior and posterior portion of the fundus were previously sutured together. This is dissected and divided using an energy device (*right*)

of the fundoplication opening to develop a plane (Fig. 16.6). After this plane is developed and enlarged, the fundus to fundus connection can be divided. If there is a clear demarcation, an energy device can be used for the division. If there is difficulty identifying the fundo-fundal plane with high risk of a gastric injury, a linear cutting stapler may be used. After division, the remaining fundal attachments are taken down carefully to avoid the vagus nerves which will run deep to the fundal wings anteriorly and posteriorly. The most difficult dissection is often in taking down the attachments between posterior fundus and lesser curvature. There are often additional subtle adhesions in the region of the angle of His which must be divided.

Once all adhesions and bands have been divided, the greater curvature is stretched outward to the left to assure restoration of normal anatomy and the stomach is investigated for any injury or remaining adhesions. If there is a remaining hernia sac, it should be truncated and removed from the abdomen [26]. It may be advisable to perform intraoperative endoscopy at this time to check for injury and to precisely locate the GEJ, which can be quite difficult with these complex cases.

16.4.3 Crural Closure

Now the hiatus is ready for closure. There are several types of hiatal opening configurations, including the slit, the oval, the teardrop and the "D". The shape of the configuration is a predictor of the degree of tension being applied to crural closure and may hint at the necessity of further intervention. Although there are devices to successfully assess crural tension intra-operatively, they are not yet commercially available and the surgeon must rely on feel, as well as the predictability of greater or lesser tension based on the configuration [27]. The tension on the crural pillars can be tested by grasping each side and pulling towards each other (Fig. 16.7). If they come together easily, then further intervention is unlikely to be needed. If there is scar tissue, fibrosis, attenuated muscle or undue tension, then further maneuvers must be used to decrease tension. Insufflation can be lowered from 15 mmHg to 10 or 12, and the liver retractor can be loosened. Meticulous adhesiolysis must be performed around the hiatus, especially on the right side near the liver. Oftentimes releasing these adhesions will free up the right crus enough to successfully complete the closure. Left pleurotomy lowers the pressure gradient between the left hemi-diaphragm and the abdomen and can also reduce tension during closure [28].

A relaxing incision may be employed if primary closure appears to be under too much tension by making a full thickness incision in the right crus 3 cm parallel to the vena cava. While the right side is preferable, if there is not enough space between the inferior vena cava and the right crus or if there are too many adhesions, a left-sided curvilinear incision may be made. In this case the incision starts to the left of the hiatus and continues laterally following the course of the 7th rib in order to avoid the phrenic nerve [28]. These full-thickness incisions must be

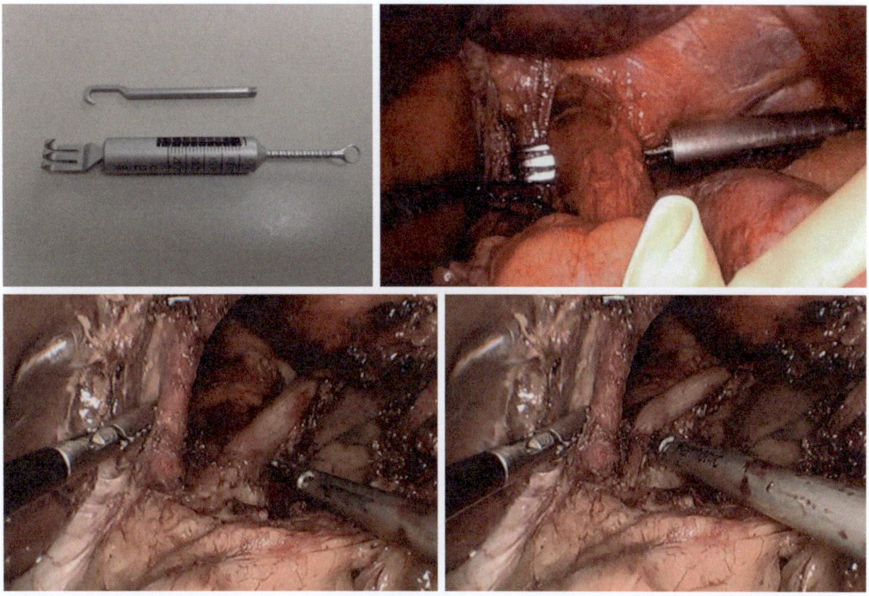

Fig. 16.7 Different methods of assessing diaphragmatic tension. A tensiometer (*top*) objectively measures the force required to bring the crus together. A subjective method of measuring tension is shown (*bottom*) by using graspers to feel the amount of tension on the crus after approximating the two pillars

bridged with permanent mesh, usually with a 1 mm polytetrafluoroethylene (PTFE) mesh sutured in place. Using absorbable mesh will result in difficult paraesophageal herniation. The primary cruroplasty can then be achieved using interrupted permanent braided suture.

For additional strength we typically utilize at least 1 or 2 pledgeted horizontal mattress sutures for closure of the large or recurrent hernia in addition to simple interrupted suture closure. The opening should be tight enough to not allow herniation to occur but not too tight so as to impinge on the esophagus. A grasper may be placed in the hiatal opening and a "twang" can be felt upon opening and removing the grasper against the rim of the anterior diaphragm.

The question of whether or not to use mesh to reinforce the crural closure remains unanswered. There is even less data regarding its use in re-operative hernia repair than for primary repair [29]. Short term results seem favorable towards mesh but long-term results remain inconclusive, and there is a real risk of erosion of permanent mesh into esophagus or stomach [4, 30]. In addition, there are many options when using mesh for crural enhancement including the type of mesh (biologic or permanent), the configuration of mesh (posterior U-shaped, circular, keyhole) and the attachment method (suture or tacking). Given the paucity of data, no definitive recommendations can be made. It is our practice to reinforce the hiatal closure with biologic mesh and avoid permanent mesh in contact with the esophagus.

16.4.4 Intra-operative Endoscopy

Intra-operative endoscopy is a valuable tool employed by the foregut surgeon during re-operative hiatal hernia repair. The true GEJ is often difficult to assess laparoscopically during re-operative repairs because of widening of the distal esophagus, poor tissue planes, and a tendency for the slipped Nissen to result in a tubular configuration of the cardia. If the GEJ is misidentified, the fundoplication will be made either too high or too low, resulting in a poorly constructed wrap, poor clinical outcomes and the need for additional interventions. Intra-operative endoscopy can help identify the true squamocolumnar junction and help guide creation of an appropriately placed fundoplication. The endoscopist identifies the squamocolumnar junction just proximal to the rugal folds while the surgeon uses a bunt grasper to intermittently apply pressure to the anterior stomach while moving upward from stomach onto presumed esophagus. In this manner, the endoscopist can correlate external laparoscopic landmarks with intra-luminal findings. When the true GEJ is identified, a clip or other mark can be placed to aid in later identification.

Endoscopy can also be helpful to identify gastric or esophageal injuries. A leak test can be performed to rule out any suspicious injuries. The stomach and esophagus are insufflated and the surgeon irrigates the GEJ and stomach to look for any bubbles. Leaks can be repaired via a sutured or stapled technique and are rarely a source of morbidity. After the fundoplication is completed, endoscopic evaluation of the valve is helpful to ensure a proper configuration of the wrap. Findings such as asymmetry, poor Hill grade, spiraling or a wrap placed too inferiorly should prompt a re-inspection of the fundoplication and consideration of revision.

16.4.5 Short Esophagus

Short esophagus can be caused by any number of conditions including congenital or acquired short esophagus. It is most commonly caused by long-term reflux disease resulting in constant inflammation and fibrosis leading to contraction of the esophageal smooth muscle and resultant shortening [31]. Other factors contributing to short esophagus include the presence of Barrett's esophagus, large type III paraesophageal hernias and esophageal strictures. Its frequency and the need for a lengthening procedure are hotly debated among surgeons but it is commonly defined as less than 2.5–3 cm of intra-abdominal esophagus between the anterior rim of the hiatus and the GE junction following high mediastinal dissection and its presence leads to failure from axial tension [32]. The length of intra-abdominal esophagus is best measured by retracting the GEJ anterior towards the anterior diaphragmatic hiatus and using a grasper or other measuring device to measure the distance between the anterior diaphragm and the previously identified GEJ. If this distance is less than 2.5 cm, then the surgeon must consider employing techniques to mitigate axial tension.

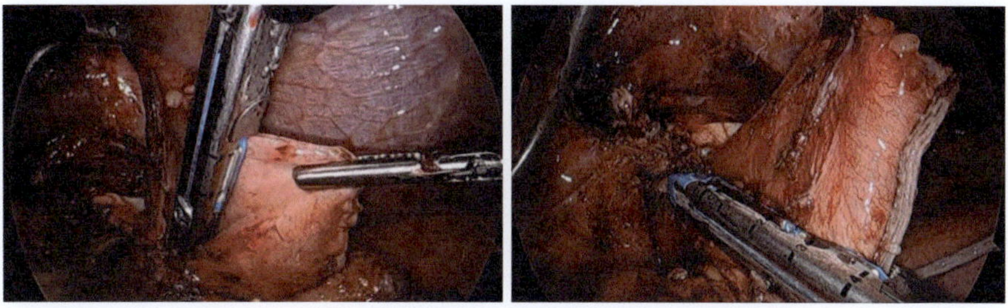

Fig. 16.8 Laparoscopic Collis-Nissen gastroplasty being performed for short esophagus. A wedge fundectomy is performed using a linear stapler over a 46 Fr bougie creating a segment of neo-esophagus. A Nissen fundoplication is then constructed using the remaining fundus

The first maneuver is to complete the hiatal dissection. An extensive mediastinal dissection to at least the inferior pulmonary vein must be undertaken to obtain the maximal amount of esophageal length, and in our experience this will usually suffice. Dividing the anterior vagus nerve in order to gain more esophageal length has been reported and is an option if no further length can be obtained otherwise [33]. Another approach to short esophagus is intra-thoracic mobilization utilizing either a thoracoscopic or open approach [34]. The esophagus can be mobilized upward above the azygous vein in order to gain intra-abdominal length. If these maneuvers are inadequate then a lengthening procedure should be considered.

The standard lengthening procedure for short esophagus is the Collis-Nissen gastroplasty. The procedure involves fashioning a short length of neo-esophagus from the proximal stomach and performing the fundoplication around the neo-esophagus [35]. There are several different approaches including the right or left chest, intra-abdominal circular stapler and the wedge fundectomy using a linear cutting stapler (Fig. 16.8). A 46–48 Fr bougie is inserted into the esophagus before creating the Collis, and the fundoplication is performed over a 56–58 Fr dilator. Care must be taken before performing this procedure in patients with esophageal stricture, the elderly, or patients with poor tissue quality as these conditions can lead to increased trauma and increased rate of post-operative leaks. Long-terms results of the Collis-Nissen are satisfactory with no difference in recurrence rate from that of the Nissen alone but there is an increased leak rate and risk of post-operative dysphagia [36, 37]. In addition the mucosa of the neo-esophagus is acid-secreting and may result in the need for chronic PPI's [31].

Another option involves a recently described technique called the Nissen-Hill Hybrid. Using the principles of the Hill repair, the GEJ is anchored to the pre-aortic fascia and combined with a Nissen fundoplication (Fig. 16.9). This is not the same as simply fixing the fundoplication to the diaphragm as it is the GEJ itself which is anchored. In the setting of short esophagus, it has been shown to be at least equivalent in recurrence to the Collis-Nissen gastroplasty without the need to create a neo-esophagus [38].

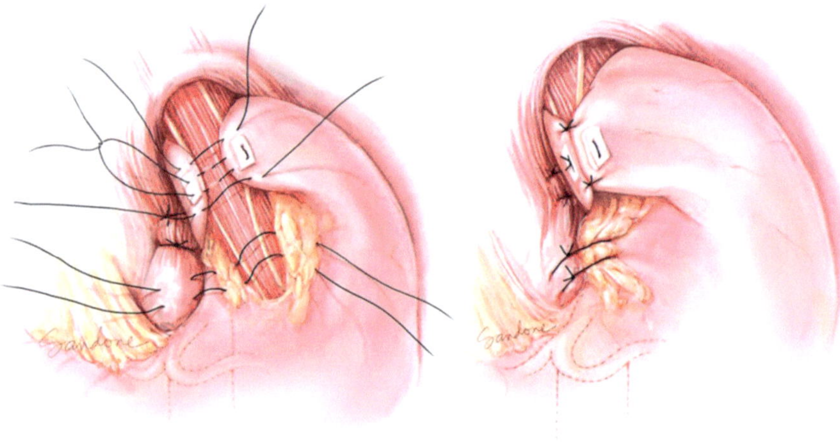

Fig. 16.9 The Nissen-Hill hybrid repair. The Hill sutures are placed through the anterior and posterior collar sling musculature at the GEJ then through the pre-aortic fascia. These sutures keep the GEJ anchored in place below the diaphragm and has shown long-term durability. A short floppy anterior-posterior Nissen fundoplication is then constructed in the standard fashion

16.4.6 Fundoplication

Once proper anatomy has been restored and adequate intra-abdominal esophageal length has been obtained, a fundoplication should be performed in order to reduce reflux [39]. During the pre-operative workup, either before the index operation or after recurrence, a manometric evaluation should be obtained. There are no clear contra-indications guiding complete versus partial fundoplication and the decision is best left to the surgeon's experience and comfort with a particular repair [40]. If a Nissen fundoplication is to be used, the short floppy variant measuring approximately 3 cm in length is appropriate [41]. The use of a bougie to create the fundoplication has been shown to reduce the rate of post-operative dysphagia [10, 42].

16.4.7 Gastropexy/Gastrostomy Tube

While it is not our common practice, the addition of an anterior gastropexy either in the form of a gastrostomy tube or an anterior gastropexy suture has been advocated to help reduce recurrence after large paraesophageal hernia repair. Some studies have shown a benefit, while others have found no significant difference [43, 44]. In high-risk patients undergoing urgent repair for incarceration, an anterior gastropexy without fundoplication can be performed but carries with it an increased rate of radiographic recurrence up to 22% at 3 months [45].

16.4.8 Conversion to Roux-en-Y Bypass

The above approaches are generally successful for a first time re-operation and even for most second time re-operations [46]. For second or third-time re-operations and in several additional situations, however, conversion to Roux-en-Y gastric bypass should be considered as the final and definitive operation for a failed GEJ. Though seemingly drastic, repeated failure of paraesophageal hernia repair is discouraging both for patient and physician and leaves few options. The decision to convert to gastric bypass can be made pre-operatively or intra-operatively. There are several different described variations of bypass to consider, including gastrojejunostomy with or without concomitant gastrectomy, gastrojejunostomy with the fundoplication in place, or esophagojejunostomy [47]. If the patient has experienced multiple operative failures, they are at high risk for subsequent failure and pre-operative planning should favor a bypass operation [48]. If the patient has a BMI of over 35 and has recurrence of a hernia, a consultation with the bariatric surgeons should be made, especially in the setting of comorbidities [49]. A two-stage procedure may even be considered where the hernia is repaired first, then a weight loss procedure is performed second in order to reduce the likelihood of intra-operative injury [50]. Another indication for bypass is very poor or absent esophageal motility in the setting of recurrence. In addition, if there are extensive or multiple intraoperative injuries with poor tissue quality and concern for the adequacy of repair, thought should be given to a bypass procedure.

16.4.9 Conversion to Open

Though uncommon, open conversion is a safe option if the laparoscopic approach proves too difficult [21]. Dense adhesions, bleeding, esophageal or bowel injury, or failure to progress should prompt the surgeon to consider continuing the case via open laparotomy. It is important for surgeons taking on a re-operative laparoscopic repair to be comfortable with the open approach should the need arise.

16.4.10 Post-operative Considerations

It is important to optimize the patient in the early post-operative period as this is the most critical time for early recurrence. Care must be taken to avoid any increase in intra-abdominal pressure such as emesis, retching or straining with defecation. This pressure puts undue tension on both the crural closure and the fundoplication and can lead to early wrap migration. To this end, aggressive anti-nausea treatment strategies are undertaken beginning with pre-operative anxiolytics, steroids and pre-hydration [51]. Post-operatively, scheduled anti-emetics are given and multimodal pain control such as acetaminophen, non-steroidal anti-inflammatory drugs and gabapentin are administered to limit the usage of nausea-inducing opioids. In addition, stool softeners and laxatives are given in order to avoid constipation and resultant straining. Activity limitations during the first 6 weeks including the proscription of heavy lifting and strenuous exercise are implemented in order to avoid recurrence and port-site hernia.

The routine use of nasogastric tube placement is unproven, but in the presence of injury, staple line or other concerns it can be useful for gastric drainage. It is our practice to perform postoperative video esophagogram on the first or second postop day for all re-operative repairs and Collis-Nissen gastroplasties. A clear liquid diet is then started and advanced to a full-liquid diet as tolerated for a 2-week period. Patients are instructed to avoid drinking liquids through a straw and to avoid carbonated beverages or cold liquids as these can increase gastric distension and contribute to recurrence [52]. In the early post-operative period, the patient should always take liquids by mouth while sitting upright in a chair and remain upright for at least 30 min afterward to assist esophageal emptying and decrease the likelihood of aspiration.

16.4.11 Long-Term Post-operative Care

As revisional GEJ surgery is complex and performed on patients who have already experienced an undesirable outcome, we believe it is the surgeon's responsibility to assume primary care for all issues related to the operation for at least the first 6 months. As symptoms correlate very imperfectly with objective findings, we also routinely recommend postoperative testing at 6–12 months to include video esophagogram and endoscopy with pH testing. This provides a postoperative baseline which can be quite helpful in the future care of the patient should new or recurrent symptoms develop.

16.5 Summary

Failure of laparoscopic paraesophageal hernia repair is a complex and often frustrating entity. With its increasing prevalence and the ever-growing need for re-operative intervention, it is important for the foregut surgeon to understand the guiding principles behind revisional hiatal hernia surgery. Because of the complex nature of re-operative paraesophageal hernia repair, it is advisable that these operations be performed in experienced specialty centers. The surgeon must be aware of mechanisms of recurrence and how to address these issues peri-operatively so as not to repeat the same mistakes that led to recurrence after the index operation. In addition, the pre-operative workup must be carefully prepared in order to identify recurrence and ensure the correct operative intervention is planned. Finally, correct surgical strategies must be employed in order to optimize clinical outcomes and avoid future recurrences.

What Is the Current Knowledge and What Future Direction Is Required

- Results of re-operative paraesophageal hernia repair are superior in experienced centers, and these operations should be performed by surgeons experienced in re-operative repair.
- Regardless of the technique used, over half of surgically repaired paraesophageal hiatal hernias will demonstrate long-term radiographic recurrence.
- Radial and axial tension are two major forces acting on the repair of the hiatal hernia that lead to disruption of the repair and ultimate failure.
- In cases of suspected recurrence, objective studies are needed to determine the presence and correlation of anatomic defects with symptoms.
- Further studies must be undertaken to determine the best way to mitigate factors leading to recurrence, including long-term effectiveness of mesh placement at the hiatus and usage of esophageal lengthening procedures.
- Long-term outcomes of re-operative paraesophageal hiatal hernia surgery must be more closely studied in order to better understand patient outcomes.

References

1. Stilson WL, Sanders I, Gardiner GA, Gorman HC, Lodge DF. Hiatal hernia and gastroesophageal reflux. Radiology. 1969;93(6):1323–7. doi:10.1148/93.6.1323.
2. Mittal RK. Hiatal hernia: myth or reality? Am J Med. 1997;103(5A):33S–9S.
3. Luketich JD, Raja S, Fernando HC, et al. Laparoscopic repair of giant paraesophageal hernia: 100 consecutive cases. Ann Surg. 2000;232(4):608–18. doi:10.1097/00000658-200010000-00016.
4. Oelschlager BK, Pellegrini CA, Hunter JG, et al. Biologic prosthesis to prevent recurrence after laparoscopic paraesophageal hernia repair: long-term follow-up from a multicenter, prospective, randomized trial. J Am Coll Surg. 2011;213(4):461–8. doi:10.1016/j.jamcollsurg.2011.05.017.
5. Furnée E, Hazebroek E. Mesh in laparoscopic large hiatal hernia repair: a systematic review of the literature. Surg Endosc. 2013;27(11):3998–4008. doi:10.1007/s00464-013-3036-y.
6. Anvari M, Allen C, Pellegrini C. Five-year comprehensive outcomes evaluation in 181 patients after laparoscopic Nissen fundoplication. J Am Coll Surg. 2003;196(1):51–9. doi:10.1016/S1072-7515(02)01604-6.
7. Byrne JP, Smithers BM, Nathanson LK, Martin I, Ong HS, Gotley DC. Symptomatic and functional outcome after laparoscopic reoperation for failed antireflux surgery. Br J Surg. 2005;92(8):996–1001. doi:10.1002/bjs.4914.
8. Kahrilas PJ, Kim HC, Pandolfino JE. Approaches to the diagnosis and grading of hiatal hernia. Best Pract Res Clin Gastroenterol. 2008;22(4):601–16. doi:10.1016/j.bpg.2007.12.007.

9. Kahrilas PJ, Wu S, Lin S, Pouderoux P. Attenuation of esophageal shortening during peristalsis with hiatus hernia. Gastroenterology. 1995;109(6):1818–25. doi:10.1016/0016-5085(95)90748-3.
10. Patterson EJ, Herron DM, Hansen PD, Ramzi N, Standage BA, Swanström LL. Effect of an esophageal bougie on the incidence of dysphagia following nissen fundoplication: a prospective, blinded, randomized clinical trial. Arch Surg. 2000;135(9):1055–61. discussion 1061–1062
11. Stefanidis D, Hope WW, Kohn GP, et al. Guidelines for surgical treatment of gastroesophageal reflux disease. Surg Endosc. 2010;24(11):2647–69. doi:10.1007/s00464-010-1267-8.
12. Morgenthal CB, Lin E, Shane MD, Hunter JG, Smith CD. Who will fail laparoscopic Nissen fundoplication? Preoperative prediction of long-term outcomes. Surg Endosc. 2007;21(11):1978–84. doi:10.1007/s00464-007-9490-7.
13. Lidor AO, Steele KE, Stem M, Fleming RM, Schweitzer MA, Marohn MR. Long-term quality of life and risk factors for recurrence after laparoscopic repair of paraesophageal hernia. JAMA Surg. 2015;150(5):424–31. doi:10.1001/jamasurg.2015.25.
14. Fornari F, Gurski RR, Navarini D, Thiesen V, Mestriner LHB, Madalosso CAS. Clinical utility of endoscopy and barium swallow X-ray in the diagnosis of sliding hiatal hernia in morbidly obese patients: a study before and after gastric bypass. Obes Surg. 2010;20(6):702–8. doi:10.1007/s11695-009-9971-y.
15. Lidor AO, Kawaji Q, Stem M, et al. Defining recurrence after paraesophageal hernia repair: correlating symptoms and radiographic findings. Surgery. 2013;154(2):171–8. doi:10.1016/j.surg.2013.03.015.
16. Hamrick MC, Davis SS, Chiruvella A, et al. Incidence of delayed gastric emptying associated with revisional laparoscopic paraesophageal hernia repair. J Gastrointest Surg. 2013;17(2):213–7. doi:10.1007/s11605-012-1989-0.
17. Clarke JO, Snape WJ. Pyloric sphincter therapy: botulinum toxin, stents, and pyloromyotomy. Gastroenterol Clin N Am. 2015;44(1):127–36. doi:10.1016/j.gtc.2014.11.010.
18. Schauer PR, Ikramuddin S, McLaughlin RH, et al. Comparison of laparoscopic versus open repair of paraesophageal hernia. Am J Surg. 1998;176(6):659–65. doi:10.1016/S0002-9610(98)00272-4.
19. Oelschlager BK, Pellegrini CA. Paraesophageal hernias: open, laparoscopic, or thoracic repair? Chest Surg Clin N Am. 2001;11(3):589–603.
20. Haider M, Iqbal A, Salinas V, Karu A, Mittal SK, Filipi CJ. Surgical repair of recurrent hiatal hernia. Hernia. 2006;10(1):13–9. doi:10.1007/s10029-005-0034-6.
21. Symons NRA, Purkayastha S, Dillemans B, et al. Laparoscopic revision of failed antireflux surgery: a systematic review. Am J Surg. 2011;202(3):336–43. doi:10.1016/j.amjsurg.2011.03.006.
22. Markar SR, Mackenzie H, Huddy JR, et al. Practice patterns and outcomes after hospital admission with acute para-esophageal hernia in England. Ann Surg. 2016;264(5):854–61. doi:10.1097/SLA.0000000000001877.
23. Bawahab M, Mitchell P, Church N, Debru E. Management of acute paraesophageal hernia. Surg Endosc. 2009;23(2):255–9. doi:10.1007/s00464-008-0190-8.
24. Muntz JE, Michota FA. Prevention and management of venous thromboembolism in the surgical patient: options by surgery type and individual patient risk factors. Am J Surg. 2010;199(1):S11–20. doi:10.1016/j.amjsurg.2009.10.007.
25. Ahmad G, O'Flynn H, Duffy JMN, Phillips K, Watson A. Laparoscopic entry techniques. Ahmad G, editor. Cochrane database Syst Rev. 2012;(2):CD006583. doi:10.1002/14651858.CD006583.pub3.
26. Edye M, Salky B. Posner a, Fierer a. Sac excision is essential to adequate laparoscopic repair of paraesophageal hernia. Surg Endosc. 1998;12(10):1259–63. doi:10.1007/s004649900832.
27. Bradley DD, Louie BE, Farivar AS, Wilshire CL, Baik PU, Aye RW. Assessment and reduction of diaphragmatic tension during hiatal hernia repair. Surg Endosc. 2015;29(4):796–804. doi:10.1007/s00464-014-3744-y.
28. Greene CL, DeMeester SR, Zehetner J, Worrell SG, Oh DS, Hagen JA. Diaphragmatic relaxing incisions during laparoscopic paraesophageal hernia repair. Surg Endosc. 2013;27(12):4532–8. doi:10.1007/s00464-013-3107-0.

29. Granderath FA, Granderath UM, Pointner R. Laparoscopic revisional fundoplication with circular hiatal mesh prosthesis: the long-term results. World J Surg. 2008;32(6):999–1007. doi:10.1007/s00268-008-9558-0.
30. Granderath FA, Schweiger UM, Kamolz T, Asche KU, Pointner R. Laparoscopic nissen fundoplication with prosthetic hiatal closure reduces postoperative intrathoracic wrap herniation. Arch Surg. 2005;140(1):40. doi:10.1001/archsurg.140.1.40.
31. Horvath KD, Swanstrom LL, Jobe BA. The short esophagus: pathophysiology, incidence, presentation, and treatment in the era of laparoscopic antireflux surgery. Ann Surg. 2000;232(5):630–40.
32. Low DE. The short esophagus—recognition and management. J Gastrointest Surg. 2001;5(5):458–61. doi:10.1016/S1091-255X(01)80082-2.
33. Oelschlager BK, Yamamoto K, Woltman T, Pellegrini C. Vagotomy during hiatal hernia repair: a benign esophageal lengthening procedure. J Gastrointest Surg. 2008;12(7):1155–62. doi:10.1007/s11605-008-0520-0.
34. DeMeester SR, Sillin LF, Lin HW, Gurski RR. Increasing esophageal length: a comparison of laparoscopic versus transthoracic esophageal mobilization with and without vagal trunk division in pigs. J Am Coll Surg. 2003;197(4):558–64. doi:10.1016/S1072-7515(03)00481-2.
35. Collis JL. An operation for hiatus hernia with short oesophagus. Thorax. 1957;12(3):181–8. doi:10.1136/thx.12.3.181.
36. Luketich JD, Nason KS, Christie NA, et al. Outcomes after a decade of laparoscopic giant paraesophageal hernia repair. J Thorac Cardiovasc Surg. 2010;139(2):395–404, 404.e1. doi:10.1016/j.jtcvs.2009.10.005.
37. Légner A, Tsuboi K, Bathla L, Lee T, Morrow LE, Mittal SK. Reoperative antireflux surgery for dysphagia. Surg Endosc. 2011;25(4):1160–7. doi:10.1007/s00464-010-1333-2.
38. Bellevue OC, Louie BE, Jutric Z, Farivar AS, Aye RW. Su1156 a hill gastropexy combined with nissen fundoplication appears to mitigate the shortcomings of collis-nissen in the management of short esophagus. Gastroenterology. 2016;150(4):S1206. doi:10.1016/S0016-5085(16)34079-3.
39. Swanstrom LL, Jobe BA, Kinzie LR, Horvath KD. Laparoscopic paraesophageal hernia repair and fundoplication. Surgery. 1999;9610(99):359–63.
40. Strate U, Emmermann A, Fibbe C, Layer P, Zornig C. Laparoscopic fundoplication: Nissen versus Toupet two-year outcome of a prospective randomized study of 200 patients regarding preoperative esophageal motility. Surg Endosc. 2008;22(1):21–30. doi:10.1007/s00464-007-9546-8.
41. DeMeester TR, Bonavina L, Albertucci M. Nissen fundoplication for gastroesophageal reflux disease. Evaluation of primary repair in 100 consecutive patients. Ann Surg. 1986;204(1):9–20.
42. Somasekar K, Morris-Stiff G, Al-Madfai H, Barton K, Hassn A. Is a bougie required for the performance of the fundal wrap during laparoscopic Nissen fundoplication? Surg Endosc. 2010;24(2):390–4. doi:10.1007/s00464-009-0592-2.
43. Poncet G, Robert M, Roman S, Boulez JC. Laparoscopic repair of large hiatal hernia without prosthetic reinforcement: late results and relevance of anterior gastropexy. J Gastrointest Surg. 2010;14(12):1910–6. doi:10.1007/s11605-010-1308-6.
44. Diaz S, Brunt LM, Klingensmith ME, Frisella PM, Soper NJ. Laparoscopic paraesophageal hernia repair, a challenging operation: medium-term outcome of 116 patients. J Gastrointest Surg. 2003;7(1):59–66. discussion 66-67
45. Rosenberg J, Jacobsen B, Fischer A. Fast-track giant paraoesophageal hernia repair using a simplified laparoscopic technique. Langenbecks Arch Surg. 2006;391(1):38–42. doi:10.1007/s00423-005-0008-2.
46. Wennergren J, Levy S, Bower C, et al. Revisional paraesophageal hernia repair outcomes compare favorably to initial operations. Surg Endosc. 2016;30(9):3854–60. doi:10.1007/s00464-015-4688-6.
47. Makris KI, Lee T, Mittal SK. Roux-en-Y reconstruction for failed fundoplication. J Gastrointest Surg. 2009;13(12):2226–32. doi:10.1007/s11605-009-0994-4.
48. Williams VA, Watson TJ, Gellersen O, et al. Gastrectomy as a remedial operation for failed fundoplication. J Gastrointest Surg. 2007;11(1):29–35. doi:10.1007/s11605-006-0048-0.

49. Chaudhry UI, Marr BM, Osayi SN, et al. Laparoscopic Roux-en-Y gastric bypass for treatment of symptomatic paraesophageal hernia in the morbidly obese: medium-term results. Surg Obes Relat Dis. 2014;10(6):1063–9. doi:10.1016/j.soard.2014.02.004.
50. Patel AD, Lin E. The intersection of foregut and bariatric surgeries: treating the whole, not the parts. Surg Obes Relat Dis. 2014;10(6):1067–9. doi:10.1016/j.soard.2014.02.016.
51. Chandrakantan A, Glass PSA. Multimodal therapies for postoperative nausea and vomiting, and pain. Br J Anaesth. 2011;107(SUPPL. 1):27–40. doi:10.1093/bja/aer358.
52. Hamoui N, Lord RV, Hagen JA, Theisen J, DeMeester TR, Crookes PF. Response of the lower esophageal sphincter to gastric distention by carbonated beverages. J Gastrointest Surg. 2006;10(6):870–7. doi:10.1016/j.gassur.2005.11.010.
53. Horgan S, Pohl D, Bogetti D, et al. Failed antireflux surgery: what have we learned from reoperations? Arch Surg. 1999;134(8):809–15. discussion 815–7.

Chapter 17
Long-Term Results After Laparoscopic Reoperation for Failed Antireflux Procedure

Giuspeppe Quero, Alfonso Lapergola, Ludovica Guerriero, and Bernard Dallemagne

17.1 Introduction

Laparoscopic antireflux surgery [1] was first introduced in 1991. Since then, it has rapidly shown significant benefits over the conventional approach, and it is now well accepted as the gold standard treatment for severe gastroesophageal reflux [2]. Most of the published clinical series show excellent outcomes in terms of symptoms in 85–90% of cases up to 10 years after surgery [3–6].

Both the number of procedures and the need for reinterventions due to failure have increased. The rate of fundoplication failure after laparoscopic treatment ranges from 3 to 30% [7]. This extensive range is mainly due to the lack of standardized definition for failure, to the lack of methods of evaluation and to differences in surgical techniques as well as patient selection [8]. Failures can be defined as GERD recurrence and/or the development of new symptoms, frequently associated with more or less substantial anatomical changes in the esophagogastric anatomy. Although many patients with mild clinical symptoms can be successfully managed nonoperatively, almost 3–6% of them require revisional surgery [9].

It is essential to consider that redo fundoplications are much more challenging than primary surgery, regardless of the surgical access, especially in the presence of adhesions, anatomical distortion and the frequent need to dismantle the previous fundoplication. The success rate for reoperations usually ranges from 50 to 89%, and has to be compared with the success rate after a primary surgery [10]. In addition, it has been shown that there is an approximate 20% decrease in the success rate after reoperations at each subsequent operation [11].

Original article: The authors have no financial disclosure to report.

G. Quero, M.D. • A. Lapergola, M.D. • L. Guerriero, M.D. • B. Dallemagne, M.D. (✉)
IRCAD and Institute of Image Guided Surgery (IHU Strasbourg),
1 Place de l'Hôpital, 67091 Strasbourg Cedex, France
e-mail: bernard.dallemagne@ircad.fr

M.A. Memon (ed.), *Hiatal Hernia Surgery*,
https://doi.org/10.1007/978-3-319-64003-7_17

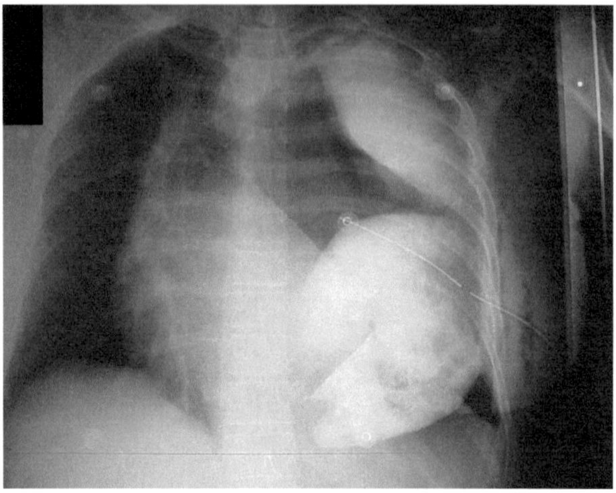

Fig. 17.1 Gastrographin swallow demonstrating an acute postoperative paraesophageal herniation

Today, there is no standardized algorithm for surgical reoperation, even if the laparoscopic approach has been shown to be safe and effective [12]. Good to excellent results were reported after short-term postoperative follow-up. However, the evaluation of long-term outcomes has shown that the selection and the quality of the redo procedure is fundamental to provide sustainable results.

17.2 Pattern of Failure and Surgical Procedures

Fundoplication failures include the recurrence of GERD symptoms or the development of new symptoms which did not exist preoperatively. Recurrent GERD (60%) and dysphagia (30%) are the most frequent symptoms of failure [7]. Chest pain, nausea, bloating, and shortness of breath can be associated with gross anatomical abnormalities such as hiatal hernia.

Failures can be observed in the early postoperative period, with the most frequent pattern being acute paraesophageal hernia or intrathoracic migration of the antireflux valve (Fig. 17.1) [13]. This type of failure is also the most frequently observed at later stages, and is accountable for 45 to 74% of reoperations [12, 14]. Disrupted (15%) and slipped/misplaced wraps (17%) come next regarding the frequency of anatomical failure patterns, which also include tight fundoplication/crural repair and loose wraps among the most common ones (Fig. 17.2). Additionally, it has been shown that esophageal motility disorders or erroneous diagnosis at primary surgery account for causes of failure in 1–2% of patients [12].

A correlation between the cause of recurrence and the interval between the primary procedure and the symptomatic failure has been reported. In the first three years, recurrence is generally due to wrap slippage while wrap breakdown is usually the most frequent cause beyond three years [15]. The probability of failure significantly increases over time. After 20 years, the probability of failure requiring remedial surgery is estimated at 30% [16].

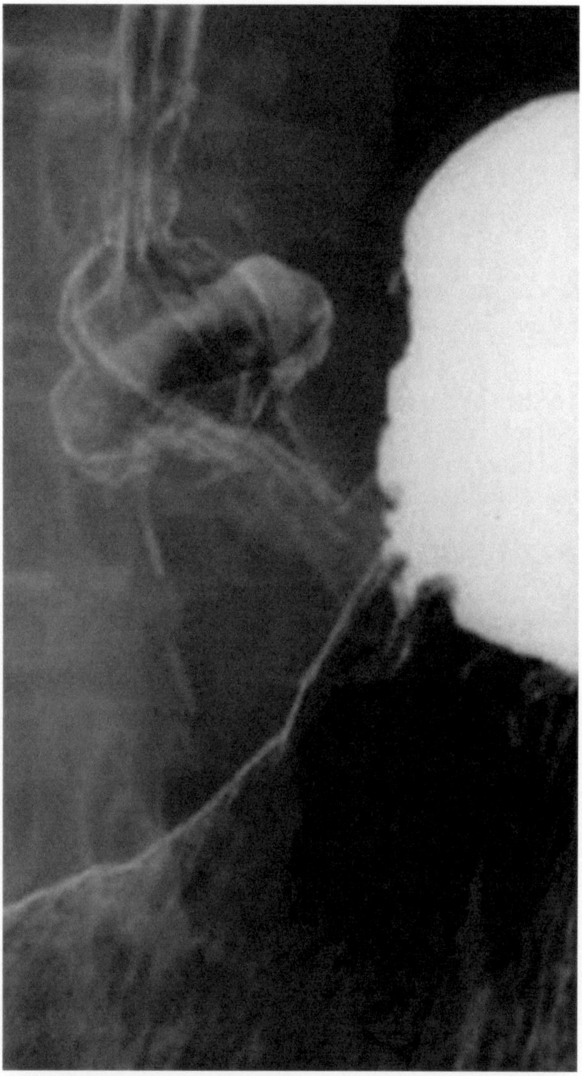

Fig. 17.2 Slipped fundoplication

Although the laparoscopic approach in revisional surgery for failed antireflux [16, 17] first met skepticism, results obtained after the initial learning curve have established minimally invasive surgery as the first management option. From a technical standpoint, the key points for an adequate surgical revision include the identification of complex anatomy, the evaluation of failure mechanisms, and the choice of the appropriate surgical procedure to correct the problems. Herniation and slippage are usually induced by an inadequate crural closure and/or excessive traction on the gastroesophageal junction and an unrecognized short esophagus. Repair under tension, which is axial on the esophagus and radial on the crura, is probably the main cause of failure. Regarding crural closure, some groups advocate the use of a mesh. However, mesh use is still a matter of debate, with heterogeneous results and complications rates [18–20]. The reality of shortened esophagus is still discussed [21].

In our series of laparoscopic reoperations, recurrent GERD (41.7%) and dysphagia (16.6%) were the most frequent indications for redo, followed by a combination of reflux and dysphagia (4%) and gas bloating. Most frequent anatomical patterns of failure were herniation and slippage, followed by a valve or cruroplasty, which was too tight, and a twisted or bilobed stomach [22].

17.3 Reoperation Techniques

The strategy in reoperations must be tailored to the patient's symptoms, patterns of failure, type and quality of the previous procedure, and number of previous operations. Recent reports on long-term outcomes provided additional information on the sustainability of different types of redo procedures.

One fundamental requirement in redo surgery is to dismantle the first fundoplication and restore the esophagogastric anatomy [22] (Fig. 17.3). The second step is to understand the mechanism of failure, which, besides surgical mistakes, is mostly related to some mechanical tension on the elements of the repair, fundoplication wrap, esophagus or crural muscles. The third and most important step is to select the appropriate redo procedure.

Recurrent GERD caused by a disruption of the wrap is probably the easiest symptom to treat. Indeed, it is usually associated with a poor surgical technique at the primary operation, in terms of suturing capabilities and/or of the suture material used. Tension on the fundoplication is usually associated with a wrap created without gastric fundus mobilization. The redo procedure has to take into account these elements and usually consists in a refundoplication using a Nissen or a partial wrap, which provides good long-term results [22]. A valve under tension is also frequently observed in the new onset of persisting dysphagia, and the treat-

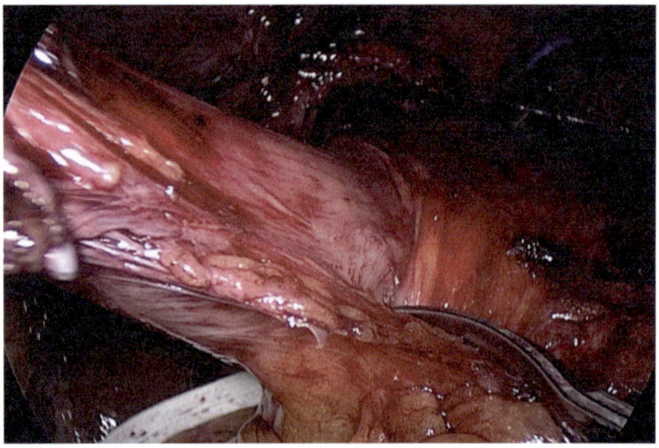

Fig. 17.3 Dismantling of fundoplication

ment is also focused on a tension-free fundoplication, with excellent results. A partial valve is usually recommended, as secondary esophageal motility disorders (pseudo-achalasia) can develop in long-standing esophageal obstruction (Fig. 17.4). Recurrent GERD, whether associated or not with dysphagia, due to wrap slippage can be more challenging. In its simplest form, it is caused by a wrong valve placement at the primary procedure and it requires a new, well-positioned fundoplication. In its more complex form, it can be related to a progressive cephalad slippage of the esophagogastric junction (EGJ) through the wrap. The main causing factor is most commonly the esophageal tension, which pulls the EGJ upwards, or more rarely the fixation of the wrap on the EGJ. In the first case,

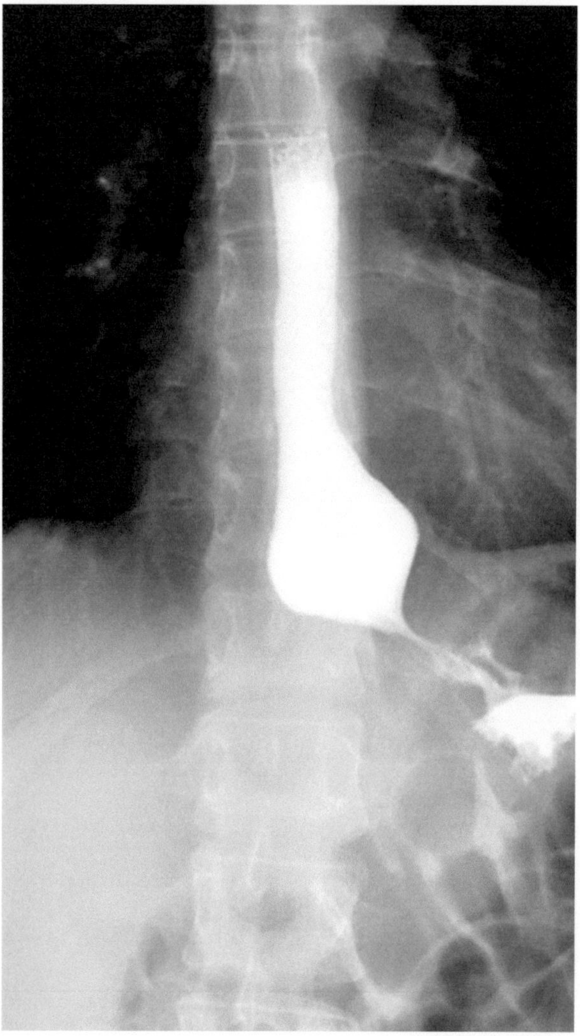

Fig. 17.4 Tight fundoplication with esophageal outlet obstruction

a high intramediastinal dissection or esophageal lengthening procedure may allow for a tension-free repositioning of the EGJ in an infra-diaphragmatic position and for the creation of a new fundoplication [22] (Fig. 17.5). A careful intraoperative assessment of the anatomical position of the endoscopic EGJ is mandatory (Fig. 17.6). Indeed, visual assessment is unreliable, due to tissue alterations. The third most common failure pattern is the intrathoracic migration of the fundoplication, or recurrent hiatal hernia, which can be associated with slippage (Fig. 17.7). Reoperation is complex as it has to take into account axial and radial tension on the antireflux repair. Axial tension can be managed similarly to slippage. Radial tension is challenging since crural repair addresses crural muscles which have been previously manipulated, sutured or reinforced with a mesh in the most difficult cases.

Dealing with more than one prior surgery is even more challenging, and the quality of the last repair is fundamental. If it was performed following the standard recommendations, one should consider alternative methods, such as Roux-en-Y bypass, fundoplication dismantling, esophageal myotomy or esophagectomy in the worst-case scenario [22].

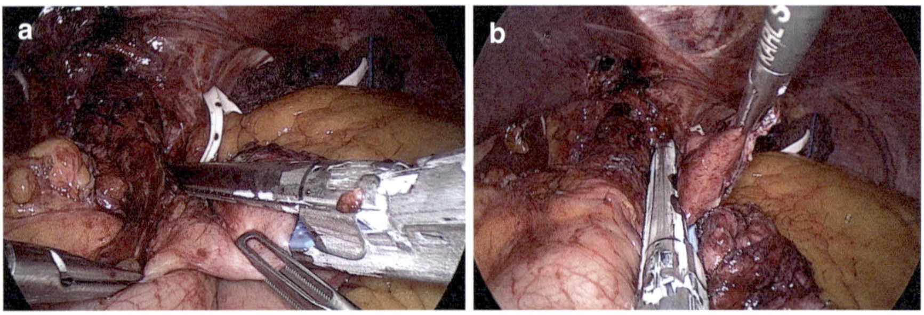

Fig. 17.5 Collis lengthening procedure. The first staple line defines the appropriate level of transection of the great curvature (**a**). The last staple line complete the partial fundectomy (**b**)

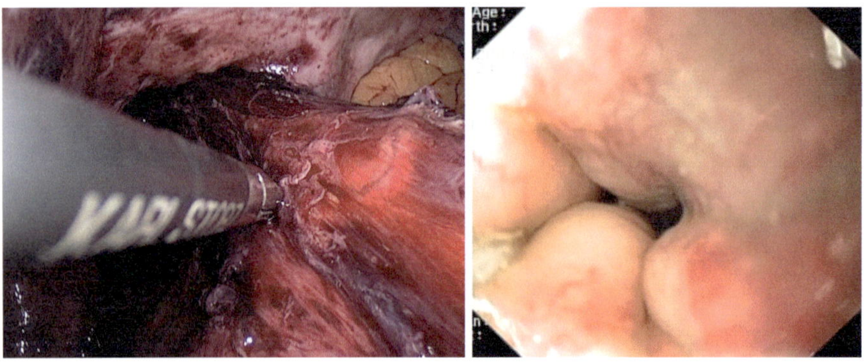

Fig. 17.6 Intraoperative control of the GEJ position

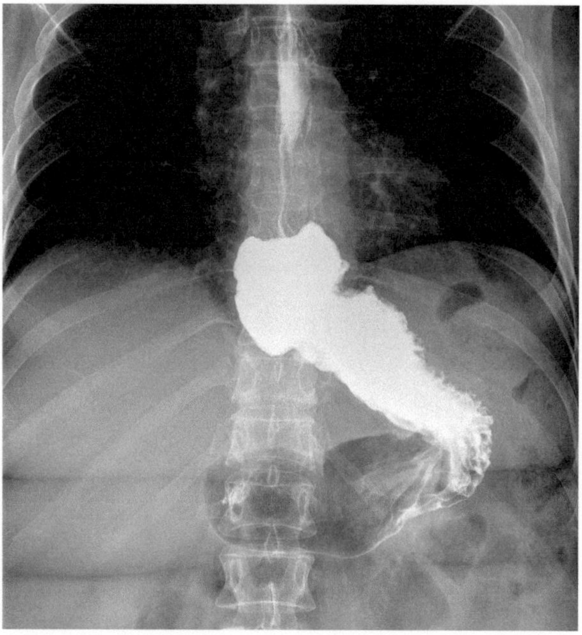

Fig. 17.7 Intrathoracic migration of the valve

In our experience [22], herniation was detected in 50 patients out of 129 laparoscopic redo surgeries. Early postoperative paraesophageal herniation required immediate laparoscopic redo, with hernia reduction and a new crural repair. In case of late presentation, one Collis-Nissen procedure was performed, while the remaining procedures varied from redo Nissen (39 patients) to partial wrap in four cases. Sutured crural repair was performed in 58% of patients, reinforced with pledgets or a mesh in other patients. In case of slipped wrap (n = 45), the previous fundoplication was taken down along with esophageal mobilization. Crural repair and a new fundoplication (32 Nissen, 8 Toupet, and 3 Collis-Nissen procedures) were performed. In the remaining two patients, the fundoplication was completely dismantled.

17.4 Intraoperative Complications and Postoperative Outcomes

In one of the most comprehensive summary of outcomes after reoperative antireflux surgery including more than 1500 patients, perioperative mortality was nil, a significant finding considering the complexity of these operations [7]. Intraoperative complications occurred in approximately 19% of cases, with perforation of either the esophagus or the stomach (14%) and accounting for 76% of total intraoperative morbidity. Conversion was required in 1–20% of patients, and was mainly caused by a loss of anatomical landmarks, adhesions, and intraoperative complications [7, 23–25]. In our series of 129 patients undergoing laparoscopic reoperations, the conversion rate due to excessive adhesions was 1.5%, the postoperative complication rate was 7%, and early reoperation was required in three patients due to cardia and pyloromyotomy leaks and to early wrap migration [22]. Those findings compare favorably with the results of one of the largest series of open redo surgeries, with a 10% reoperation rate and a 25.4% postoperative complication rate [16].

17.5 Long-Term Outcomes

Good to excellent long-term outcomes after primary laparoscopic antireflux surgery have been reported up to 90% of patients [26]. The success rate after reoperative antireflux surgery depends on the indication for redo (dysphagia, recurrent GERD mostly), on the anatomical failure pattern; which can make the redo procedure more or less challenging, and on the type of procedure performed. The need for re-reoperation is a good indicator of success. While the satisfaction rate after the first redo surgery for failure remains valuable at short-term follow-up (>80%), this rate tends to drop with the duration of follow-up and the number of previous operations [27–29].

At a short-term follow-up period (<2 years), good to excellent results were obtained in 74–81% of patients [7, 27, 30]. Better results for the laparoscopic approach were reported in the short run in a comparative study with the open approach, 94 versus 74% respectively, while similar results (70% success rate) were obtained in the long run with laparoscopy, laparotomy or thoracotomy [31].

Few studies in the literature report results with a long-term follow-up period (>3 years) [32–34] and only one at more than 5 years [22]. Long-term results are more disappointing than short-term ones, even if a group reported an excellent 90% success rate [13, 21].

In a case series by Vignal et al. (median follow-up: 4.5 years, completed in 29 patients) [32], 2 out of 47 patients required further surgery after a first reoperation at 3 and 7 months respectively, in the first case for wrap herniation and in the second case for complicated recurrent reflux, requiring a total duodenal diversion with truncal vagotomy. The authors also provided a comparison between the redo surgery group and a group of patients who underwent a single antireflux procedure during the same period. The GIQLI score was higher in patients after primary surgery (103 ± 27 versus 82 ± 23 in the redo surgery group). However, the satisfaction rate and the need for proton pump inhibitors (PPIs) were equivalent.

Granderath et al. [33] reported a satisfaction rate of 93% in their cohort of 27 patients, up to 5 years after surgery. The GIQLI score was significantly higher than the preoperative score, and increased significantly at interval reports at 3 years and 5 years, reaching values comparable to the score of healthy populations. In terms of symptoms, heartburn recurrence was reported in two patients at 3 and 5 years of follow-up, without any evidence of anatomical or morphological failure and successfully treated with low-dose PPIs. Dysphagia persisted in seven cases of patients who underwent a Nissen fundoplication as a redo surgery.

In the extensive retrospective analysis by Awais et al. [34], a long-term evaluation was performed with the GERD-HRQOL test and the SF36 test in a total of 186 patients available at a median follow-up of 3.3 years. The GERD-HRQOL was excellent in 52.2%, satisfactory in 33.3%, and poor in 14.5% of patients.

Finally, in our long-term study (mean follow-up: 76 months) [22], resolution of dysphagia was obtained in 68% of patients while recurrent GERD was treated in 73% of patients referred for index symptoms. After a redo procedure for herniation, the probability of being free-from-failure at 5 years was 83 versus 93% in case of slippage. After 10 years, the probabilities were 37 and 50% in case of herniation and slippage respectively. Failure of the repair was found in 41% of patients who underwent redo surgery for herniation, and four of them necessitated an additional operation. After reoperation for wrap slippage, failure was demonstrated in 27% of patients, three of them requiring additional surgery.

Failure after a reoperative antireflux surgery is challenging. Almost 10% of patients failed again and required another redo procedure [16, 34]. The best illustration of this problem was put forward by Smith et al. who reported a large series of 285 patients who underwent 307 reoperations for failed antireflux surgery [35]. Two hundred and forty-one patients underwent 1 redo, 59 patients 2 redos, 6 patients 3 redos, and 1 patient 4 redos. Transdiaphragmatic wrap migration was the main indication for multiple redo surgeries. The mean interval between the first and second redo was 24 ± 33 months and 12 ± 7 months between the second and the third redo. The failure rate was 7.1% after the first redo and 17% after the third redo. The type of procedure performed successively was iterative fundoplication. Based on this experience, the authors did not consider redoing the primary operation after three prior attempts, but instead, they planned to perform a different operation.

There is no consensus in the literature regarding the anatomical or symptomatic failure pattern nor regarding the number of previous antireflux reoperations, which could lead the surgeon to opt for an alternative procedure. It was previously reported that morbid obesity, esophageal dysmotility, short esophagus, severe preoperative dysphagia, and extraesophageal GERD symptoms were factors which contributed to poor outcomes after refundoplication [31]. Among the different options, there has been an increasing trend towards conversion to a Collis lengthening procedure with fundoplication, Roux-en-Y (RNY) reconstruction with an esophagojejunostomy or gastrojejunostomy [34, 36–38], esophageal myotomy or esophagectomy for end-stage pseudo-achalasia [34, 38].

Roux-en-Y reconstruction is progressively expanding, and if it was initially considered for overweight patients, it is also gradually offered to patients with a normal weight but with 1 or more previous operations. In a retrospective study comparing refundoplication (RF) and RNY reconstruction after a mean follow-up of 53.5 months, results were favorable, even though operative morbidity and long-term complications (anastomotic strictures) are higher than after a simple fundoplication [39]. The reoperation rate was similar between the two groups (7.2 and 9.5% in case of redo surgery and Roux-en-Y reconstruction respectively). However, long-term anastomotic strictures occurred in 28% of patients, who were managed with endoscopic dilatation. All assessed symptoms, heartburn, chest pain, dysphagia, and regurgitation significantly improved in both groups except for dysphagia, which was significantly improved only in the refundoplication group. Eighty patients (65.6%) had a complete resolution of symptoms or had only minimal symptoms at follow-up. There was no significant difference in symptom control among patients who underwent RF or RNY reconstruction. In a subset analysis, patients with morbid obesity, esophageal dysmotility, or additional risk factors have a better satisfaction with RNY reconstruction as compared to RF (18.2 versus 66.7%, $p = 0.031$). Among patients who had esophageal dysmotility, the incidence of postoperative dysphagia in patients who underwent RF was higher than in those who had RNY (58 versus 31%, $p = 0.07$).

The option of RNY reconstruction has to be appended to the armamentarium of procedures put forward to patients with fundoplication failure. The selected technique must be individualized taking into account the risk factors of failure that were identified. The refundoplication may remain the first choice for most patients, at least for the first reoperation.

17.6 Conclusions

Our experience and the reports published in the literature clearly demonstrate that antireflux failures should be managed laparoscopically, which provides substantial benefits over an open approach with an acceptable complication rate, at the cost of a higher conversion rate when compared to primary antireflux procedures. Good to excellent short-term results are obtained in almost 80% of patients undergoing a first reoperation. However, the long-term assessment of objective and subjective outcomes has revealed a significant failure rate, which increases with follow-up duration. Risk factors for failure have been identified, and multiple reoperations have led to poor results. These findings call for a change in the operative procedures, even if there is currently no formal algorithm for the management of failures. Preliminary, yet substantial results have shown that incorporation of Collis gastroplasty and Roux-en-Y reconstruction in the surgical armamentarium may change the long-term outcome after reoperation for failed antireflux surgery.

What Is the Current Knowledge and What Future Direction Is Required

- The most common causes of failure after fundoplication are the intrathoracic migration of the valve and slippage of the valve.
- Any repair performed in tension, axial on the esophagus and radial on the diaphragm can lead to rupture of the architecture of the valve.
- The long-term results of reoperations for failure are difficult to interpret given the paucity of detailed reports and the heterogeneity of the evaluation methods.

- The repetition of the reoperations leads to a significant reduction in the chances of success.
- After two consecutive failures, it seems logical to change the type of surgical assembly to hope for a stable result.
- The reason for placing a prosthesis to avoid the risk of re-migration seems simplistic and does not prevent a new recurrence while increasing the risk of complication related to the prosthesis.
- Detailed studies of reoperation results based on the indication and failure pattern would help establish a decisional algorithm.

References

1. Dallemagne B, Weerts JM, Jehaes C, et al. Laparoscopic Nissen fundoplication: preliminary report. Surg Laparosc Endosc. 1991;1:138–43.
2. Morton J, Lucktong T, Behrns KE, et al. National trends in fundoplication utilization and outcomes from 1989 and 1999. J Am Coll Surg. 2002;195:S55.
3. Fein M, Bueter M, Thalheimer A, et al. Ten-year outcome of laparoscopic antireflux surgery. J Gastrointest Surg. 2008;12:1893–9. https://doi.org/10.1007/s11605-008-0659-8.
4. Dallemagne B, Weerts J, Markiewicz S, et al. Clinical results of laparoscopic fundoplication at ten years after surgery. Surg Endosc. 2006;20:159–65. https://doi.org/10.1007/s00464-005-0174-x.
5. Lundell L, Miettinen P, Myrvold HE, et al. Seven-year follow-up of a randomized clinical trial comparing proton-pump inhibition with surgical therapy for reflux oesophagitis. Br J Surg. 2007;94:198–203. https://doi.org/10.1002/bjs.5492.
6. Lafullarde T, Watson DI, Jamieson GG, et al. Laparoscopic Nissen fundoplication: five-year results and beyond. Arch Surg. 2001;136:180–4.
7. van Beek DB, Auyang ED, Soper NJ. A comprehensive review of laparoscopic redo fundoplication. Surg Endosc. 2011;25:706–12. https://doi.org/10.1007/s00464-010-1254-0.
8. Dallemagne B, Weerts JM, Jehaes C, Markiewicz S. Causes of failures of laparoscopic antireflux operations. Surg Endosc. 1996;10:305–10.
9. Morse C, Pennathur ALJ. Laparoscopic techniques in reoperation for failed antireflux repairs. Philadelphia, PA: Churchill Livingstone; 2008.
10. Hunter JG, Smith CD, Branum GD, et al. Laparoscopic fundoplication failures: patterns of failure and response to fundoplication revision. Ann Surg. 1999;230:595–604. discussion 604-6.
11. Little AG, Ferguson MK, Skinner DB. Reoperation for failed antireflux operations. J Thorac Cardiovasc Surg. 1986;91:511–7.
12. Symons NRA, Purkayastha S, Dillemans B, et al. Laparoscopic revision of failed antireflux surgery: a systematic review. Am J Surg. 2011;202:336–43. https://doi.org/10.1016/j.amjsurg.2011.03.006.
13. Watson DI, Jamieson GG, Devitt PG, et al. Paraoesophageal hiatus hernia: an important complication of laparoscopic Nissen fundoplication. Br J Surg. 1995;82:521–3.
14. Luketich JD, Fernando HC, Christie NA, et al. Outcomes after minimally invasive reoperation for gastroesophageal reflux disease. Ann Thorac Surg. 2002;74:328–31. discussion 331-2.
15. Avaro J-P, D'Journo X-B, Trousse D, et al. Long-term results of redo gastro-esophageal reflux disease surgery. Eur J Cardiothorac Surg. 2008;33:1091–5. https://doi.org/10.1016/j.ejcts.2008.01.066.
16. Deschamps C, Trastek VF, Allen MS, et al. Long-term results after reoperation for failed antireflux procedures. J Thorac Cardiovasc Surg. 1997;113:545–50. https://doi.org/10.1016/S0022-5223(97)70369-6. discussion 550-1.

17. Ohnmacht GA, Deschamps C, Cassivi SD, et al. Failed antireflux surgery: results after reoperation. Ann Thorac Surg. 2006;81:2050–3. https://doi.org/10.1016/j.athoracsur.2006.01.019. discussion 2053-4.
18. Granderath FA, Kamolz T, Schweiger UM, Pointner R. Laparoscopic refundoplication with prosthetic hiatal closure for recurrent hiatal hernia after primary failed antireflux surgery. Arch Surg. 2003;138:902–7. https://doi.org/10.1001/archsurg.138.8.902.
19. Koch OO, Asche KU, Berger J, et al. Influence of the size of the hiatus on the rate of reherniation after laparoscopic fundoplication and refundopilication with mesh hiatoplasty. Surg Endosc. 2011;25:1024–30. https://doi.org/10.1007/s00464-010-1308-3.
20. Zügel N, Lang RA, Kox M, Hüttl TP. Severe complication of laparoscopic mesh hiatoplasty for paraesophageal hernia. Surg Endosc. 2009;23:2563–7. https://doi.org/10.1007/s00464-009-0456-9.
21. Swanstrom LL, Marcus DR, Galloway GQ. Laparoscopic Collis gastroplasty is the treatment of choice for the shortened esophagus. Am J Surg. 1996;171:477–81. https://doi.org/10.1016/S0002-9610(96)00008-6.
22. Dallemagne B, Arenas Sanchez M, Francart D, et al. Long-term results after laparoscopic reoperation for failed antireflux procedures. Br J Surg. 2011;98:1581–7. https://doi.org/ 10.1002/bjs.7590.
23. Funch-Jensen P, Bendixen A, Iversen MG, Kehlet H. Complications and frequency of redo antireflux surgery in Denmark: a nationwide study, 1997-2005. Surg Endosc. 2008;22:627–30. https://doi.org/10.1007/s00464-007-9705-y.
24. Granderath FA, Kamolz T, Schweiger UM, et al. Is laparoscopic refundoplication feasible in patients with failed primary open antireflux surgery? Surg Endosc. 2002;16:381–5. https://doi.org/10.1007/s00464-001-9102-x.
25. Floch NR, Hinder RA, Klingler PJ, et al. Is laparoscopic reoperation for failed antireflux surgery feasible? Arch Surg. 1999;134:733–7.
26. Dallemagne B, Taziaux P, Weerts J, et al. Laparoscopic surgery of gastroesophageal reflux. Ann Chir. 1995;49:30–6.
27. Khajanchee YS, O'Rourke R, Cassera MA, et al. Laparoscopic reintervention for failed antireflux surgery: subjective and objective outcomes in 176 consecutive patients. Arch Surg. 2007;142:785–901. https://doi.org/10.1001/archsurg.142.8.785. discussion 791-2.
28. Byrne JP, Smithers BM, Nathanson LK, et al. Symptomatic and functional outcome after laparoscopic reoperation for failed antireflux surgery. Br J Surg. 2005;92:996–1001. https://doi.org/10.1002/bjs.4914.
29. Horgan S, Pohl D, Bogetti D, et al. Failed antireflux surgery: what have we learned from reoperations? Arch Surg. 1999;134:809–15. discussion 815-7.
30. Bathla L, Legner A, Tsuboi K, Mittal S. Efficacy and feasibility of laparoscopic redo fundoplication. World J Surg. 2011;35:2445–53. https://doi.org/10.1007/s00268-011-1250-0.
31. Furnée EJB, Draaisma WA, Broeders IAMJ, Gooszen HG. Surgical reintervention after failed antireflux surgery: a systematic review of the literature. J Gastrointest Surg. 2009;13:1539–49. https://doi.org/10.1007/s11605-009-0873-z.
32. Vignal JC, Luc G, Wagner T, et al. Re-operation for failed gastro-esophageal fundoplication. What results to expect? J Visc Surg. 2012;149:e61–5. https://doi.org/10.1016/j.jviscsurg.2011.12.004.
33. Granderath FA, Kamolz T, Schweiger UM, Pointner R. Long-term follow-up after laparoscopic refundoplication for failed antireflux surgery: quality of life, symptomatic outcome, and patient satisfaction. J Gastrointest Surg. 2002;6:812–8.
34. Awais O, Luketich JD, Schuchert MJ, et al. Reoperative antireflux surgery for failed fundoplication: an analysis of outcomes in 275 patients. Ann Thorac Surg. 2011;92:1083–9. https://doi.org/10.1016/j.athoracsur.2011.02.088. discussion 1089-90.
35. Smith CD, McClusky DA, Rajad MA, et al. When fundoplication fails: redo? Ann Surg. 2005;241(6):861–9.

36. Stefanidis D, Navarro F, Augenstein VA, et al. Laparoscopic fundoplication takedown with conversion to Roux-en-Y gastric bypass leads to excellent reflux control and quality of life after fundoplication failure. Surg Endosc. 2012;26:3521–7. https://doi.org/10.1007/s00464-012-2380-7.
37. Makris KI, Panwar A, Willer BL, et al. The role of short-limb Roux-en-Y reconstruction for failed antireflux surgery: a single-center 5-year experience. Surg Endosc. 2012;26:1279–86. https://doi.org/10.1007/s00464-011-2026-1.
38. Awais O, Luketich JD, Tam J, et al. Roux-en-Y near esophagojejunostomy for intractable gastroesophageal reflux after antireflux surgery. Ann Thorac Surg. 2008;85:1954–9. doi:10.1016/j.athoracsur.2008.01.072. discussion 1959-61.
39. Mittal SK, Légner A, Tsuboi K, et al. Roux-en-Y reconstruction is superior to redo fundoplication in a subset of patients with failed antireflux surgery. Surg Endosc. 2013;27:927–35. https://doi.org/10.1007/s00464-012-2537-4.

Chapter 18
Utility of the Robot in Revisional Paraosophageal Hiatus Hernia

Maamoun Harmouch, Erik B. Wilson, Peter A. Walker, and Shinil K. Shah

18.1 Introduction

Diaphragmatic hernias are broadly divided into hiatal and parahiatal hernia. The incidence and prevalence of hiatal hernias increase with age [1]. Hiatal hernias are typically a "wear and tear" phenomenon. They occur secondary to disruption and or laxity of the ligamentous complex (phrenoesophageal, gastrocolic, and gastrosplenic ligaments) that maintain the esophagus and stomach in their normal anatomical locations [2, 3]. Disruption of this complex allow for varying degrees of abdominal organs to shift into the mediastinum causing a wide spectrum of clinical manifestations that range from mild reflux as seen with small type I hiatal hernias to gastric necrosis secondary to gastric volvulus [4]. Parahiatal hernias most commonly occur secondary to traumatic injury to the diaphragm or a congenital anomaly such as Bochadlek and Morgagni hernias [1].

M. Harmouch, M.D. • E.B. Wilson, M.D. • P.A. Walker, M.D.
Department of Surgery, McGovern Medical School, University of Texas Health Science Center at Houston, 6431 Fannin Street, MSB 4.156, Houston, TX 77030, USA

S.K. Shah, D.O. (✉)
Department of Surgery, McGovern Medical School, University of Texas Health Science Center at Houston, 6431 Fannin Street, MSB 4.156, Houston, TX 77030, USA

Michael E. DeBakey Institute of Comparative Cardiovascular Science and Biomedical Devices, Texas A&M University, College Station, TX, USA
e-mail: shinil.k.shah@uth.tmc.edu

M.A. Memon (ed.), *Hiatal Hernia Surgery*,
https://doi.org/10.1007/978-3-319-64003-7_18

18.2 Classification and Clinical Manifestations

Traditional classification of hiatal hernia include types I to IV. A more clinically relevant distinction includes sliding hiatal hernia (Type I) and paraesophageal hernias (Types II–IV) (Fig. 18.1). Sliding hiatal hernias account for more than 95% of all hiatal/paraesophageal hernias. Type III hernias are the most common type of paraesophageal hernia (PEH). Clinically, about 50% of patients are asymptomatic [5, 6]. When symptoms are present, they are typically a result of a dysfunctional lower esophageal sphincter and or mechanical obstruction of the distal esophagus or stomach.

Patients can experience a wide array of signs and symptoms such as heartburn, regurgitation, epigastric pain, postprandial fullness, dysphagia, dyspnea, aspiration

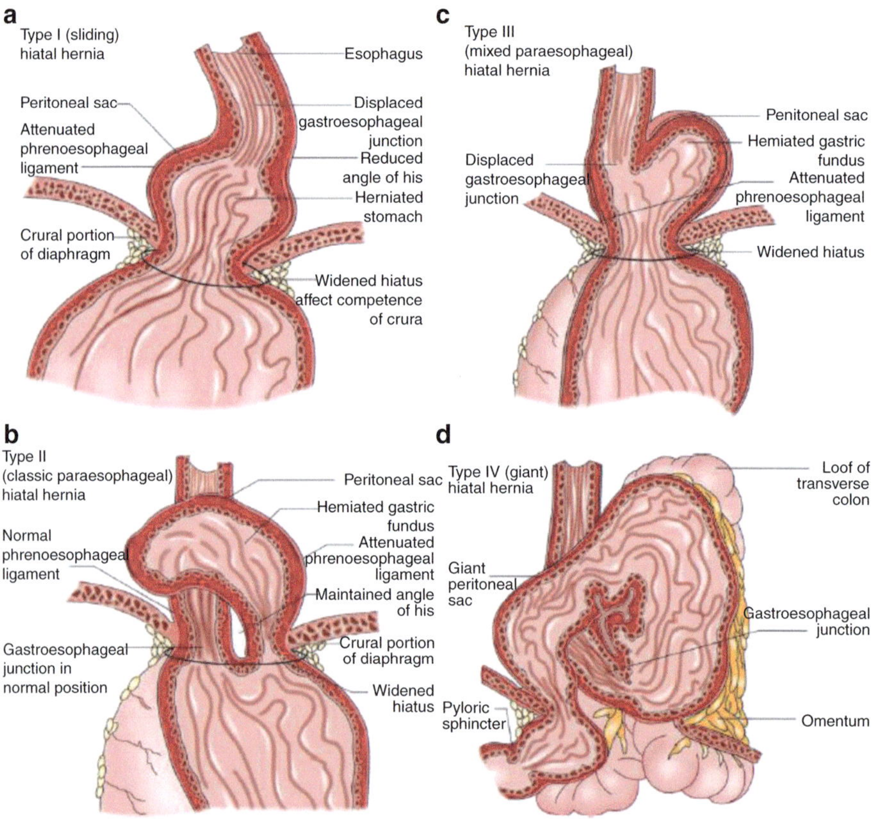

Fig. 18.1 Types of hiatal/paraesophgeal hernias. (**a**) Type 1 (sliding hernia) (**b**) Type 2 (normal location of the gastroesophageal junction with herniation of the fundus (**c**) Type 3 (combination of Types 1 and 2) (**d**) Type 4 (herniation of additional intra abdominal organ). Figure reproduced with permission [43]

pneumonia, and iron deficiency anemia that occur secondary to Cameron ulcers [5–7]. The majority of patients will have a chronic intermittent presentation and can be managed electively. Rarely gastric necrosis, perforation, and bleeding occur secondary to acute gastric obstruction. This devastating complication has an operative mortality of 17–56% and is considered a surgical emergency [4, 8].

Indications for operative repair, surgical approach, and surgical technique are all areas of current debate. In general, older patients with multiple co-morbidities and high peri-operative risk and patients with mild symptoms can be managed non-operatively. On the other hand, symptomatic patients at reasonable surgical risk should be offered surgical repair. With current technology, the minimally invasive approach has become the standard of care [7, 9]. Irrespective of the approach, keys to successful repair include adequate mobilization of the esophagus to achieve tension free intra-abdominal esophageal length of at least 2–3 cm, excision of hernia sac, tension free closure of hiatus defect, and an antireflux procedure (fundoplication) [5, 6, 10].

18.3 Evolution of Operative Treatment

Gastrointestinal surgery entered a new era with the introduction of laparoscopic surgery in the late 1980s and robotic surgery in the early 1990s [11, 12]. These minimally invasive techniques have revolutionized operative medicine in the majority of surgical specialties. Compared to open surgery, conventional laparoscopy (CL) offer multiple advantages including decreased postoperative pain and post operative morbidity, improved cosmesis, faster recovery, and decreased length of hospital stay [13]. Despite these advantages, CL carries with it multiple disadvantages and limitations such as reduced surgical dexterity, poor surgical ergonomics, translation of natural tremors, 2-dimensional visualization, and a steep learning curve to master most complex gastrointestinal operations [14–16]. These limitations along with advancement in computer technology and robotics led to the birth of surgical robotic systems. This novel technology started in 1985 with the Puma 560 platform that was used in the field of neurosurgery. Over the next decade, multiple other platforms were introduced into the market to assist in different specialties such as orthopedics and urology. The automated endoscopic system of optimal positioning (AESOP) was the first robotic platform used in abdominal surgery in the 1990s. Over the next few years, this technology underwent multiple phases of refinement to give rise to da Vinci surgical system (Intuitive Surgical, Inc., Sunnyvale, CA). This new platform was FDA approved in July of 2000 for use in general surgery procedures. While maintaining most of the advantages offered by CL, surgical robots were designed to provide promising solutions for most of the limitations and drawbacks encountered with CL [15].

18.4 Da Vinci Surgical System

Currently, the most widely used robotic system in gastrointestinal surgery is the da Vinci surgical system. There are several other platforms either in development or soon to enter the market, including systems developed by Titan Medical (Toronto, Ontario, Canada), Verb Surgical (Mountain View, CA), Medtronic (Minneapolis, MN), and Transenterix (Morrisville, NC).

The da Vinci system consists of a surgeon console, patient side-cart, and a vision system. The console consists of a stereoscopic viewer, controllers, and pedals that allow the surgeon to be comfortably seated and engrossed in the surgical field in order to minimize fatigue and distraction. The side cart consists of three or four robot arms that translate the surgeon's movements at the console. Multiple endowrist instruments that carry different functions have been designed. These instruments are designed with seven degrees of motion, a range of motion similar to human wrist. The vision system consists of a high definition 3D endoscope and a large vision cart that provide enhanced visualization for the operating surgeon, as well as the rest of the OR team. In addition, the surgeon's movements are digitalized which allow exclusion of surgical tremors and improve motion scaling up to five times, which may result in increased operative precision [17–19].

18.5 Surgical Repair of Paraesophagael Hernias

Historically, PEH repair was done through an open transthoracic or transabdominal approach. However, with the development of laparoscopic techniques, large acceptance and adoption of minimally invasive techniques have been seen by most surgeons. This enthusiasm was further boosted by multiple early reports demonstrating the ability to perform large PEH repairs using laparoscopic techniques safely and with good symptomatic results [9, 10]. Although CL offered its inherent set of advantages that is seen in the perioperative course, most initial series reported higher recurrence rates. The recurrence rate ranged from 16 to 57% with the laparoscopic approach compared to 2 to 15% with the open approach. Despite this higher recurrence rates, multiple studies showed that this recurrence is often a radiographic finding that lacks any clinical implications. In addition, the majority of these patients with a documented radiographic recurrence had excellent clinical outcomes and improved quality of life with very few that required reoperation [20, 21]. The introduction of robotic surgical system into foregut surgery was believed to improve upon CL and potentially yield better operative outcomes.

The first robotic assisted laparoscopic (RAL) Nissan fundoplication was done by Cadiere and colleagues (1999, France). Cadiere went on to conduct a prospective randomized trial comparing the outcome of robotic versus laparoscopic Nissan fundoplication in 21 patients. Both approaches had similar outcomes although operative time was significantly longer in the robotic group (72 vs. 52 min, $p < 0.01$) [22]. Multiple other studies were then carried out comparing robotics to CL. These studies demonstrated an average of a 30 min longer operative time and a total of 2000 US dollar higher cost with the robotic platform [19]. On the other hand, robotic surgery was proven to be a safe alternative with comparable clinical outcomes to CL. Despite the thoughts that robotic surgery would yield better patient outcomes in antireflux and hiatal hernia surgery, this was not seen in clinical studies when it was compared to CL [23–25]. Of note, most of the studies were performed on patients with symptomatic GERD and/or small type I hiatal hernia. Perhaps, if CL was compared to robotic platforms with large and more complex PEH that require more dissection and precision of movements in the narrow hiatus, then significant clinical advantages may be seen. The role of robotics continues to represent an area ripe for research and prospective trials.

18.6 Failure of Primary Repair

The operative management for GERD and treatment of PEHs increased dramatically in the past decade. This increase occurred with the introduction and advancement in the minimally invasive techniques which was demonstrated to be safe, effective, and with a low risk of operative morbidity and mortality [26]. This led to more patients with failed primary surgical repair being encountered in the clinical setting. Most studies report recurrence rates of around 28% after primary repair. The pathogenesis of PEH recurrence is multi-factorial and includes patient characteristics, physiologic factors such as repetitive movement of the diaphragm, and technical factors. Patient related factors include obesity, presence of atypical symptoms, poor response to medications, pulmonary disease, smoking, prior abdominal surgeries, and size of the PEH [27]. Technical factors that have been associated with increased rates of recurrence include inadequate dissection of hiatus, failure to recognize short esophagus or inadequate dissection of the esophagus, false identification of GE junction, sub-optimally constructed wrap, and vagal nerve injury. Upon reoperation, transdiaphragmatic migration of wrap and disruption of wrap were the two most common causes for failure [28–30]. Despite the relatively high recurrence rate of laparoscopic PEH, only a minority of patients are symptomatic and require reoperation. The most common indication for reoperation includes reflux, dysphasia, and bloating along with a documented radiographic abnormality [31].

18.7 Redo Paraesophageal Hernia Repair

Patients with failed PEH repair embody a complicated clinical picture and a technical challenge for surgeons. Reoperations are often more complex due to dense adhesions, scarred surgical planes, and altered anatomy [32]. Not surprisingly, these challenges are greater if the primary repair was done via an open approach. Compared to primary repair, redo surgery has higher mortality, higher intraoperative and postoperative complication rate, and lower satisfactory symptomatic outcomes [27, 31–37]. Further, clinical outcomes become less satisfactory if more than one reoperation is needed [27, 34–37]. The satisfaction rate drops to 42% with patients requiring three or more operations [34]. Therefore, studies suggest that patients have best outcomes with their primary surgical repair followed by the first reoperation.

Patients being considered for reoperation should have a thorough evaluation. One must obtain a detailed history regarding their initial preoperative symptoms, response to the operation, and whether these symptoms persisted after the primary repair or new symptoms arise. A complete workup for esophageal and gastric disorders should be undertaken, with comprehensive testing with radiographs, barium esophagogram, pH study, endoscopy, esophageal manometry, and gastric emptying studies [27, 35–37].

These tests may reveal an undiagnosed underlying problem such as abnormal esophageal motility, abnormal stomach emptying, and/or a short esophagus. With this preoperative information, surgeons can often tailor their operative plans to the individual patients. As an example, patients with dysphasia might need a partial fundoplication during their reoperation, those having true shortened esophagus might benefit from an esophageal lengthening procedure and/or more aggressive mediastinal dissection, and patients that are obese or have major esophageal dysmotility might benefit from roux-en-y (RNY) gastrojejunostomy or esophagojejunostomy. In carefully selected patients, an even more aggressive operation such as esophagectomy may be required [27, 31–37].

Traditionally, patients being evaluated for redo PEH repair are referred to thoracic and or gastrointestinal surgeons and a majority of the redo operations are done via an open approach. Around 66% of patients are done via transabdominal approach and 25% are done via transthoracic approach. However, up to one third of patients are currently being done via laparoscopy due to the increased experience and skills in minimally invasive techniques.

Outcomes after the first reoperation for a failed antireflux surgery are satisfactory with long term satisfaction rates of about 80% as compared to 95% seen after a primary repair [33]. Intraoperative and postoperative complication rates are far more common after redo surgery (21.4% and 15.6%, respectively) [31]. Postoperative complications and mortality are higher with an open approach. On the other hand, intraoperative complications were much higher in the laparoscopic group and rate for conversion to open surgery was around 8.7% [31]. Reasons for conversion include dense adhesions, intraoperative bleeding, and poor visualization. In addition, current literature demonstrates that failure of laparoscopic redo operation is as high as 11% and these patients required additional revisional operations [32, 33, 35].

These factors along with the known advantages of the robotic surgical system have led many investigators to revisit the role of robotic surgery in redo antireflux and hiatal hernia surgery. Currently there is paucity of studies looking at the role of robotic surgical system in redo antireflux and hiatal hernia repair. Tolboom et al., in a single cohort study, included 75 patients who underwent either CL or RAL redo surgery. He found that median hospital stay was reduced by 1 day in the robotic group. In addition there was less conversion to open surgery in the RAL group. There was no difference in mortality rates, complications, and outcomes between the two groups [38]. There is some data that can be gleaned from robotic revisional bariatric surgery that may point to a role for robotics in re-do antireflux surgery and the basis for additional future trials. Although small, series of robotic revisional bariatric surgery demonstrate decreased conversion rates to open surgery, complication rates, hospital length of stay, as well as major complication rates approaching that of primary bariatric surgical options [39–42].

18.8 Description of Redo Robot Assisted Laparoscopic Paraesophageal Herina Repair

The set up for RAL primary and/or revisional PEH repair is similar to that of other foregut operations. The set-up used by the authors is similar, with minor modifications, to techniques described by others. Patients are positioned in steep reverse Trendelenburg with care taken to pad all pressure points. Using either the SI or XI system, four robotic arms are utilized with or without an accessory port. Port configuration is noted in Fig. 18.2. A parallel side dock technique is utilized for positioning of the patient side cart (Figs. 18.3 and 18.4).

Typically, two bowel graspers, two needle drivers, as well as monopolar shears and an energy device (Harmonic scalpel) are utilized for the case (Fig. 18.5). An accessory port may be utilized to introduce sutures/and or mesh, as well as aid in retraction, exposure, and suctioning. An internal (Freehold Surgical, New Hope, PA) or external

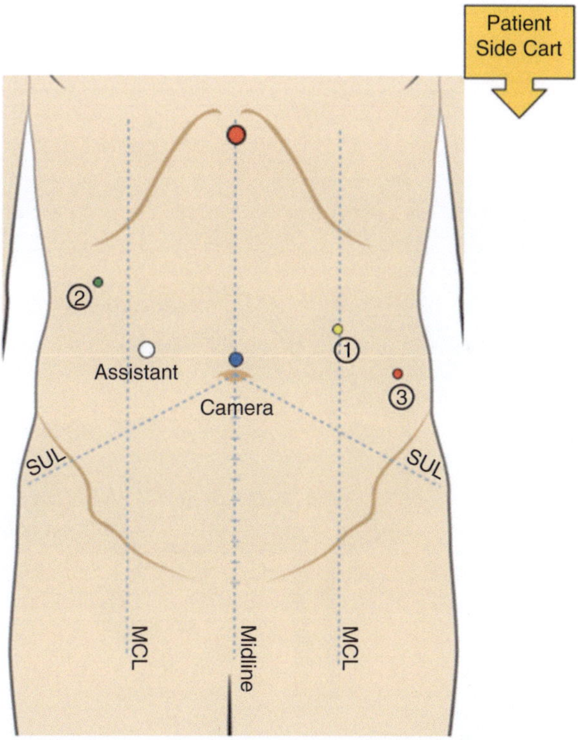

Fig. 18.2 Port placement for robotic assisted laparoscopic redo paraesophageal hernia repair. Utilizing the SI system, typically a 5 mm robotic port (Instrument arm 2), 8 mm robotic port (Instrument arm 1), 5 mm robotic port (Instrument arm 4), 10/30 robotic camera, and a 8–12 mm accessory port are utilized. The position of the port corresponding to Instrument arm 1 may need to be placed higher for very large paraesophageal hernias for high mediastinal dissection. A subxiphoid 5 mm incision is utilized for external liver retractor insertion; if an internal liver retractor is utilized this port can be eliminated. Port placement for the XI system is similar. All ports are 8 mm ports aside from the accessory port and ports are placed in a more horizontal fashion. Docking can be performed from any position due to the differences in the patient side cart

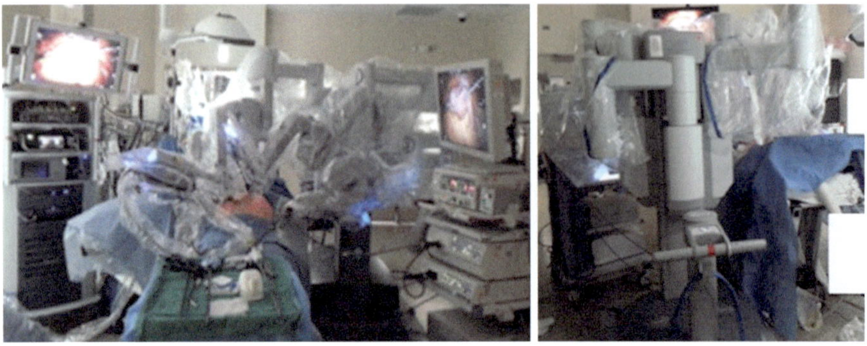

Fig. 18.3 Robotic patient side cart. Demonstrated is an intra operative photograph demonstrating the da Vinci SI system. Note the parallel side dock technique which allows for easy access to the head of the patient for anesthesia as well as for intra operative endoscopy. Figure reproduced from: **Shah SK**, Walker PA, Snyder BE, Wilson EB. Chapter 6: Essentials and future directions of bariatric surgery. In: Kroh M, Chalikonda S (eds) Essentials of Robotic Surgery, Springer Science + Business Media, New York. 2015

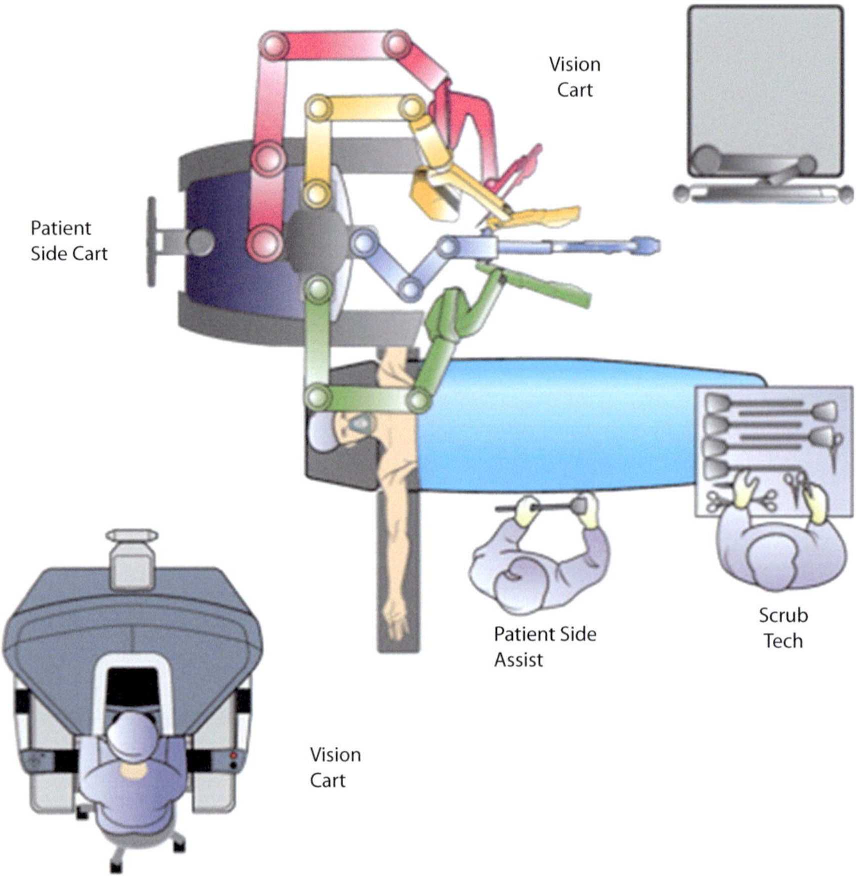

Fig. 18.4 Operating room set-up. Demonstrated is a representation of the operating room set up for robotic foregut surgery

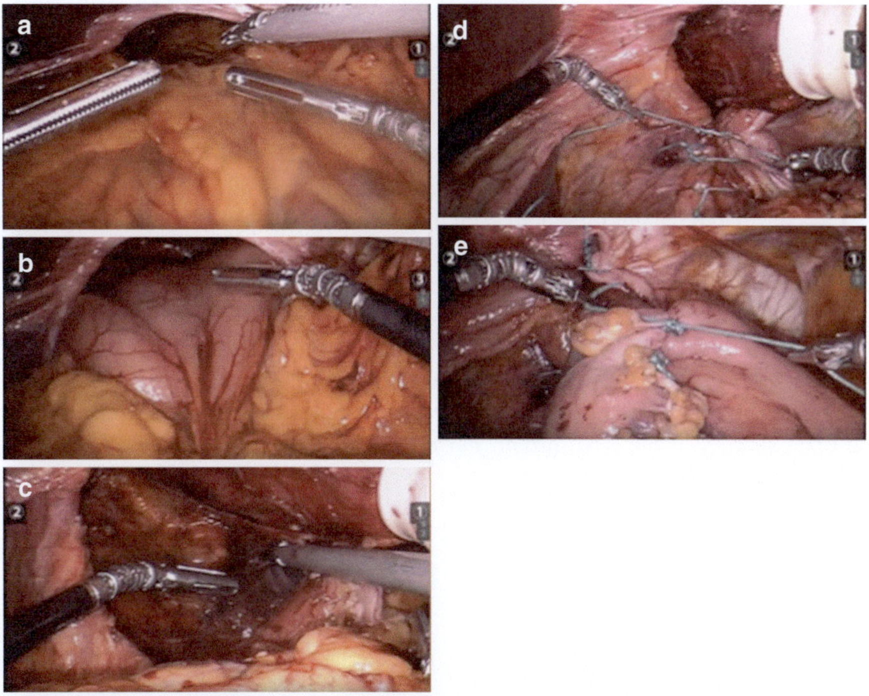

Fig. 18.5 Robotic repair of a type 4 paraesophageal hernia. Demonstrated are intra operative photographs from a robotic assisted laparoscopic repair of a type 4 paraesophageal hernia containing stomach, colon, and omentum. (**a**) Initial appearance. Typically, dissection is initiated with two robotic bowel graspers and an energy device. (**b**) Appearance after reduction of colon and omentum. Atraumatic bowel graspers are utilized for handling of intra abdominal viscera. (**c**) Appearance during final esophageal mobilization. A penrose drain is placed around the esophagus to assist with retraction. (**d**) Appearance during posterior crural repair. Two robotic needle drivers are utilized. (**e**) Appearance during completion of the Nissen fundoplication

(laparoscopic Nathanson liver retractor, introduced through a 5 mm subxiphoid incision) liver retractor is utilized to facilitate anterior retraction of the left lobe.

Key operative steps in redo-PEH repair include takedown of adhesions, identification of the left and right crus, takedown of short gastric vessels (if not done previously), complete dissection and excision of the hernia sac, identification and preservation of vagus nerves (can be very difficult in redo operations), adequate mediastinal dissection to achieve at least 2–3 cm of tension free intra abdominal esophagus, primary crural repair, mesh placement (surgeon preference), and takedown and re-do fundoplication (if necessary).

Choice of partial or complete fundoplication is typically based on history and pre operative workup and any evidence of possible esophageal dysfunction. Gastropexy and/or gastrostomy tube placement may be performed. In very large re-do PEHs, gastrostomy tube may help prevent retching/nausea caused by immediate post operative gas bloat. All dissection of the esophagus is done around a bougie to adequately size the crural closure, fundoplication, as well as to aid in identification of the esophagus during dissection. At the conclusion of the case, intra operative endoscopy may be useful.

18.9 Conclusion

Patients with failed primary antireflux surgery and hiatal hernia repair present a major challenge to the surgical community. These patients should have a thorough preoperative evaluation in conjunction with a gastroenterologist to obtain critical information that can tailor the redo operation to the individual patient. Currently, CL is considered the gold standard even in redo cases. However, many studies demonstrated higher intra-operative complications and higher conversion rates, which are believed to occur secondary to dense adhesions, scarred surgical planes, poor visualization, and obscured anatomy. These challenges seemed to be better overcome with the robotic surgical system due to the aforementioned advantages. Currently, there is a single study comparing RAL to CL in redo antireflux surgery and hiatal hernia repair which showed decreased hospital stay and less conversion to open surgery in the RAL group. Further study is needed to clarify the role of robotics in redo PEH repair.

Summary: What Is the Current Knowledge and What Future Direction Is Required

- Minimally invasive surgical approaches currently represent the gold standard for repair of paraesophageal hernia in both primary and revisional cases.
- Patients undergoing revisional paraesophageal hernia repair should undergo a complete pre operative workup to exclude co-existing esophageal and or gastric pathology.
- Most studies demonstrate higher intra-operative complications and higher conversion rates in laparoscopic redo paraesophageal hernia secondary to dense adhesions, scarred surgical planes, poor visualization, and obscured anatomy.
- Robotic assisted laparoscopy may offer promise in decreasing complication and conversion rates in re-do paraesophageal hernia repair
- There is limited data comparing robotic to conventional laparoscopy in re-do paraesophageal hernia and further studies comparing the two modalities are needed.

References

1. Ilves R. Hiatus hernia. The condition. Chest Surg Clin N Am. 1998;8(2):401–9.
2. Weston AP. Hiatal hernia with cameron ulcers and erosions. Gastrointest Endosc Clin N Am. 1996;6(4):671–9.
3. Hill LD, et al. The gastroesophageal flap valve: in vitro and in vivo observations. Gastrointest Endosc. 1996;44(5):541–7.
4. Hill LD. Incarcerated paraesophageal hernia. A surgical emergency. Am J Surg. 1973;126(2):286–91.

5. Peridikis G, Hinder RA. Paraesophageal hiatal hernia. In: Nyhus LM, Condon RE, editors. Hernia. Philadelphia: JB Lippincott; 1995. p. 544–54.
6. Maish MS, DeMeester SR. Paraesophageal hiatal hernia. In: Cameron J, editor. Current surgical therapy. Philadelphia: Elsevier Mosby; 2004. p. 38–42.
7. Stylopoulos N, Gazelle GS, Rattner DW. Paraesophageal hernias: operation or observation? Ann Surg. 2002;236(4):492–500. discussion 500–1
8. Skinner DB, Belsey RH. Surgical management of esophageal reflux and hiatus hernia. Long-term results with 1,030 patients. J Thorac Cardiovasc Surg. 1967;53(1):33–54.
9. Schieman C, Grondin SC. Paraesophageal hernia: clinical presentation, evaluation, and management controversies. Thorac Surg Clin. 2009;19(4):473–84.
10. Zehetner J, et al. Laparoscopic versus open repair of paraesophageal hernia: the second decade. J Am Coll Surg. 2011;212(5):813–20.
11. Maeso S, et al. Efficacy of the Da Vinci surgical system in abdominal surgery compared with that of laparoscopy: a systematic review and meta-analysis. Ann Surg. 2010;252(2):254–62.
12. Mouret P. How I developed laparoscopic cholecystectomy. Ann Acad Med Singap. 1996;25(5):744–7.
13. Peters MJ, et al. Meta-analysis of randomized clinical trials comparing open and laparoscopic anti-reflux surgery. Am J Gastroenterol. 2009;104(6):1548–61. quiz 1547, 1562
14. Watson DI, Baigrie RJ, Jamieson GG. A learning curve for laparoscopic fundoplication. Definable, avoidable, or a waste of time? Ann Surg. 1996;224(2):198–203.
15. Lunca S, Bouras G, Stanescu AC. Gastrointestinal robot-assisted surgery. A current perspective. Rom J Gastroenterol. 2005;14(4):385–91.
16. Byrn JC, et al. Three-dimensional imaging improves surgical performance for both novice and experienced operators using the da Vinci Robot System. Am J Surg. 2007;193(4):519–22.
17. Berguer R, Smith W. An ergonomic comparison of robotic and laparoscopic technique: the influence of surgeon experience and task complexity. J Surg Res. 2006;134(1):87–92.
18. Toro JP, Lin E, Patel AD. Review of robotics in foregut and bariatric surgery. Surg Endosc. 2015;29(1):1–8.
19. Ito F, Gould JC. Robotic foregut surgery. Int J Med Robot. 2006;2(4):287–92.
20. Furnee E, Hazebroek E. Mesh in laparoscopic large hiatal hernia repair: a systematic review of the literature. Surg Endosc. 2013;27(11):3998–4008.
21. Draaisma WA, et al. Controversies in paraesophageal hernia repair: a review of literature. Surg Endosc. 2005;19(10):1300–8.
22. Cadiere GB, et al. Nissen fundoplication done by remotely controlled robotic technique. Ann Chir. 1999;53(2):137–41.
23. Owen B, et al. How does robotic anti-reflux surgery compare with traditional open and laparoscopic techniques: a cost and outcomes analysis. Surg Endosc. 2014;28(5):1686–90.
24. Mi J, et al. Whether robot-assisted laparoscopic fundoplication is better for gastroesophageal reflux disease in adults: a systematic review and meta-analysis. Surg Endosc. 2010;24(8):1803–14.
25. Wang Z, Zheng Q, Jin Z. Meta-analysis of robot-assisted versus conventional laparoscopic Nissen fundoplication for gastro-oesophageal reflux disease. ANZ J Surg. 2012;82(3):112–7.
26. Richter JE. Gastroesophageal reflux disease treatment: side effects and complications of fundoplication. Clin Gastroenterol Hepatol. 2013;11(5):465–71. quiz e39
27. Wilshire CL, et al. Clinical Outcomes of Reoperation for Failed Antireflux Operations. Ann Thorac Surg. 2016;101(4):1290–6.
28. Lidor AO, et al. Defining recurrence after paraesophageal hernia repair: correlating symptoms and radiographic findings. Surgery. 2013;154(2):171–8.
29. Patti MG, Allaix ME, Fisichella PM. Analysis of the causes of failed antireflux surgery and the principles of treatment: a review. JAMA Surg. 2015;150(6):585–90.
30. Hunter JG, et al. Laparoscopic fundoplication failures: patterns of failure and response to fundoplication revision. Ann Surg. 1999;230(4):595–604. discussion 604-6
31. Furnee EJ, et al. Surgical reintervention after failed antireflux surgery: a systematic review of the literature. J Gastrointest Surg. 2009;13(8):1539–49.

32. van Beek DB, Auyang ED, Soper NJ. A comprehensive review of laparoscopic redo fundoplication. Surg Endosc. 2011;25(3):706–12.
33. Dallemagne B, et al. Laparoscopic surgery of gastroesophageal reflux. Ann Chir. 1995;49(1):30–6.
34. Little AG, Ferguson MK, Skinner DB. Reoperation for failed antireflux operations. J Thorac Cardiovasc Surg. 1986;91(4):511–7.
35. Awais O, et al. Reoperative antireflux surgery for failed fundoplication: an analysis of outcomes in 275 patients. Ann Thorac Surg. 2011;92(3):1083–9. discussion 1089-90
36. Symons NR, et al. Laparoscopic revision of failed antireflux surgery: a systematic review. Am J Surg. 2011;202(3):336–43.
37. Yamamoto SR, et al. Long-term outcomes of reintervention for failed fundoplication: redo fundoplication versus Roux-en-Y reconstruction. Surg Endosc. 2014;28(1):42–8.
38. Tolboom RC, Draaisma WA, Broeders IA. Evaluation of conventional laparoscopic versus robot-assisted laparoscopic redo hiatal hernia and antireflux surgery: a cohort study. J Robot Surg. 2016;10(1):33–9.
39. Ayloo SM, Choudhury N. Robotic revisional bariatric surgery: single-surgeon case series. Int J Med Robotics Comput Assist Surg. 2015;11:284–9.
40. Bindal V, Gonzalez-Heredia R, Elli EF. Outcomes of robot-assisted Roux-en-Y gastric bypass as a reoperative bariatric procedure. Obes Surg. 2015;25(10):1810–5.
41. Buchs NC, et al. Robotic revisional bariatric surgery: a comparative study with laparoscopic and open surgery. Int J Med Robot. 2014;10(2):213–7.
42. Snyder B, et al. Robotically assisted revision of bariatric surgeries is safe and effective to achieve further weight loss. World J Surg. 2013;37(11):2569–73.
43. Zaman JA, Lidor AO. The optimal approach to symptomatic paraesophageal hernia repair: important technical considerations. Curr Gastroenterol Rep. 2016;18(10):53.

Chapter 19
Quality of Life Following Laparoscopic Antireflux Surgery for Primary and Recurrent Gastroesophageal Reflux Disease

Ilmo Kellokumpu and Eero Sihvo

19.1 Introduction

GERD is prevalent worldwide, and the disease burden seems to be increasing. The range of GERD prevalence estimates are 18.1–27.8% in North America, 8.8–25.9% in Europe, 2.5–7.8% in East Asia, 8.7–33.1% in the Middle East, 11.6% in Australia and 23.0% in South America [1, 2]. Prior use of non-steroidal anti-inflammatory drugs, smoking, excess body weight and gastrointestinal and cardiac conditions are associated with an increased risk of gastro-oesophageal reflux disease [3].

Patients suffering from gastro-oesophageal reflux disease (GERD) seek relief for heartburn, regurgitation and dysphagia. Patients with frequent and severe symptoms require targeted therapy with the most effective treatment strategies. The efficacy of proton pump inhibitors (PPI)s in the control of acid reflux has been proven [4]. However, these medications do not stop reflux or cure GERD, while fundoplication restores competence to the gastroesophageal junction.

Surgical treatment of GERD in properly selected patients has demonstrated its efficacy in reducing symptoms and the need for proton-pump inhibitor therapy. The introduction of laparoscopic techniques has reduced perioperative complications and facilitated postoperative recovery, without compromising the level of GERD control [5–14]. Good short-term cure of GERD symptoms is reported in 90–97% [5–14], and mid-term cure (up to 5 years) in 85–90% of patients [15–18] who have laparoscopic fundoplication. Partial fundoplication is associated with a lower rate of postoperative side effects but may have a higher rate of reoperation for recurrence of GERD. Side effects of Nissen fundoplication such as dysphagia, increased bloating and flatulence, and inability to belch or vomit may limit the success of antireflux surgery.

I. Kellokumpu (✉) • E. Sihvo
Department of Surgery, Central Hospital of Central Finland,
Keskussairaalantie 19, Jyväskylä 40620, Finland
e-mail: ilmo.kellokumpu@ksshp.fi

M.A. Memon (ed.), *Hiatal Hernia Surgery*,
https://doi.org/10.1007/978-3-319-64003-7_19

Long term follow-up studies suggest that antireflux surgery can cause failures and side-effects, and therefore is not a durable solution for all patients. A Swedish nationwide survey reported long-term treatment failure in 25.4% and 29.0% of patients operated on 1995–96 and 2000, respectively , demonstrating that approximately a quarter of patients experience some sort of treatment failure [19]. The level of impairment and types of problems experienced by GERD patients relate to symptom severity, the type and effectiveness of the treatment, side-effects of surgery, and non-disease related factors such as the presence of other medical conditions, sex, or anxiety. Some patients may revert to the use of long-term medical therapy, or need revision surgery to improve symptom control following recurrent symptoms.

19.2 Measuring the Effectiveness of Antireflux Surgery

Evaluating the impact of antireflux surgery has usually relied on scales assessing reflux symptom severity, such as heartburn, regurgitation, or pain, together with the endoscopic appearance of the oesophageal mucosa and patient's perception of overall success. Twenty-four hour pH monitoring, although useful in selected subjects is generally not used to assess therapeutic response. However, these assessment methods, even when used collectively, still fail to reflect the functional status of patients. Moreover, no standard, universally accepted definition of what constitutes failure of antireflux surgery exists.

In the contemporary health care environment outcome and quality of life constructs are seen as relevant end points for the evaluating the success of treatment and justifying continued intervention. Pope first discussed the relevance of quality of life in the assessment of antireflux surgery in 1992 [20]. Health related quality of life (HRQoL) can be defined as the functional effect of an illness and its therapy on an individual, as perceived by the individual himself or herself [21]. It is determined by both disease and non-disease related factors. The domains that determine HRQoL include physical and occupational function, emotional state, social interactions, and somatic sensation. These determinants can also be further classified as disease related, including symptom severity, treatment efficacy, and adverse effects of treatment, or disease independent factors, such as sex or age, education and knowledge, personality and coping skills, culture, and beliefs. Several QoL instruments have been developed to assess QoL in upper gastrointestinal disease. The two most extensively examined are the GSRS and the QOLRAD scale (Table 19.1).

19.3 The Impact of Gastroesophageal Reflux Disease on Patients Health Related Quality of Life (HRQoL)

A number of studies [22–24] have demonstrated that HRQoL in patients presenting with reflux disease is significantly impaired in comparison to the general population, and patients perceive themselves to be as affected by their condition as patients

Table 19.1 Instruments to assess QoL in gastroesophageal reflux disease

VAS (visual analog scale) of patient satisfaction with symptom control score range from 0 (no relief) to 100 (complete symptom relief), more than 70 equals symptom control
De Mester symptom score to evaluate GERD symptoms (heartburn, regurgitation, and dysphagia) total range from 0 (no GERD symptoms) to 9 (maximum symptoms)
EQ-5D (EuroQol-5-dimension) score of five dimensions (mobility, self-care, pain, usual activities, psychological status), range from 0 (equivalent to being dead) to 1 (best health state imaginable)
GERSS (gastroesophageal reflux symptom score) product of severity and frequency of five symptoms (heartburn, regurgitation, bloating, dysphagia and epigastric/retrosternal pain) scale range from 0 to 60, less than 18 equals symptom control
GRACI (gastrooesophageal reflux disease activity index) score of certain GERD symptoms ranging from 74 (no symptoms) to 172 (worst symptoms)
GSRS (gastrointestinal symptom rating scale) 15 symptoms producing five subscales (reflux, diarrhea, constipation, abdominal pain, indigestion), mean subscale scores range from 1 (no discomfort) to 7 (very severe discomfort)
QOLRAD (quality-of-life in reflux and dyspepsia) 25 questions comprising five dimensions (emotional stress, sleep disturbance, food and drink, physical and social functionality, vitality) the higher the score, the higher the quality-of-life
REFLUX quality-of-life score assessment of gastrointestinal symptoms, side effects, and complications of both treatments; score range from 0 to 100; the higher the score, the better the patients feel
SF-36 (36-item short form general health and well-being survey) score of eight dimensions (limitations in physical and social activity, physical and emotional role limitations, bodily pain, vitality, general health, general mental health); score range from 0 to 100
PGWBI (psychological general well-being index) 22 items combining into six dimensions (anxiety, depressed mood, sense of positive well-being, self-control, general health, vitality) the higher the score, the better the well-being
GIQLI (36 items, including 5 subitems: gastrointestinal symptoms, emotional status, physical functions, social functions, and stress by medical treatment); score range from 0 to 144

with other serious chronic conditions [24]. Disease severity correlates strongly with HRQoL. Increasing symptom frequency and symptom severity in patients with GERD both lead to lower physical and mental health, and higher levels of work absenteeism. Nocturnal symptoms have an additional negative impact on HRQoL leading to further worsening of physical health [24]. From the patient's standpoint the QoL will be improved to the extent that reflux symptoms are relieved and surgery-related major side-effects are not acquired.

19.4 The Impact of Laparoscopic Antireflux Surgery on Quality of Life in the Short and Medium Term

In the last two decades laparoscopic antireflux surgery has been shown to improve QoL in patients with GERD. Several randomized trials comparing PPI therapy with laparoscopic antireflux surgery have been conducted, particularly over short-medium terms [6–18]. Some of these trials [6–11, 14, 17] showed an advantage for surgical therapy in outcome and cost-effectiveness after a few years, whereas The LOTUS-trial showed an advantage for PPI therapy after 5 years [12, 13, 15, 16].

Mahon et al. [6] randomized 217 patients, 109 to LNF and 108 to PPI therapy. The two groups were well matched for age, sex, weight and severity of reflux. Twenty-four-hour pH monitoring and manometry were performed 3 months after treatment, and quality of life was assessed in both groups using the Psychological General Well-being Index (PGWBI) and the Gastrointestinal Symptom Rating Scale (GSRS) at 3 and 12 months after treatment. The mean gastrointestinal symptom and general well-being scores improved from 31.7 and 95.4 respectively before treatment to 37.0 and 106.2 at 12 months after laparoscopic Nissen fundoplication (LNF), compared with changes from 34.3 and 98.5 to 35.0 and 100.4 respectively in the PPI group. The differences in both of these scores were significant between the two groups at 12 months (P = 0.003). This study showed that LNF leads to significantly less acid exposure of the lower oesophagus at 3 months and significantly greater improvements in both gastrointestinal and general well-being after 12 months compared with PPI treatment.

In a randomized trial conducted by Anvari et al. [10, 11, 14], the patients randomized to medical therapy received optimized treatment with proton pump inhibitors (PPIs) using a standardized management protocol based on best evidence and published guidelines. The surgical patients underwent LNF. Symptom evaluation was done using the GERD symptom scale (GERSS) and the global visual analog scale (VAS) for overall symptom control. At 3 years, surgery was associated with more heartburn-free days, and a significantly lower VAS score than medical management. Surgical patients also reported improved quality of life on the general health subscore of the Medical Outcomes Survey Short Form 36 (SF-36) at 3 years. The groups did not differ significantly in terms of GERSS or acid exposure on 24-h esophageal pH monitoring at 3 years. The authors concluded that for patients whose GERD symptoms are stable and controlled with PPI, continuing medical therapy and laparoscopic antireflux surgery are equally effective, although surgery may result in better symptom control and quality of life.

The LOTUS trial [12, 13, 15, 16] demonstrated that with modern forms of antireflux therapy, either by PPI-induced acid suppression or after laparoscopic Nissen fundoplication, the estimated remission rates at 5 years were higher in the esomeprazole group (92%) than in the LARS group (85%), log-rank $P = 0.048$. There was more regurgitation with esomeprazole than with LARS. In contrast, dysphagia, bloating, and flatulence were more common after LARS than with esomeprazole. Both treatments were well tolerated, with no surgery-related mortality. With regard to HRQoL, quality-of-life in reflux and dyspepsia (QOLRAD) scores on the food and drink and vitality dimensions as well as scores on the Gastrointestinal Symptom Rating Scale (GSRS) reflux dimension were the most abnormal at entry and the most sensitive to improve with treatment. The mean scores for all dimensions improved in both groups and remained close to values observed in a healthy population.

In the REFLUX trial [8, 9, 17, 18], a high proportion of patients (53%) had a partial fundoplication in contrast to a standardised, protocol specified total Nissen fundoplication in the LOTUS trial. The main outcome in the REFLUX trial was the score from the REFLUX questionnaire, a validated measure of HRQoL incorporating assessment of reflux related and other gastrointestinal symptoms and side effects and complications of both treatment modalities. Other measures were the overall health status (SF-36 and EuroQoL EQ-5D). Among responders differences in reflux scores at 5 years significantly favored the surgery group. SF-36 scores favored the surgical group in all domains at all time points. However, differences decreased over time, and at 5 years only the norm-based general health and role emotional domains were significantly better in the surgical arm. Mean EQ-5D scores showed a similar pattern—differences all favoring the surgical group within 2–3 years after surgery but at later time points scores were not significantly different. Long term rates of dysphagia, flatulence, and inability to vomit were similar in the medical and surgical groups.

All these trials are consistent in showing small numbers of operations needing to be converted to an open procedure, visceral injuries associated with the procedure, postoperative problems, and a small number of patients requiring dilatation of the wrap. However, quality has varied across these studies, with all trials having limitations in terms of design, duration of follow-up and reporting [25]. Due to these limitations the most recent Cochrane review [25] including four controlled trials concluded that the difference between laparoscopic fundoplication and medical treatment was imprecise for overall short- and medium-term HRQOL, medium-term GERD-specific QoL, percentage of people with adverse events, long-term dysphagia (difficulty in swallowing), and long-term acid regurgitation. The short-term GERD-specific quality of life, however, was better in the laparoscopic fundoplication group than in the medical treatment group.

19.5 The Impact of Laparoscopic Fundoplication on Quality of Life in Partial Responders to PPI-Therapy

Most studies in the surgical literature have included only patients who respond adequately to PPIs. Patients who do not respond adequately to PPI treatment, however, are often referred to surgery. The available evidence for efficacy of laparoscopic fundoplication in patients who do not respond adequately to PPI treatment was reviewed by Lundell et al. [26]. Across the included studies, LF offered a substantial and clinically relevant improvement in GERD symptoms, physiological measures of GERD and QoL parameters in partial responders beyond that provided by PPI treatment alone [26]. Particularly, four trials compared QoL before LF while patients were taking a PPI with that after LF. Of these, three found that GERD-HRQL scores improved 1 year after LF, two reported improvements in VAS scores, including a substantial increase at 1 year and at 10 years after LF. Only one study used the GIQLI scores and reported improved values at 1 year after LF. Symptoms recurred, however, in around 30–35% of patients a decade after LF in those studies reporting long-term follow-up data.

19.6 Impact of Antireflux Surgery on QoL in Patients with Non-erosive Reflux Disease (NERD)

GERD can be subdivided into erosive (ERD) and non-erosive reflux disease (NERD) depending upon endoscopy findings. Decreased QoL and symptom severity are similar in both ERD and NERD. Less is known about the long-term surgical outcome in NERD patients.

The study by Kamolz et al. [27] evaluated the surgical outcome in a well-selected group of EGD-negative patients compared to that of EGD-positive patients. Of more than 500 patients who underwent LARS, 89 EGD-negative patients were treated surgically because of persistent reflux-related symptoms despite medical therapy. In all cases, preoperative 24-h pH monitoring showed pathological values. To perform a comparative analysis, a matched sample of EGD-positive patients was selected from the database. Surgical outcome included objective data (e.g., manometry and pH data and endoscopy), quality of life evaluation with GIQLI), as well as patients' satisfaction with surgery.

Based on the data of a complete 5-year follow-up there were no significant differences in symptomatic improvement, percentage of persistent surgical side-effects, or objective parameters. In general, patients' satisfaction with surgery was comparable in both groups: 95% rated long-term outcome as excellent or good and would undergo surgical treatment again if necessary. Quality of life improvement was significantly better ($p < 0.05$) in the EGD-negative group because of the fact that GIQLI was more impaired before surgery. Five years after surgery, GIQLI in both groups showed comparable values to healthy controls. The authors concluded that LARS is an excellent treatment option for well-selected patients with persistent GERD-related symptoms who have no endoscopic evidence of esophagitis.

In a similar study by Broeders et al. [28] the relief of reflux symptoms at 5 years was similar (EGD negative 89% *versus* EGD positive 96%). PPI uses showed a similar reduction (82% to 21% *versus* 81% to 15% respectively; both $P < 0.001$). QoL score measured by Visual analogue scale (VAS) improved equally 50.3 to 65.2 ($P < 0.001$) *versus* 52.0 to 60.7 ($P = 0.016$). Five patients with NERD developed erosions after surgery; oesophagitis healed in 87% of patients with ERD. Reduction in total acid exposure time and increase in LOS pressure were similar. The reintervention rate was comparable (EGD negative15% *versus* EGD positive 12.8%).

19.7 The Impact of Laparoscopic Antireflux Surgery on Quality of Life in the Long Term (10 Years)

Up until now, there have only been a few studies comparing postoperative early and late (10 years) results after antireflux surgery, and reporting long-term control of reflux in some 74–90% of patients [29–36]. None of the randomized trials comparing laparoscopic fundoplication with PPI therapy has reported long-term (more than 5 years) health-related quality of life (HRQoL) or GERD-specific quality of life QoL.

In a randomized trial by Mardani et al. [29] 99 patients with chronic gastro-oesophageal reflux disease were referred for antireflux surgery and enrolled in the trial. Short gastric vessels were divided completely in 52 patients (group 1) and left intact in 47 (group 2). Quality of life was assessed before surgery and at 1 and 6 months, and 1 and 10 years after operation, using the Psychological General Well-Being (PGWB) index and the Gastrointestinal Symptom Rating Scale (GSRS).

No statistically significant differences were found between the two study groups for symptoms of heartburn, acid regurgitation, postfundoplication complaints such as gas bloat, and ability to belch or vomit. Scores for dysphagia were identical in the two groups. Health-related quality of life, as assessed by the generic PGWB index, was normal and similar in the two groups, with a mean (s.e.m.) total score of 100.0(17.2) in group 1 and 92.7(21.4) in group 2. The disease-specific GSRS scores also showed the same normal profile in the two study groups. The authors conclusion was that with total fundoplication it makes no difference whether the fundus is mobilized or not. Both types of repair provide lasting control of reflux.

Broeders et al. [30] reported 10 years outcome of a multicenter randomized controlled trial on laparoscopic (LNF) and conventional Nissen fundoplication (CNF), with focus on effectiveness and reoperation rate. A total of 148 patients (79 LNF, 69 CNF) participated in this 10-year follow-up study. GERD symptoms were relieved in 92.4% and 90.7% (NS) after LNF and CNF, respectively. The effect of surgery on self-rated change in general health was measured on a 3-point scale that ranges from "improved," to "unchanged," to "worsened." A visual analogue scale (VAS), validated for QoL assessment after esophageal surgery, was used to measure the impact on quality of life. The scale ranged from 0 to 100, where zero represented worst possible health and 100 represented perfect health. General health (74.7% vs. 72.7%; NS) and quality of life (visual analogue scale score: 65.3 vs. 61.4; NS) improved similarly in both groups. The percentage of patients who would have opted for surgery again was similar as well (78.5% vs. 72.7%; NS). The authors concluded that the 10-year effectiveness of LNF and CNF is comparable in terms of improvement of GERD symptoms, PPI use, quality of life, and objective reflux control.

Long-term HRQoL and GERD-specific quality of life QoL have been reported also in some observational studies. Dallemagne et al. [31] performed a laparoscopic Nissen fundoplication for 68 patients by tailoring a floppy 360° wrap with routine division of the short gastric vessels and crural repair. A laparoscopic partial posterior fundoplication (Toupet fundoplication) was performed for other 32 patients by tailoring a posterior wrap with routine division of the short gastric vessels and crural repair. At 10 years after antireflux surgery, 89.5% of the patients still were free of significant reflux (93.3% after Nissen, 81.8% after Toupet). Using the Gastrointestinal quality of life index (GIQLI) the authors demonstrated that GIQLI scores at 10 years were significantly better than the preoperative scores of the patients under PPI therapy. The global score, however, remained inferior to the score for a control group of healthy patients. The major difference was found in the "gastrointestinal symptoms" subdivision of the index.

Another observational study by Fein et al. [32] reported 120 patients who had primary laparoscopic fundoplication with a "tailored approach" (type of wrap chosen according to esophageal peristalsis): 88 received a Nissen, 22 an anterior, and 10 a Toupet fundoplication. Follow-up examinations were completed by 99 of 114 patients (87%) at 10 years after surgery, and included disease-related questions and the gastrointestinal quality-of-life index (GIQLI). Of these, 89% would select surgery again. Heartburn was reported by 30% of the patients. Regurgitations were noted from 15% of patients after a Nissen, 44% after anterior fundoplication, and 10% after a Toupet (P = 0.04). Twenty-eight percent of patients were on acid-suppressive drugs again. Following Nissen fundoplication, proton pump inhibitors were less frequently used (P = 0.01) and pH-metry was less likely to be abnormal. The GIQLI was 110 ± 24 without significant differences between the type of fundoplication. Ten years after laparoscopic fundoplication, overall outcome was good. A quarter of the patients were on acid suppressive drugs. Nissen fundoplication appeared to control reflux better than a partial fundoplication.

In the study by Gee et al. [33], a validated survey instrument, the Gastroesophageal Reflux Disease–Health-Related Quality-of- Life Scale (GERD-HRQL) was mailed to all patients who underwent laparoscopic fundoplications from 1997 to 2006. Additional information was obtained regarding reintervention, satisfaction, and medication use. Median follow-up was 60 months (range, 4–75 months). In patients who underwent primary LF, the mean (SD) GERD-HRQL score was 5.71 (7.99) (range, 0–45, with 0 representing no symptoms). Seventy-one percent of patients were satisfied with long-term results. Forty-three percent of patients took antireflux medications at some point following surgery; half of these patients had no diagnostic testing to document GERD recurrence. Only three patients (1.2%) required reoperation. These results demonstrate that patients undergoing primary LF by an experienced surgical team have near-normal GERD-HRQL scores at long-term follow-up.

In the study by Sgromo et al. [34] the long-term outcome of total (Nissen) and partial (Toupet) fundoplication, performed in a single institution was examined. The QOLRAD questionnaire was used as the quality-of-life measurement. Completed questionnaires were received from 161 patients (61%) of whom 99 had a laparoscopic Nissen fundoplication and 62 laparoscopic Toupet fundoplication. Both procedures were equivalent in improving reflux symptom scores in the long term, 79 of 99 (80%) and 56 of 62 (90%) patients were either symptom free or had obtained significant symptomatic relief. Both groups had equivalent QoL scores on the QOLRAD questionnaire. An equivalent number of patients (86% and 83.9% after Nissen and Toupet, respectively, were sufficiently satisfied to recommend antireflux surgery to a friend or relative complaining of reflux symptoms. The authors conclusion was that long-term satisfaction, general symptom scores, and quality of life are equivalent after laparoscopic Nissen (complete) or Toupet (partial) fundoplication. There is, however, an increased prevalence of persistent heartburn after laparoscopic Toupet fundoplication.

Kellokumpu et al. [35] performed laparoscopic Nissen fundoplication for 249 patients. Short- and long-term (at 10 years) outcomes were examined by several domains affected by the operation. Antireflux surgery was considered a failure based on the following criteria: moderate to severe heartburn or regurgitation; moderate to severe dysphagia reported in combination with heartburn or regurgitation; regular proton pump inhibitor medication use; endoscopic evidence of erosive esophagitis Savary-Miller grade 1–4; pathological 24-h pH monitoring; or necessity to undergo an additional surgery. Gastroesophageal reflux disease was cured in 98.4% of patients in the short-term. Cumulative long-term cure rates were 87.7% (81.0–92.2%) at 5 years and 72.9% (64.0–79.9%) at 10 years. Of the 139 patients available for 10-year follow-up, 83% rated their operation a success, and 85% were willing to undergo surgery again under similar preoperative conditions. Gastrointestinal symptom rating scores and SF-36 quality of life scores of patients with treatment success were similar to those of the general population but significantly lower in those with failed antireflux surgery (Figs. 19.1). In this study, the GSRS reflected well the long-term success of antireflux surgery as well as the side effects of antireflux surgery; it differentiated patients experiencing treatment failure from those being cured and from healthy controls [35]. Certain side effects, including increased bloating and rectal flatulence, manifest as indigestion syndrome and seem to be inevitable for most patients following fundoplication. This study demonstrated that failed antireflux surgery and symptom recurrence significantly worsened quality of life in most dimensions.

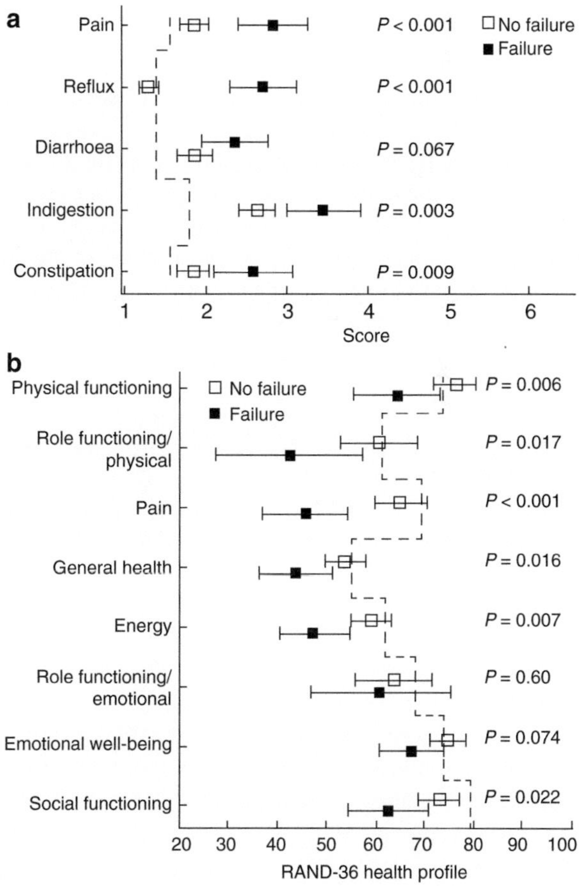

Fig. 19.1 (**a**) Gastrointestinal symptom rating scores (GSRS) according to treatment success or failure (*dotted line* = healthy controls). (**b**) SF-36 (RAND-36) scores according to treatment success or failure (*dotted line* = age-matched and sex-matched general population). P-values were age- and sex-adjusted for treatment success or failure. With permission of Baishideng Publishing Group (ref. [35])

19.8 The Impact of Redo Surgery for Failed Antireflux Operation on Quality of Life

Redo fundoplications are generally carried out for failure of improvement of existing symptoms or new symptoms of GERD [36–39]. Both patient and technical factors may contribute to failed antireflux surgery. Common technical reasons at the time of initial operation include inadequate crural closure or a too loose or too tight or misplaced fundoplication wrap [36–42]. Patient-related factors are morbid obesity, preoperative poor esophageal peristalsis, large hiatal hernia, old age, retching and coughing.

Options for redo surgery include reversal of fundoplication, redo fundoplication with hiatal hernia repair if needed, conversion to Roux-en-Y anatomy, or, as a last resort, esophagectomy. A review of a US database including 13,050 patients who had undergone laparoscopic fundoplication reported a reoperation rate of approximately 5% at 5 years and 7% at 10 years [43]. The majority of these reoperations were 'redo' fundoplications (87%) while the remaining 13% of reoperations were reversals of fundoplication [44]. Reversal of fundoplication is usually performed because of symptoms such as bloating and dysphagia caused by overly tight wrap or excessive, overly tight crural repair [44]. Dysphagia can also be due to initially unrecognized esophageal motility disorders such as achalasia.

Overall, surgery for failed antireflux procedures is technically more demanding than primary fundoplication, and the success rate does not equal that of the primary procedures [41, 42]. In a single-institution series of 275 redo operations by Awais et al. [45], the most common pattern of failure of the initial operation was transmediastinal migration-recurrent hernia in 177 patients (64%). Other identified causes included short esophagus (43%), misplaced wrap (16%), wrap too loose or too tight (14%), and a disrupted wrap (4%). Redo surgery included Nissen fundoplication in 200 (73%), Collis gastroplasty in 119 (43%), and partial fundoplication in 41 (15%). Laparoscopic surgery was attempted in 266 of these patients, with a rate of conversion to open surgery of 3%. With a median follow-up of 3.3 years, 11% of patients had failure of the redo operation, necessitating another surgical intervention. From the GERD-HRQL questionnaire, 85% of patients were satisfied with their results. The authors concluded that minimally invasive redo antireflux procedures can be safely performed in an experienced center. Overall, results following redo LF are not as good as after primary fundoplication, highlighting the importance of proper patient selection and surgical technique when performing primary LF.

Wilshire et al. [46] retrospectively reviewed patients who underwent revision after failed antireflux operations from 2004 to 2014. Patients were divided into two groups: first reoperation (Reop 1) and more than one reoperation (Reop >1). For comparison, a control group of patients who underwent primary antireflux operations was included. Patients underwent quality of life assessment preoperatively and postoperatively. The primary reason for failure was combined fundoplication herniation and slippage. Morbidity, mortality, and readmission rates were similar in all groups. Postoperative outcomes were improved in all groups but to a lesser degree in subsequent reoperations. Gastroesophageal Reflux Disease Health-Related Quality of Life was as following: controls, 20.0 to 2.0; Reop(1), 26.5 to 4.0; and Reop(>1), 13.0 to 2.0. Quality of Life in Reflux and Dyspepsia: controls, 4.5 to 7.0; Reop(1), 3.7 to 6.7; and Reop(>1), 3.5 to 5.8. Dysphagia Severity Score: controls, 44.0 to 45.0; Reop(1), 36.0 to 45.0; and Reop(>1), 30.8 to 45.0. Patients undergoing redo antireflux surgery had improved quality of life, relatively normal swallowing, and primary symptom resolution at a median of 20 months postoperatively. However, patients who underwent more than one reoperation had lower quality of life scores and less improvement in dysphagia, suggesting that other procedures such as Roux-en-Y or short colon interposition, should be considered after a failed initial reoperation.

The results of Roux-en-Y esophagojejunostomy for recurrent GERD after antireflux operations were analyzed in the study by Awais et al. [47]. Perioperative outcomes, dysphagia , and HRQoL were examined. Over a 12-year period, 105 patients with body mass index (BMI) greater than 25 underwent Roux-en-Y esophagojejunostomy for failed antireflux operations. Most were obese [BMI > 30; 82 patients (78%)]; esophageal dysmotility was demonstrated in more than one-third of patients. Forty-eight (46%) patients had multiple antireflux operations before Roux-en-Y esophagojejunostomy, and 27 patients had undergone a previous Collis gastroplasty. During mean follow-up of 23 months, median BMI decreased from 35 to 27.6 ($p < 0.0001$), and the mean dysphagia score decreased from 2.9 to 1.5 ($p < 0.0001$). The median GERD HRQOL score, assessed in a subset of patients, was classified as excellent. This study demonstrated that Roux-en-Y esophagojejunostomy for persistent GERD after antireflux operations in appropriately selected patients can be performed safely with good results in experienced centers. Roux-en-Y esophagojejunostomy should be considered an important option for the treatment of intractable recurrent symptoms after antireflux operations, particularly in obese patients.

19.9 Conclusion

Overall, it is the symptom response experienced by the patients that determines the success or failure of laparoscopic Nissen fundoplication. Quality of life response closely follows the clinical outcome of surgical treatment reflecting its side-effects as well. Based on available studies, it can be concluded that in the short-medium term, laparoscopic antireflux surgery effectively alleviates symptoms of gastroesophageal reflux disease, cures erosive esophagitis and improves quality of life. Postoperative adverse effects are usually mild and patient satisfaction good. For the long-term (10 years), limited data indicate decreasing effectiveness of laparoscopic antireflux surgery. HRQoL of patients with long term treatment success seems to be similar to that of general population. On the other hand, failed antireflux surgery and symptom recurrence significantly worsens the QoL in most dimensions. Disease-specific QoL instruments may differentiate patients experiencing treatment failure from those being cured and from healthy controls. The presence of several QoL instruments used in different studies, however, limits the interpretation and comparison of results. Moreover, an accurate and universally accepted definition of treatment failure to evaluate the clinical outcome after antireflux surgery is a critical issue. Given the scarcity of long-term data, longer follow-up of randomized trials is needed to determine whether antireflux surgery is an equivalent alternative to lifelong medication.

What Is the Current Knowledge and What Future Direction Is Required

- In the short-medium term (≤5 years), laparoscopic antireflux surgery effectively alleviates symptoms of gastroesophageal reflux disease, cures erosive esophagitis and improves quality of life. Longer follow-up of randomized trials is needed to determine whether antireflux surgery is an equivalent alternative to lifelong medication.
- For the long-term (10 years), limited data indicate decreasing effectiveness of laparoscopic antireflux surgery. HRQoL of patients with long term treatment success, however, seems to be similar to that of general population. Failed antireflux surgery and symptom recurrence significantly worsens the QoL in most dimensions.
- Disease-specific QoL instruments may differentiate patients experiencing treatment failure from those being cured and from healthy controls. The presence of several QoL instruments used in different studies, however, limits the interpretation and comparison of results.
- There is a need for an accurate and universally accepted definition of treatment failure to evaluate the clinical outcome after antireflux surgery.

Appendix

GERD-Health Related QualityofLife Questionnaire(GERD-HRQL)

Institution:________________ PatientID: ________________________ Date ___/___/___

□ On PPIs □ Off PPIs If off, forhow long? _________________ days/ months

Scale:
0 = No symptom
1 = Symptoms noticeable but not bother some
2 = Symptoms noticeable and bother some but not every day
3 = Symptoms bother some every day
4 = Symptoms affect daily activity
5 = Symptoms are in capacitatingto do daily activities

Please check the box to the right of each question which best describes your experience over the past ***2 weeks***

1. How bad is the heartburn? □0 □1 □2 □ 3 □4 □5
2. Heartburn when lying down? □0 □1 □2 □ 3 □4 □5
3. Heartburn when standing up? □0 □1 □2 □ 3 □4 □5
4. Heartburn after meals? □0 □1 □2 □ 3 □4 □5
5. Does heartburn change your diet? □0 □1 □2 □ 3 □4 □5
6. Does heartburn wakeyou from sleep? □0 □1 □2 □ 3 □4 □5
7. Do you have difficulty swallowing? □0 □1 □2 □ 3 □4 □5
8. Do you have pain with swallowing? □0 □1 □2 □ 3 □4 □5
9. If you take medication, does this affect your daily life? □0 □1 □2 □ 3 □4 □5
10. How bad is there gurgitation? □0 □1 □2 □ 3 □4 □5
11. Regurgitation when lying down? □0 □1 □2 □ 3 □4 □5
12. Regurgitation when standing up? □0 □1 □2 □ 3 □4 □5
13. Regurgitation after meals? □0 □1 □2 □ 3 □4 □5
14. Does regurgitation change your diet? □0 □1 □2 □ 3 □4 □5
15. Does regurgitation wake you from sleep? □0 □1 □2 □ 3 □4 □5
16. How satisfied are you with your present condition?
    □ Satisfied □ Neutral □ Dissatisfied

________________________ ________________________
Administered by Monitored by

________________________ ________________________
Date (mm/dd/yy) Date (mm/dd/yy)

GERD-HRQLQuestionnaire Page 1of 2

GERD-HRQL Questionnaire–Instructions

The GERD-HRQL questionnaire was developed and validated to measure changes of typical GERD symptoms such as heartburn and regurgitationin response to surgical or medical treatment.[1]

When comparing GERD-HRQL scores post-TIFto scores pre-TIF, it is important to take medication use into consideration.It is recommended to request patients take this questionnaire twice at screening (once off PPIs and the other time on PPIs) for fair comparison at follow-upspost-TIF

Total Score: Calculated by summing the individual scores to questions 1-15.

- Greatest possible score (worst symptoms) = 75
- Lowest possible score (no symptoms) = 0

HeartburnScore: Calculated by summing the individual scores to questions 1-6 .

- Worst heartburn symptoms = 30
- No heartburn symptoms = 0
- Scores of ≤ 12 with each individual question not exceeding 2 indicate heartburn elimination.[2]

RegurgitationScore: Calculated by summing the individual scores to questions10-15.

- Worst regurgitation symptoms = 30
- No regurgitation symptoms = 0
- Scores of ≤ 12 with each individual question not exceeding 2 indicate regurgitation elimination.[2]

References Cited

[1] VelanovichV. The development of the GERD-HRQL symptom severity instrument. *Dis Esophagus* 2007;20:130-4.
[2] Hunter JG, TrusTL, BranumGD, WaringJP, WoodWC. Aphysiologic approach to laparoscopic fundoplication for gastroesophageal reflux disease. *Ann Surg* 1996;223:673-85.

SF-36 QUESTIONNAIRE

Name:____________________ **Ref. Dr:**____________________ **Date:** _______

ID#: _______________ **Age:** _______ **Gender: M / F**

Please answer the 36 questions of the **Health Survey** completely, honestly, and without interruptions.

GENERAL HEALTH:
In general, would you say your health is:
○ Excellent ○ Very Good ○ Good ○ Fair ○ Poor

Compared to one year ago, how would you rate your health in general now?
○ Much better now than one year ago
○ Somewhat better now than one year ago
○ About the same
○ Somewhat worse now than one year ago
○ Much worse than one year ago

LIMITATIONS OF ACTIVITIES:
The following items are about activities you might do during a typical day. Does your health now limit you in these activities? If so, how much?

Vigorous activities, such as running, lifting heavy objects, participating in strenuous sports.
○ Yes, Limited a lot ○ Yes, Limited a Little ○ No, Not Limited at all

Moderate activities, such as moving a table, pushing a vacuum cleaner, bowling, or playing golf
○ Yes, Limited a Lot ○ Yes, Limited a Little ○ No, Not Limited at all

Lifting or carrying groceries
○ Yes, Limited a Lot ○ Yes, Limited a Little ○ No, Not Limited at all

Climbing several flights of stairs
○ Yes, Limited a Lot ○ Yes, Limited a Little ○ No, Not Limited at all

Climbing one flight of stairs
○ Yes, Limited a Lot ○ Yes, Limited a Little ○ No, Not Limited at all

Bending, kneeling, or stooping
○ Yes, Limited a Lot ○ Yes, Limited a Little ○ No, Not Limited at all

Walking more than a mile
○ Yes, Limited a Lot ○ Yes, Limited a Little ○ No, Not Limited at all

Walking several blocks
○ Yes, Limited a Lot ○ Yes, Limited a Little ○ No, Not Limited at all

Walking one block
○ Yes, Limited a Lot ○ Yes, Limited a Little ○ No, Not Limited at all

Bathing or dressing yourself
○ Yes, Limited a Lot ○ Yes, Limited a Little ○ No, Not Limited at all

PHYSICAL HEALTH PROBLEMS:
During the past 4 weeks, have you had any of the following problems with your work or other regular daily activities as a result of your physical health?

Cut down the amount of time you spent on work or other activities
○ Yes ○ No

Accomplished less than you would like
○ Yes ○ No

Were limited in the kind of work or other activities
○ Yes ○ No

Had difficulty performing the work or other activities (for example, it took extra effort)
○ Yes ○ No

EMOTIONAL HEALTH PROBLEMS:
During the past 4 weeks, have you had any of the following problems with your work or other regular daily activities as a result of any emotional problems (such as feeling depressed or anxious)?

Cut down the amount of time you spent on work or other activities
○ Yes ○ No

Accomplished less than you would like
○ Yes ○ No

Didn't do work or other activities as carefully as usual
○ Yes ○ No

SOCIAL ACTIVITIES:
Emotional problems interfered with your normal social activities with family, friends, neighbors, or groups?

○ Not at all ○ Slightly ○ Moderately ○ Severe ○ Very Severe

PAIN:
How much bodily pain have you had during the past 4 weeks?

○ None ○ Very Mild ○ Mild ○ Moderate ○ Severe ○ Very Severe

During the past 4 weeks, how much did pain interfere with your normal work (including both work outside the home and housework)?

○ Not at all ○ A little bit ○ Moderately ○ Quite a bit ○ Extremely

ENERGY AND EMOTIONS:
These questions are about how you feel and how things have been with you during the last 4 weeks. For each question, please give the answer that comes closest to the way you have been feeling.

Did you feel full of pep?
- All of the time
- Most of the time
- A good Bit of the Time
- Some of the time
- A little bit of the time
- None of the Time

Have you been a very nervous person?
- All of the time
- Most of the time
- A good Bit of the Time
- Some of the time
- A little bit of the time
- None of the Time

Have you felt so down in the dumps that nothing could cheer you up?
- All of the time
- Most of the time
- A good Bit of the Time
- Some of the time
- A little bit of the time
- None of the Time

Have you felt calm and peaceful?
- All of the time
- Most of the time
- A good Bit of the Time
- Some of the time
- A little bit of the time
- None of the Time

Did you have a lot of energy?
- All of the time
- Most of the time
- A good Bit of the Time
- Some of the time
- A little bit of the time
- None of the Time

Have you felt downhearted and blue?

- ◯ All of the time
- ◯ Most of the time
- ◯ A good Bit of the Time
- ◯ Some of the time
- ◯ A little bit of the time
- ◯ None of the Time

Did you feel worn out?

- ◯ All of the time
- ◯ Most of the time
- ◯ A good Bit of the Time
- ◯ Some of the time
- ◯ A little bit of the time
- ◯ None of the Time

Have you been a happy person?

- ◯ All of the time
- ◯ Most of the time
- ◯ A good Bit of the Time
- ◯ Some of the time
- ◯ A little bit of the time
- ◯ None of the Time

Did you feel tired?

- ◯ All of the time
- ◯ Most of the time
- ◯ A good Bit of the Time
- ◯ Some of the time
- ◯ A little bit of the time
- ◯ None of the Time

SOCIAL ACTIVITIES:
During the past 4 weeks, how much of the time has your physical health or emotional problems interfered with your social activities (like visiting with friends, relatives, etc.)?

- ◯ All of the time
- ◯ Most of the time
- ◯ Some of the time
- ◯ A little bit of the time
- ◯ None of the Time

GENERAL HEALTH:
How true or false is each of the following statements for you?

I seem to get sick a little easier than other people
◯ Definitely true ◯ Mostly true ◯ Don't know ◯ Mostly false ◯ Definitely false

I am as healthy as anybody I know
◯ Definitely true ◯ Mostly true ◯ Don't know ◯ Mostly false ◯ Definitely false

I expect my health to get worse
◯ Definitely true ◯ Mostly true ◯ Don't know ◯ Mostly false ◯ Definitely false

My health is excellent
◯ Definitely true ◯ Mostly true ◯ Don't know ◯ Mostly false ◯ Definitely false

References

1. El-Serag HB, Sweet S, Winchester CC, Dent J. Update on the epidemiology of gastro-oesophageal reflux disease: a systematic review. Gut. 2014;63(6):871–80.
2. Peery AF, Dellon ES, Lund J, Crockett SD, McGowan CE, Bulsiewicz WJ, et al. Burden of gastrointestinal disease in the United States: 2012 update. Gastroenterology. 2012;143(5):1179–87.
3. Ruigomez A, Garcia Rodrıguez LA, Wallander MA, Johansson S, Graffner H, Dent J. Natural history of gastro-oesophageal reflux disease diagnosed in general practice. Aliment Pharmacol Ther. 2004;20:751–60.
4. Malfertheiner P, Nocon M, Vieth M, Stolte M, Jaspersen D, Koelz HR, Labenz J, Leodolter A, Lind T, Richter K, Willich SN. Evolution of gastro-oesophageal reflux disease over 5 years under routine medical care—the ProGERD study. Aliment Pharmacol Ther. 2012;35(1):154–64.
5. Peters JH, DeMeester TR, Crookes P, et al. The treatment of gastroesophageal reflux disease with laparoscopic Nissen fundoplication: prospective evaluation of 100 patients with “typical” symptoms. Ann Surg. 1998;228:40–50.
6. Mahon D, Rhodes M, Decadt B, Hindmarsh A, Lowndes R, Beckingham I, et al. Randomized clinical trial of laparoscopic Nissen fundoplication compared with proton-pump inhibitors for treatment of chronic gastro-oesophageal reflux. Br J Surg. 2005;92:695–9.
7. Mehta S, Bennett J, Mahon D, Rhodes M. Prospective trial of laparoscopic Nissen fundoplication versus proton pump inhibitor therapy for gastroesophageal reflux disease: seven-year follow-up. J Gastrointest Surg. 2006;10:1312–7.
8. Grant A, Wileman S, Ramsay C, Bojke L, Epstein D, Sculpher M, et al. The effectiveness and cost-effectiveness of minimal access surgery amongst people with gastro-oesophageal reflux disease—a UK collaborative study. The REFLUX trial. Health Technol Assess. 2008;12(31):1–181.
9. Grant AM, Wileman SM, Ramsay CR, Mowat NA, Krukowski ZH, Heading RC, et al. Minimal access surgery compared with medical management for chronic gastro-oesophageal reflux disease: UK collaborative randomised trial. BMJ. 2008;337:a2664.
10. Anvari M, Allen C, Marshall J, Armstrong D, Goeree R, Ungar W, et al. A randomized controlled trial of laparoscopic Nissen fundoplication versus proton pump inhibitors for treatment of patients with chronic gastroesophageal reflux disease: one-year follow-up. Surg Innov. 2006;13:238–49.
11. Anvari M, Allen C, Marshall J, Armstrong D, Goeree R, Ungar W, et al. A randomized controlled trial of laparoscopic Nissen fundoplication versus proton pump inhibitors for the treatment of patients with chronic gastroesophageal reflux disease (GERD): 3-year outcomes. Surg Endosc. 2011;25:2547–54.
12. Attwood SE, Lundell L, Hatlebakk JG, Eklund S, Junghard O, Galmiche JP, et al. Medical or surgical management of GERD patients with Barrett’s Esophagus: the LOTUS trial 3-year experience. J Gastrointest Surg. 2008;12(10):1646–54.
13. Lundell L, Attwood S, Ell C, Fiocca R, Galmiche JP, Hatlebakk J, et al. Comparing laparoscopic antireflux surgery with esomeprazole in the management of patients with chronic gastro-oesophageal reflux disease: a 3-year interim analysis of the LOTUS trial. Gut. 2008;57(9):1207–13.
14. Anvari M, Allen C. Five-year comprehensive outcomes evaluation in 181 patients after laparoscopic Nissen fundoplication. J Am Coll Surg. 2003;196(1):51–7.
15. Galmiche JP, Hatlebakk JG, Attwood SE, Ell C, Fiocca R, Eklund S, et al. Laparoscopic antireflux surgery vs long-term esomeprazole treatment for chronic GERD. Final results after 5 years of follow up in the LOTUS study. Gastroenterology. 2010;138(5 Suppl):S53.
16. Galmiche J, Hatlebakk J, Attwood S, Ell C, Fiocca R, Eklund S, et al. Laparoscopic antireflux surgery vs esomeprazole treatment for chronic GERD. The LOTUS randomized clinical trial. JAMA. 2011;305:1969–77.

17. Grant AM, Cotton SC, Boachie C, Ramsay CR, Krukowski ZH, Heading RC, et al. Minimal access surgery compared with medical management for gastro-oesophageal reflux disease: five year follow-up of a randomised controlled trial (REFLUX). BMJ. 2013;346:f1908.
18. Grant AM, Boachie C, Cotton SC, Faria R, Bojke L, Epstein DM, et al. Clinical and economic evaluation of laparoscopic surgery compared with medical management for gastro-oesophageal reflux disease: 5-year follow-up of multicentre randomised trial (the REFLUX trial). Health Technol Assess. 2013;17(22):1–167.
19. Sandbu R, Sundbom M. Nationwide survey of long-term results of laparoscopic antireflux surgery in Sweden. Scand J Gastroenterol. 2010;45:15–20.
20. Pope CE II. The quality of life following antireflux surgery. World J Surg. 1992;16:355–8.
21. Irvine EJ. Quality of life assessment in gastro-oesophageal reflux disease. Gut. 2004;53(Suppl 4):iv35–9.
22. Kulig M, Leodolter A, Vieth M, Schulte E, Jaspersen D, Labenz J, Lind T, Meyer-Sabellek W, Malfertheiner P, Stolte M, Willich SN. Quality of life in relation to symptoms in patients with gastro-oesophageal reflux disease—an analysis based on the PROGERD initiative. Aliment Pharmacol Ther. 2003;18(8):767–76.
23. Gisbert JP, Cooper A, Karagiannis D, Hatlebakk J, Agréus L, Jablonowski H, Zapardiel J. Impact of gastroesophageal reflux disease on patients' daily lives: a European observational study in the primary care setting. Health Qual Life Outcomes. 2009;7:60.
24. Tack J, Becher A, Mulligan C, Johnson DA. Systematic review: the burden of disruptive gastro-oesophageal reflux disease on health-related quality of life. Aliment Pharnmacol Ther. 2012;35(11):1257–66.
25. Garg KS, Gurusamy KS. Laparoscopic fundoplication surgery versus medical management for gastro-oesophageal reflux disease (GORD) in adults. Cochrane Database Syst Rev. 2015. https://doi.org/10.1002/14651858.CD003243.pub3.
26. Lundell L, Bell M, Ruth M. Systematic review: laparoscopic fundoplication for gastroesophageal reflux disease in partial responders to proton pump inhibitors. World J Gastroenterol. 2014;20(3):804–13. https://doi.org/10.3748/wjg.v20.i3.804.
27. Kamolz T, Granderath FA, Schweiger UM, Pointner R. Laparoscopic Nissen fundoplication in patients with nonerosive reflux disease. Long-term quality-of-life assessment and surgical outcome. Surg Endosc. 2005;19(4):494–500. Epub 2005 Feb 3.
28. Broeders JA, Draaisma WA, Bredenoord AJ, Smout AJ, Broeders IA, Gooszen HG. Long-term outcome of Nissen fundoplication in non-erosive and erosive gastro-oesophageal reflux disease. Br J Surg. 2010;97(6):845–52.
29. Mardani J, Lundell L, Lönroth H, Dalenbäck J, Engström C. Ten-year results of a randomized clinical trial of laparoscopic total fundoplication with or without division of the short gastric vessels. Br J Surg. 2009;96(1):61–5.
30. Broeders JA, Rijnhart-de Jong HG, Draaisma WA, Bredenoord AJ, Smout AJ, Gooszen HG. Ten-year outcome of laparoscopic and conventional Nissen fundoplication: randomized clinical trial. Ann Surg. 2009;250:698–706.
31. Dallemagne B, Weertz J, Markiewicz S, Dewandre JM, Wahlen C, Monami B, Jehaes C. Clinical results of laparoscopic fundoplication ten years after surgery. Surg Endosc. 2006;20:159–65.
32. Fein M, Bueter M, Thalheimer A, Pachmayer V, Heimbucher J, Freys SM, Fuchs KH. Ten year outcome of laparoscopic antireflux procedures. J Gastrointest Surg. 2008;12:1893–9.
33. Gee DW, Andreoli MT, Rattner DW. Measuring the effectiveness of laparoscopic antireflux surgery long-term results. Arch Surg. 2008;143(5):482–7.
34. Sgromo B, Irvine LA, Cuschieri A, Shimi SM. Long-term comparative outcome between laparoscopic total Nissen and Toupet fundoplication: symptomatic relief, patient satisfaction and quality of life. Surg Endosc. 2008;22(4):1048–53. Epub 2007 Nov 20
35. Kellokumpu I, Voutilainen M, Haglund C, Färkkilä M, Roberts P, Kautiainen H. Quality of life following laparoscopic Nissen fundoplication: assessing short-term and long-term outcomes. World J Gastroenterol. 2013;19(24):3713–914.

36. Furnée EJ, Draaisma WA, Broeders IA, Gooszen HG. Surgical reintervention after failed antireflux surgery: a systematic review of the literature. J Gastrointest Surg. 2009;13:1539–49.
37. Dallemagne B, Arenas Sanchez M, Francart D, Perretta S, Weerts J, Markiewicz S, Jehaes C. Long-term results after laparoscopic reoperation for failed antireflux procedures. Br J Surg. 2011;98(11):1581–7. Epub 2011 Jun 28.
38. Pessaux P, Arnaud JP, Delattre JF, Meyer C, Baulieux J, Monier H. Laparoscopic antireflux surgery: five-year results and beyond in 1340 patients. Arch Surg. 2005;140:946–51.
39. Hunter JG, Smith CD, Branum GD, Waring JP, Trus TL, Cornwell M, et al. Laparoscopic fundoplication failures: patterns of failure and response to fundoplication revision. Ann Surg. 1999;230:595–604.
40. Smith CD, McClusky DA, Rajad MA, Lederman AB, Hunter JG. When fundoplication fails: redo? Ann Surg. 2005;241(6):861–9.
41. Grover BT, Kothari SN. Reoperative antireflux surgery. Surg Clin N Am. 2015;95:629–40.
42. Hashimi S, Bremner RM. Complications following surgery for gastroesophageal reflux disease and achalasia. Thorac Surg Clin. 2015;25:485–98.
43. Zhou T, Harnsberger C, Broderick R, Fuchs H, Talamini M, Jacobsen G, et al. Reoperation rates after laparoscopic fundoplication. Surg Endosc. 2015;29(3):510–4.
44. Stefanidis D, Navarro F, Augenstein VA, et al. Laparoscopic fundoplication takedown with conversion to Roux-en-Y gastric bypass leads to excellent reflux control and quality of life after fundoplication failure. Surg Endosc. 2012;26(12):3521–7.
45. Awais O, Luketich JD, Schuchert MJ, Morse CR, Wilson J, Gooding WE, Landreneau RJ, Pennathur A. Reoperative antireflux surgery for failed fundoplication: an analysis of outcomes in 275 patients. Ann Thorac Surg. 2011;92(3):1083–9.
46. Wilshire CL, Louie BE, Shultz D, Jutric Z, Farivar AS, Aye RW. Clinical outcomes of reoperation for failed antireflux operations. Ann Thorac Surg. 2016;101(4):1290–6.
47. Awais O, Luketich JD, Reddy N, Bianco V, Levy RM, Schuchert MJ, Gooding WE, Crist LR, Landreneau RJ, Pennathur A. Roux-en-Y near esophagojejunostomy for failed antireflux operations: outcomes in more than 100 patients. Ann Thorac Surg. 2014;98(6):1905–11.

Erratum to: Hiatal Hernia Surgery

Muhammed Ashraf Memon

Erratum to:
M.A. Memon, Hiatal Hernia Surgery, An Evidence Based Approach, DOI 10.1007/978-3-319-64003-7

In the original version of the book, the first name of the editor was incorrectly spelled as Muhammad Ashraf Memon in the Cover and Front matter.

The correct version of the editor name is Muhammed Ashraf Memon.

The online version of the original book can be found under DOI 10.1007/978-3-319-64003-7

M.A. Memon
Faculty of Health Sciences and Medicine, Department of Surgery,
University of Queensland Mayne Medical School, Brisbane, Queensland, Australia

M.A. Memon (ed.), *Hiatal Hernia Surgery*,
https://doi.org/10.1007/978-3-319-64003-7_20

Index

M.A. Memon (ed.), *Hiatal Hernia Surgery*,
https://doi.org/10.1007/978-3-319-64003-7

MIX
Papier aus verantwortungsvollen Quellen
Paper from responsible sources
FSC® C105338

If you have any concerns about our products,
you can contact us on
ProductSafety@springernature.com

In case Publisher is established outside the EU,
the EU authorized representative is:
Springer Nature Customer Service Center GmbH
Europaplatz 3, 69115 Heidelberg, Germany

Printed by Libri Plureos GmbH
in Hamburg, Germany